KT-476-664

▶ Except where otherwise stated, drug doses and recommendatio
for the non-pregnant adult who is not breast-feeding.

Diabetes Care:

A practical manual

Dr Rowan Hillson MBE, MD, FRCP

Consultant Physician,
Diabetes and Endocrine Unit,
The Hillingdon Hospital, UK

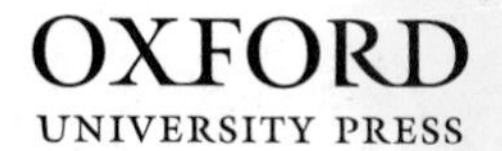

OXFORD
UNIVERSITY PRESS

Great Clarendon Street, Oxford OX2 6DP

Oxford University Press is a department of the University of Oxford.
It furthers the University's objective of excellence in research, scholarship,
and education by publishing worldwide in

Oxford New York

Auckland Cape Town Dar es Salaam Hong Kong Karachi
Kuala Lumpur Madrid Melbourne Mexico City Nairobi
New Delhi Shanghai Taipei Toronto

With offices in

Argentina Austria Brazil Chile Czech Republic France Greece
Guatemala Hungary Italy Japan Poland Portugal Singapore
South Korea Switzerland Thailand Turkey Ukraine Vietnam

Oxford is a registered trade mark of Oxford University Press
in the UK and in certain other countries

Published in the United States
by Oxford University Press Inc., New York

First published 2008

British Library Cataloguing in Publication Data
Data available

Library of Congress Cataloguing in Publication Data
Data available

Typeset by Cepha Imaging Private Ltd., Bangalore, India
Printed by L. E. G. O. S. p. A

ISBN 978–0–19–921808–0

10 9 8 7 6 5 4 3 2 1

For Kay and Rodney Hillson

Acknowledgements

I wish to thank the following for their help.

This book would not have been possible without the support of my family, my patients, my colleagues in Diabeticare, and my colleagues around The Hillingdon Hospital.

I particularly wish to thank my family for their patience and encouragement, and, alphabetically, Pat Bacon, Carol Candlish, Ruth Chalmers, Anne Currie, Deb Datta, Mark Edwards, David Evans, Mary Jurd, Sandra Ross, Gill Ruane, Pat Smith, Dai Thomas, and the anonymous but most helpful GP reviewer, and the pharmacology reviewer engaged by OUP.

I thank my editor Helen Liepman, Kate Wilson, Anna Winstanley, and Susan Crowhurst, all from Oxford University Press.

I am grateful to eMIMS (electronic Monthly Index of Medical Specialties), the American Diabetes Association, and the Office of Public Sector Information for permission to use material.

Contents

Introduction

Who is this book for?

- All health care staff in any discipline, e.g. doctors, nurses, dietitians, podiatrists, physiotherapists, occupational therapists, speech and language therapists, psychologists, pharmacists, health care assistants, medical secretaries, managers and care planners—and others
- Primary, community, secondary, NHS, or private care service

For example:
- Are you a GP or practice nurse working in primary care running your own diabetic clinic?
- Do people with diabetes ask for your advice?
- Are you a diabetologist or a GP with a special interest in diabetes who teaches other staff about diabetes?
- Are you a nurse working in A&E?
- Are you working on a hospital ward or clinic caring for diabetic patients—often or sometimes?
- Are you a doctor admitting emergency patients?
- Have you just started work with a diabetes firm in a hospital?
- Are you a student of medicine, nursing, dietetics, podiatry, physiotherapy, occupational therapy?
- Are you a person with diabetes who wants to learn more—or a family member of a person with diabetes? This book is written for health staff but many patients will find it of interest

Diabetes

Diabetes is a common long-term condition. Some numbers:

- There are 246 million people with diabetes worldwide
- The International Diabetes Federation (IDF) estimates that there will be 380 million by 2025
- 53 million live in Europe
- 2.4 million live in England (4.75% prevalence including 19% with undiagnosed diabetes) (2006)
- 14–16% of hospital inpatients have diabetes
- Nationally, total expenditure on people with diabetes has been estimated at 5–10% of national health expenditure
- Primary care prescriptions for diabetes in England cost £561 million in 2005*

*http://www.yhpho.org.uk/Download/Public/1265/1/Prescribing%20for%20Diabetes%20in%20England%20Nov%202007%20FINAL.pdf

Why write this book?

There are lots of textbooks about diabetes. This is a pocket book, an *aide-memoire*, a quick guide. The aim is to help those caring for diabetes to manage most patients themselves, and to recognize and refer those who need specialist care. References will lead you to more detailed descriptions of specialist care. Each chapter has a contents index, and there is also a complete index at the end. There are duplications where it appears helpful.

Diabetes is compatible with many years of healthy living but can also be more lethal than cancer. It is a multisystem disorder of which one manifestation is raised blood glucose. Because the complications of diabetes are so varied, and present in so many ways, the underlying influence of the diabetes may be ignored. Each complication may be managed as a 'one-off'. It is crucial that people with diabetes have continuity of care from a team who know them well, and whom they can trust to monitor them to reduce risk factors for complications, and to detect and manage complications and emergencies. Please note that this book makes no assumptions about where routine diabetes care will be provided. Anyone providing diabetes care should have training in this and ensure high standards of care. Each of us should know when to refer patients to someone with more specialist knowledge of diabetes care. Many diabetes specialist services are now available in primary care or community settings.

No book or guideline can provide perfect advice for every patient. This manual is a general guide, but you must tailor the care of each diabetic patient to that person's individual condition and situation. A particular patient's condition may mean that the advice in this manual is not applicable or that the situation is not covered. Ask the district diabetes team for advice. Agree local protocols for your practice, hospital, or district. Diabetes is a very rapidly moving field and so it is important to keep up to date. All drug information and dosages should be confirmed for your particular patient using a current BNF.

References are brief and many relate to websites. The links worked at the time of writing. No responsibility can be taken for the content of websites nor for sequelae of using them (or not using them). This book expresses my personal views as an individual. For official Department of Health publications please see the Department of Health (dh) website. As an author I welcome constructive feedback—please contact me with comments or suggestions: rowan.hillson@thh.nhs.uk

National publications about diabetes:
http://www.dh.gov.uk/en/Policyandguidance/Healthandsocialcaretopics/Diabetes/index.htm

Abbreviations

🕮	this book
❗	warning
~	about/circa
<	less than
>	more than
≥	equal to or greater than
≤	equal to or less than
=	equals or equal to
×	times (e.g. 2× = two times)
999	call emergency ambulance
A&E	Accident and Emergency
ABCD	Association of British Clinical Diabetologists
ACE	angiotensin-converting enzyme
ACR	albumin-to-creatinine ratio
ACS	acute coronary syndrome(s)
ADA	American Diabetes Association
ADAG	HbA$_{1c}$-derived average glucose
AGE	advanced glycosylation end-products
ALT	alanine aminotransferase
AMI	acute myocardial infarction
antiGAD-Ab	glutamic acid decarboxylase autoantibodies
ARB	angiotensin receptor blocker
ARDS	adult respiratory distress syndrome
AST	aspartate aminotransferase
BDA	British Diabetic Association (now Diabetes UK)
BHS	British Hypertension Society
BMI	weight/height^2 (kg/m^2); body mass index
BNF	British National Formulary
BP	blood pressure
CABG	coronary artery bypass graft(ing)
CAPD	continuous ambulatory peritoneal dialysis
CEMACH	Confidential Enquiry into Maternal and Child Health
CHO	carbohydrate
CK	creatine kinase
CKD	chronic kidney disease

COPD	chronic obstructive pulmonary disease
CRP	C-reactive protein
CSII	continuous subcutaneous insulin infusion
CT scan	computed tomography scan
CVD	cardiovascular disease
CVP	central venous pressure
DCCT	Diabetes Control and Complications Trial
DDA	Disability Discrimination Act
DKA	diabetic ketoacidosis
DSN	diabetes specialist nurse
DVLA	Driver and Vehicle Licensing Agency
ECG	electrocardiogram
ED	erectile dysfunction
eGFR	estimated glomerular filtration rate
FBC	full blood count
FDA	US Food and Drug Administration
FVC	forced vital capacity
FEV1	forced expiratory volume in 1 sec
GDM	gestational diabetes mellitus
GI	gastrointestinal
GIT	gastrointestinal tract
GKI	glucose–potassium–insulin infusion
GLP-1	glucagon-like polypeptide-1
GPwSI	GP with a special interest
HbA_{1c}	Haemoglobin A_{1c}
HBGM	home finger-prick blood glucose monitoring
HDL	high-density lipoprotein cholesterol
HDU	high dependency unit
HONK	hyperosmolar non-ketotic hyperglycaemic state
HPS	Heart Protection Study
hr	hour
HRT	hormone replacement therapy
ICU	intensive care unit
IDF	International Diabetes Federation
IFCC	International Federation of Clinical Chemists
IFG	impaired fasting glucose
IGT	impaired glucose tolerance
IHD	ischaemic heart disease
IM	intramuscular or intramuscularly
INR	International Normalized Ratio

IT	information technology
ITU	intensive care unit
IUCD	intra-uterine contraceptive device
IUS	intra-uterine system
IV	intravenous or intravenously
LADA	latent autoimmune diabetes of adulthood
LDL	low-density lipoprotein cholesterol
LFT	liver function test/liver enzymes
LGV	large goods vehicle
LH	luteinizing hormone
MAC	microalbumin-to-creatinine ratio
mcg	microgram
mg	milligram
MHRA	Medicines and Healthcare Products Regulatory Agency
min	minute(s)
mmol/l	millimol/litre
MODY	maturity-onset diabetes of the young
MRI	magnetic resonance imaging
MRSA	methicillin-resistant Staphylococcus aureus
MSU	midstream urine
NaCl	sodium chloride
NAFLD	non-alcoholic fatty liver disease
NASH	non-alcoholic steatohepatitis
NG	nasogastric or nasogastrically
NSAID	non-steroidal anti-inflammatory drug
NSF	National Service Framework
NSTEMI	non-ST elevation myocardial infarction
OCP	oral contraceptive pill
OGTT	oral glucose tolerance test
PC	personal computer
PCT	primary care trust
pCO_2	arterial carbon dioxide
PCOS	polycystic ovary syndrome
PCR	protein-to-creatinine ratio
PCV	passenger-carrying vehicle
PEF	peak expiratory flow
PIL	patient information leaflet
PPAR-γ	peroxisome proliferator-activated receptor-gamma
PO	oral or orally
pO_2	arterial oxygen level

POD1	post-operative day one
QOF	Quality and Outcomes Framework
PVD	peripheral vascular disease
RCT	randomized controlled trial
RNIB	Royal National Institute for the Blind
SC	subcutaneous or subcutaneously
SPC	summary of product characteristics
SMR	standardized mortality ratio
SSRI	selective serotonin-reuptake inhibitor
STEMI	ST elevation myocardial infarction
TDD	total daily dose
TFT	thyroid function test
TIA	transient ischaemic attack
U&E	urea and electrolytes (in practice, plasma urea, sodium, potassium, and creatinine)
ULN	upper limit of normal
UTI	urinary tract infection
VC	vital capacity
WBCC	white blood cell count
WHO	World Health Organization
vs	versus (compared with)
YDC	young diabetic clinic
YHPHO	York and Humber Public Health Observatory
yr(s)	year(s)

Chapter 1

Is it diabetes?

The path to diagnosis

Diabetes presents in many forms to different people in different fields. The person to whom it presents or the place in which it is diagnosed affects initial assessment and management. Once you suspect the diagnosis of diabetes, confirm it, tell the patient the diagnosis, and explain what happens next.

Presentations

The way in which the diagnosis comes to light influences the patient's attitude to his/her condition. Those with thirst and polyuria want relief from their symptoms and may be more likely to comply with treatment than those patients who feel well (Box 1.1).

Box 1.1 Presentations of diabetes

- Patient-initiated
  - Symptoms of hyperglycaemia (e.g. thirst, polyuria)
  - Symptoms of diabetic tissue damage
  - Symptoms of conditions causing diabetes (e.g. steroid excess)
  - Unrelated symptoms leading to general biochemical screen
- Screening
  - Well-person health check (state decreed or patient request)
  - Insurance medical
  - During training in glucose testing (e.g. nurse)
  - Employment medical

Symptoms of diabetes

Thirst, polydipsia, and polyuria

- Severe thirst, including at night. A few, often elderly, ignore their thirst for fear of increasing urination. This causes dehydration and may precipitate hospital admission.
- Sugary drinks worsen hyperglycaemia.
- Polyuria (frequent passage of large volumes of urine, usually dilute).
- Nocturia with sleep disturbance.
- Urinary incontinence (elderly people), bed-wetting (children).
- Stress incontinence.
- Urinary retention in men with prostatism.
- The severity of the polyuria, or the thirst and polydipsia, may not match the degree of hyperglycaemia.
- Polyuria without glycosuria is not due to diabetes mellitus and other causes must be sought.

Weight loss

- Some weight loss is due to dehydration. The rest is due to reduction of adipose tissue by lipolysis and muscle breakdown to fuel gluconeogenesis.
- Obese patients may be pleased with their weight loss, not realizing that this is a manifestation of diabetes. On treatment, the lost weight may be regained.
- Classically, the weight loss of diabetes mellitus is associated with normal or even increased appetite. A few patients crave sweet foods.
- Cachexia may develop rapidly in patients with type 1 diabetes who were slim to start with or in whom the diagnosis has been delayed.
- Some patients with type 2 diabetes do not lose weight.
- In patients with steroid-induced diabetes the weight gain of steroid excess may balance the weight loss of untreated diabetes.

Tiredness and malaise

- Tiredness is an insidious but frequent symptom.
- Non-specific malaise may be unnoticed until the treated patient looks back.
- People may complain that the patient is irritable and hard to live with.

Bowel symptoms

- Dehydration may cause constipation, which may be severe in the elderly.
- Lack of pancreatic enzyme may cause steatorrhoea.

Recurrent or refractory infections

- Boils, cellulitis, abscesses. Consider nasal carriage of *Staphylococcus aureus*.
- Candida may recur despite antifungals—thrush or balanitis
- Recurrent urinary tract or chest infections.

Visual disturbance

- Changes in blood glucose concentrations may alter the refractive index of the lens, aqueous humour, and cornea, and cause blurred vision.
- New spectacles may be useless once the hyperglycaemia resolves.
- Additional symptoms relating to tissue damage are discussed below.

Paraesthesiae

- Pins and needles in hands and feet; may resolve on treatment of the diabetes.
- Peripheral nerve damage may persist or worsen.

Pruritus

Pruritus vulvae is a common presenting feature caused by candidal infection. Generalized pruritus is not a feature of diabetes alone. There are many minor causes. After excluding these consider pancreatic malignancy or other serious pathology.

Cramp

Patients with uncontrolled diabetes often complain of cramp, especially in the legs, probably secondary to diuresis. If persistent it can be relieved by quinine sulphate.

Symptoms of diabetic tissue damage

These will be discussed in the relevant sections below. Diabetes can remain undetected for many years and its first manifestation may be a myocardial infarction or a foot ulcer. The higher the fasting glucose at presentation of type 2 diabetes, the more likely the patient is to have tissue damage later (*Diabetes Care* 2002; **25**:1410–17)

Box 1.2 Symptoms of diabetes

- General
  - Thirst and polydipsia
  - Polyuria
  - Weight loss
  - Tiredness, malaise, irritability
  - Constipation
  - Visual disturbance, e.g. blurring
  - Parasethesiae
  - Pruritus
  - Cramp
- Tissue damage. Any form of diabetic tissue damage may present. The more common ones are:
  - Ischaemic heart disease
  - Peripheral vascular disease
  - Cerebrovascular disease
  - Neuropathy
  - Cataract or retinal disease
- Conditions causing diabetes
  - Steroid excess (iatrogenic) is the most common

No symptoms

It is estimated that 500 000 people in the UK have undiagnosed diabetes - in some areas half of those with diabetes do not know that they have it. 19% of patients with diabetes in the community remain unrecorded at their GP practice (Diabetes Audit 2004–5 www.icservices.nhs.uk/ncasp). This may not mean that the patient is unaware of the diagnosis. However, some may be undiagnosed—ignoring symptoms (Boxes 1.1 and 1.2). About 10% of type 2 patients are asymptomatic.

Diabetic tissue damage begins long before diabetes is actually diagnosed: 30–50% of patients with newly recognized type 2 diabetes (📖 p.14) have tissue damage already. Diabetes UK used linear regression analysis of an audit of 155 000 type 2 patients to calculate the number of years before diagnosis that complications (and hence diabetes) began to occur. The audit suggested a 10-yr delay in diagnosing diabetes (Diabetes UK 2000). It also indicated that large-vessel complications started 20 yrs before diagnosis. This is consistent with the known link between IGT (📖 p.11) and CVD. People with diabetes progress from IFG and/or IGT to frank diabetes over a period of years. Symptoms occur only with frank diabetes. It is essential to identify patients with all degrees of glucose intolerance as early as possible to allow risk-reduction care.

Screening

There is no single simple screening method for diabetes which fulfils requirements for a universal screening test. (See National Screening Committee Handbook reference 📖 p.017). People in whom a one-off screening opportunity is taken should be warned that the test may be inconclusive, and that a negative test may not exclude diabetes. Only laboratory venous glucose measurements should be used to diagnose diabetes.

Urine screening is not recommended. Some people with diabetes do not have glycosuria. A post-prandial urine sample is more likely to detect diabetes. 22% of those with diabetes identified in one study had post-prandial glycosuria but no glucose in a fasting sample. Use blood glucose, preferably fasting, and ideally venous laboratory.

Screening must be performed with care.

> A 10-yr-old boy was brought to a diabetes information stand at a county show. A voluntary screening group had just diagnosed diabetes on the basis of a finger-prick glucose level of 11 mmol/l. His distraught mother begged for help. She was clutching a large sticky lolly, confiscated because 'diabetics can't eat sweets'. After a thorough hand wash his finger-prick glucose was 4 mmol/l.

Box 1.3 People who should be screened for diabetes

- Symptoms of diabetes
- White people >40 yrs, non-white ethnic groups >25 yrs if overweight:
  - BMI over 25 kg/m^2 and/or
  - Waist circumference
    ≥94cm White/Black men
    ≥90cm Asian men
    ≥80cm White/Black/Asian women
- Hypertension
- Ischaemic heart disease/cerebrovascular disease/peripheral vascular disease
- Tissue damage known to be associated with diabetes
- Everyone with an acute medical problem, i.e dealt with by physicians (no evidence base but practical)
- Impaired fasting glucose or impaired glucose tolerance
- Those with conditions known to cause or to be associated with diabetes (e.g. endocrinopathies, polycystic ovarian syndrome)
- On medication known to be associated with diabetes (e.g. steroids, thiazides)
- Past gestational diabetes
- Current pregnancy (📖 p.376)
- Severe mental health disorders
- Hypertriglyceridaemia
- First-degree relatives of patients with type 2 diabetes
- First-degree family history of ischaemic heart disease

Expanded from recommendations of Diabetes UK Position Statement for Early Identification of Type 2 Diabetes, July 2006

Making the diagnosis

The diagnosis of diabetes has major implications for the individual, not only with regard to changes in lifestyle and the introduction of self-monitoring and medication, but also with regard to employment, insurance, driving, sports, and hobbies. Therefore it is essential to prove the diagnosis at the outset.

Do a random finger-prick capillary glucose in patients in front of you who are symptomatic, have a high risk of diabetes, or who are unlikely to comply with fasting/revisits. Note that there are differences between capillary and venous glucose (📖 p.110) . Follow the action plan in Table 1.1

The best test is a fasting venous laboratory glucose. However, note that a normal fasting glucose could still be associated with diabetic post-prandial levels.

If you have a clear diagnosis of diabetes on one (or two) venous laboratory glucose samples, or if the patient is known to be diabetic, there is no need to do an OGTT.

Table 1.1 Acting on one-off glucose test results (mmol/l)

	Action
Capillary whole blood	
<5.5 fasting/random	Diabetes unlikely: rescreen as indicated
≥5.5–11.0 fasting/random	Diabetes possible: do fasting venous laboratory glucose
≥11.1 fasting/random	Probable diabetes: if ill send venous laboratory glucose same day, consider urgent referral to hospital diabetes team/medical admissions If not ill, do fasting venous laboratory glucose
Venous plasma laboratory	
<5.6 fasting/random	Diabetes unlikely: rescreen as indicated
5.6–6.9 fasting	IFG or diabetes likely: do OGTT
7.0–11.0 fasting ≥11.1 random	Diabetes if classical symptoms: repeat venous plasma laboratory glucose if not symptomatic Refer children to paediatric diabetes service same day

Table 1.2 The oral glucose tolerance test (OGTT) (75 g)

Ask the patient to eat his/her normal diet. If the dietary carbohydrate is less than 125 g daily, the patient should eat 150 g daily for the three days before the test.
Fast the patient overnight for 10–14 hours. He/she should eat nothing, drink only water, and should not smoke during this time nor during the test.
The patient should be sitting at rest during the test.
Take a venous blood sample for plasma glucose estimation. Test the urine for glucose.
Give the patient 75 g glucose dissolved in 250–350 ml water to be swallowed over 5–15 min. (420 ml Original Lucozade® can be used.)
Two hours after the start of the test take another venous blood sample for plasma glucose estimation. Test the urine for glucose.
Ensure all samples are labelled with the patient's name, the time, and the date. Ensure that the request card(s) mirrors this labelling.

Table 1.3 Interpreting the results of the oral glucose tolerance test

	Venous plasma glucose concentration (mmol/l)		
	Fasting		**2 hr after glucose load**
Diabetes	≥7.0	*or*	≥11.1
Impaired glucose tolerance (IGT)	<7.0	*and*	7.8-11.0
Impaired fasting glucose (IFG)	6–6.9	*and*	<11.1

Metabolic stress

In patients whose blood glucose levels suggest diabetes but who are under a metabolic stress, such as an infection, myocardial infarction, surgery, or a course of steroid treatment, repeat the blood glucose tests at least 6 weeks after the patient has recovered to confirm the persistence of diabetes. A glycosylated haemoglobin reading may be helpful—if raised the patient is highly likely to have diabetes.

Ill patients

Do not delay treatment of severely hyperglycaemic and clinically ill patients because laboratory confirmation is unobtainable or slow. In unwell patients, if the finger-prick glucose concentration is >20 mmol/l, wash another of the patient's fingers with plain water, dry well, and repeat the finger-prick glucose. If hyperglycaemia is confirmed treat the patient accordingly, but send a pre-treatment blood sample to the laboratory for blood glucose estimation.

Pregnancy

Many authorities consider that these diagnostic criteria also apply to pregnant women. However, different criteria are sometimes used in pregnancy (📖 p.376).

Retrospective diagnosis of diabetes

Occasionally, a doctor is presented with a patient in whom oral hypoglycaemic treatment for diabetes has already been started without proper confirmation of the diagnosis. This should not occur if the guidelines above are followed. If the patient is seen within 6 weeks of starting medication, the finding of a raised haemoglobin A_{1c} (📖p.124) provides support for the diagnosis of diabetes. Sometimes oral hypoglycaemic treatment has to be stopped to allow clarification of the diagnosis.

Table 1.4 Impaired glucose tolerance (IGT)

OGTT: Fasting venous plasma glucose <7 mmol/l
Two-hour venous plasma glucose 7.8–11.0 mmol/l

Not a benign condition

This condition is associated with a substantial risk of future diabetes (about 10% per annum). In overweight people appropriate diet and exercise greatly reduce the risk of developing diabetes. IGT is also associated with increased risk of cardiovascular disease.

Check for cardiovascular disease—heart, brain, peripheries

Check and treat risk factors

Smoking
Blood pressure
Weight
Lack of exercise
Fasting cholesterol (total, HDL, LDL)
Triglyceride

Tell the patient:

'Your body is not using glucose properly. You do not have diabetes although this condition may lead to diabetes. Healthy eating, so your weight is normal for your height, with regular exercise will reduce your risk of developing diabetes.'

Give them a copy of the results. Explain the risk of diabetes and heart and circulatory disease (and what both of these are). Warn the patient to seek a blood glucose test if he/she experiences thirst, increased urination, weight loss, thrush/perineal irritation, undue tiredness; or if he/she is ill, injured, or pregnant.

Recheck fasting glucose

Venous plasma glucose at OGTT <6 mmol/l—recheck annually; repeat OGTT if 6–7 mmol/l.

Venous plasma glucose at OGTT 6–7 mmol/l—follow impaired fasting glucose pathway.

This guideline was adapted by the author from the Diabetes UK Guidelines, June 2000, with the help of Dr Dai Thomas, The Hillingdon Hospital.

Table 1.5 Impaired fasting glucose (IFG)

OGTT	Fasting venous plasma glucose 6–7 mmol/l Two-hour venous plasma glucose below 11.1 mmol/l
This new category identifies people likely to develop diabetes. Patients can have both IFG and IGT and such patients have a high risk of diabetes and should be followed closely.	
Check for cardiovascular disease—heart, brain, peripheries	
Check and treat risk factors	
Smoking Blood pressure Weight Lack of exercise Fasting cholesterol (total, HDL, LDL) Triglyceride	
Tell the patient: 'Your blood sugar is higher than normal but not in the diabetic range. You may develop diabetes although this process can be slowed by early treatment.' Explain what diabetes is. Give the patient a copy of their results. Warn the patient to seek a blood glucose test if he/she experiences thirst, increased urination, weight loss, thrush/perineal irritation, undue tiredness; or if he/she is ill, injured, or pregnant.	
Recheck fasting glucose Recheck fasting venous plasma glucose in 3 months, then every 6 months. If IFG *and* IGT, check every 3 months, long term. If IFG persists do an OGTT annually	
Consensus awaited IFG is a new category of glucose intolerance. The patient cannot be officially diagnosed as diabetic until he/she has a fasting glucose >7.0 mmol/l or a 2 hr glucose >11.0 mmol/l.	

This guideline was adapted by the author from the Diabetes UK Guidelines, June 2000, with the help of Dr Dai Thomas, The Hillingdon Hospital.

Types of diabetes

It is estimated that there are 2.4 million people with diabetes in England (4.75% prevalence). This is expected to increase to 2.6 million by 2010 (5.05% prevalence). 15–20% of all diabetic patients have type 1 diabetes. 10–25% of adults with apparent type 2 diabetes appear to have latent autoimmune diabetes of adulthood (LADA) or type 1 diabetes. 47% of type 2 diabetes can be attributed to obesity. York and Humber Public Health Observatory (YHPHO) have produced local and national prevalence estimates for total diabetes in NHS districts: http://www.yhpho.org.uk/viewResource.aspx?id=7

The same blood glucose criteria apply to the diagnosis of all types of diabetes. The two main types are type 1 (insulin-dependent diabetes or juvenile-onset diabetes previously) and type 2 (non-insulin-dependent or maturity-onset diabetes previously).

People with type 1 diabetes are usually:
- under 40 yrs of age
- slim
- ketosis-prone
- islet-cell antibody, and/or glutamic acid decarboxylase autoantibodies (antiGAD-Ab) positive
- have rapid onset of symptoms (often severe)
- unable to survive without insulin treatment.

People with type 2 diabetes are usually:
- over 40 yrs of age
- overweight
- not ketosis-prone
- islet cell or antiGAD-Ab negative
- have variable onset of symptoms (often slow and less severe)
- able to survive without insulin treatment
- have a family history of type 2 diabetes.

Type 1 diabetes

Type 1 diabetes appears to have three general forms of onset—symptoms over weeks or months, high glucose, high HbA_{1c}, ketones present, antibodies often found (**type 1a**)—usually in young people.

Type 1a may also present as late onset autoimmune diabetes (LADA) in apparent type 2 diabetic patients. Patients with LADA may manage on tablets for years but have positive anti-GAD antibodies and ultimately need insulin. Parental diabetes is uncommon.

Type 1b. Some patients have features of type 1a. but are antibody negative.

Type 1c. A few patients may have very rapid onset with normal or only slightly raised HbA_{1c} but high ketones. This is rare.

Type 2 diabetes

Most diabetic patients in the UK have type 2 diabetes as defined above. There appear to be multiple genes causing this, with significant interaction with environmental factors. Ongoing genetic projects are likely to clarify this. Variation in the gene TCF7L2 is linked to type 2 diabetes (*Diabetes* 2006; **55**:2640–4).

Most patients have metabolic syndrome. While many can be managed by diet oral hypoglycaemics, many come to need insulin. Type 2 diabetes is usually a combination of relative insulin lack and insulin resistance.

Early-onset type 2 diabetes is an unusual variant which starts between 25 and 40 yrs of age. 90% of parents and 68% of siblings have glucose intolerance. It is associated with obesity. Insulin is often needed and micro-vascular complications are common.

Monogenic diabetes/maturity onset diabetes of youth (MODY)

A subset of people with type 2 diabetes have monogenic diabetes, the preferred name for maturity-onset diabetes of the young (MODY). MODY is used here as the familiar term. This usually starts under 25 yrs old and forms 2–5% of type 2 diabetes. 50% of parents and 50% of siblings have glucose intolerance. MODY is slowly progressive and seldom needs insulin. Six gene defects have been identified (87% of all MODY patients):

- HNF1-α (70% all MODY patients, sulphonylureas very effective so worth diagnosing; 60% diabetes diagnosed <25 yrs old)
- Glucokinase: uncommon, glucose rarely needs medication
- HNF1-β (including renal cysts and diabetes)
- HNF4-α (variable age of onset, 30% will need insulin)
- IPF1
- NeuroD1

For more information, see www.diabetesgenes.org. If you think you have a patient with MODY contact them via the website or in writing before arranging tests:

Diabetes Research
Peninsula Medical School
Barrack Road
Exeter EX2 5DW
UK

Other forms of diabetes

Some patients are difficult to classify but can still be treated on clinical and biochemical assessment. African Caribbean patients presenting in DKA may have ketosis-prone type 2 diabetes or type 1b diabetes. There is a sub-Saharan variant. Tropical diabetes is rarely seen in the UK. It is associated with pancreatic calculi and, sometimes, with malnutrition.

Inheritance of diabetes

This is a more complex topic than in the past. Diabetes—a high blood glucose—is the endpoint of many different genetic and environmental interactions. Multiple variants of type 2 diabetes have now been identified, and there appear to be different versions of type 1 diabetes

Type 1 diabetes

An identical twin has a 30–40% chance of developing type 1 diabetes if his/her twin has it. The sibling of someone with type 1 diabetes has about an 8% chance of developing diabetes (this can be better predicted if HLA typing is done, but this is not performed outside research projects). A child has a 2–4% chance of developing diabetes if his/her mother has it and a 6-8% chance if his/her father has it. If both parents have type 1 diabetes, the risk is 6–12%. These figures should be compared with the frequency of type 1 diabetes in the population as a whole, which is about 1%.

Type 2 diabetes

The chance of inheriting type 2 diabetes is harder to assess as some individuals do not develop the disease until they are in their eighties. There is virtually 100% concordance of diabetes in identical twins. About 25% of the relatives of someone with type 2 diabetes have had, have, or will eventually develop diabetes. If one parent has type 2 diabetes about 15% of their children will eventually develop it; if both parents have type 2 diabetes the risk may be as high as 75%. The frequency in the population as a whole is about 4%.

MODY is dominantly inherited -i.e. 50% of children will have it.

Summary

- There are many paths to the diagnosis of diabetes and many patients are asymptomatic
- Check a finger-prick glucose immediately in symptomatic patients
- Use targeted screening, although most of the population will fulfil one or more criteria
- Remember that a one-off screening glucose test is not foolproof
- Confirm the diagnosis formally with laboratory venous glucose tests
- Differentiate between diabetes, IFG, and IGT
- Remember that IFG and IGT can progress to diabetes, and carry excess cardiovascular risk. Warn patients and advise on lifestyle measures.
- Classify diabetes into type 1 or type 2
- Remember unusual versions of diabetes. Seek advice if suspected.
- Do not delay treatment whilst trying to type the diabetes. Treat the patient and the glucose

Useful reading

IDF 2006 Diabetes Atlas Third Edition www.idf.org

Chapter 2

Assessing a person with diabetes

Emergencies

Box 2.1 Emergencies

Danger signs

Start urgent treatment. Consider hospital admission. Seek specialist/hospital advice immediately.

- Any impairment of conscious level
- Clinically ill
- Vomiting
- Hyperventilation
- Severe dehydration
- Low blood pressure
- Fever
- Foot or leg infection or gangrene
- Patients with any concomitant severe illness, especially infection
- Child
- Pregnant woman
- Blood glucose >20 mmol/l (some patients tolerate high glucose levels well but it can be difficult to decide who needs urgent help)

Urgent management

These patients need urgent assessment and management but in the absence of danger signs above can usually be managed out of hospital.

- Severe symptoms
- Profuse urinary ketones
- Marked weight loss
- Under 30 yrs of age

For both groups consider giving *adults* 4–8 units fast-acting insulin subcutaneously (intramuscularly or intravenously if shocked) immediately if the diagnosis of diabetes is secure and the blood glucose level is >20 mmol/l. (see Diabetic emergencies, 📖 p.460).

Information needed by the diabetes care team

Much of this may seem basic, but items are frequently omitted, to the detriment of patient care, and causing extra work and delays. Diabetes is lifelong and has a major impact on social and family life. Robust regularly updated information is essential. Much of this information is already available in practice or hospital records. GPs may feel that this is much too detailed, but as about half of all patients with newly diagnosed type 2 diabetes have complications at diagnosis it is important to make a thorough initial assessment.

Demographic

- Name
- Address
- Telephone (day and night) and mobile numbers (say which to try first)
- Name and contact details of carer if relevant
- E-mail address if patient wishes and understands that this may not be a confidential mode of communication
- Date of birth
- NHS number
- Practice/hospital record number
- Does patient want copies of letters? If so, delivery address

Practical

- Current occupation
- Language spoken (if not English note name and address of interpreter)
- Hearing, visual, speech, or other communication problems
- Comprehension problems (e.g. Down's syndrome)
- Mobility problems or other physical disabilities
- Religious or other beliefs which may influence treatment (e.g. vegetarian, non-beef/pork eating, no blood products, prefers to see female staff, etc.)
- Names and contact details of health or social care professionals, e.g. social worker

Clinical history

- Patient's main concerns
- Presentation of diabetes, symptoms and duration (📖 p.2)
- Previous medical history:
  - large-vessel disease, e.g. myocardial infarct, stroke
  - small-vessel disease, e.g. renal disease
  - endocrine disorders, e.g. thyroid
  - autoimmune disorders, e.g. pernicious anaemia
  - conditions likely to need steroid treatment or diuretics
  - obstetric history, e.g. gestational diabetes, big babies
  - pancreatitis
  - carcinoma pancreas
  - pancreatic or major abdominal surgery, trauma
  - other rarer linked conditions (📖 p.24)

- Family history:
  - diabetes
  - heart/arterial disease
  - endocrine
  - autoimmune disease
  - other inherited disease (📖 p.24)
- Family circle/support from friends.
- Women of child-bearing potential—are they planning pregnancy, risking it, or using contraception?
- Social history. Accommodation: stairs, council/state, residential/nursing home, detention centre/prison
- Education: to help tailor explanations and introduction of self-care
- Occupation. What does it involve? The diagnosis may have important financial implications.
  - sedentary
  - physically strenuous
  - risky, e.g. water or heights
  - shift work
  - feet at risk, e.g. building sites
  - armed forces
  - handles gun, e.g. police
  - driving—car, large goods vehicle, passenger vehicle
  - flying
- Leisure activities:
  - energetic, e.g. football, dancing
  - potentially hazardous, e.g. martial arts, sub-aqua diving, rock climbing
- Diet (in general—the dietitian will check in detail)
- Exercise
- Smoking (ask about bindi or hookah in relevant groups)
- Alcohol:
  - consider pancreatitis and malabsorption
  - check liver function and triglyceride
  - warn about hypoglycaemia with glucose-lowering medication
- Prescribed drugs:
  - steroids
  - oral contraceptives
  - thiazides
  - tricyclics
  - atypical antipsychotics
  - antiretrovirals
  - ß-blockers (impair hypoglycaemia warning)
- Street drugs: used by one in four young people. Injecting drugs increases risk of hepatitis B/C and HIV. Diabetic patients: test finger-prick glucose (📖 p.110)
- Allergy/adverse drug reactions. Sulphonamide allergy precludes sulphonylurea use. Most diabetic patients will need antibiotics sometimes
- System review—do not skimp. Consider evidence of diabetic tissue damage

Clinical examination

General observations

- Conscious level. Impaired? Consider hypoglycaemia (if on glucose-lowering medication), diabetic ketoacidosis, hyperosmolar non-ketotic state, stroke
- Personality, psychological and educational factors. These will influence impact of diabetes and ability to self-care
- Fever? (Infection common)
- Weight and height, body mass index
- Abdominal circumference
- Dehydration
- Clues to causes of secondary diabetes, or associated syndromes:
    - alcoholic pancreatic disease (common)
    - polycystic ovarian syndrome (common)
    - steroid excess, including iatrogenic (common), or lack (rarer)
    - thyroid disease (common)
    - acromegaly
    - haemochromatosis
    - Down's syndrome
    - cystic fibrosis
    - Wolfram's syndrome
    - hypogonadal syndromes, e.g. Kleinfelter's, Turner's, Prader–Willi, Laurence–Moon–Biedl
    - ataxia telangiectasia
    - dystrophia myotonica
    - congenital rubella
    - lipoatrophic conditions
    - Freidreich's ataxia
    - Huntington's chorea

Skin (📖 p.318)

- Skin infections, e.g. boils, cellulitis, ulcers, fungi (common)
- Diabetic dermopathy (quite common)
- Necrobiosis lipoidica diabeticorum (rare)
- Vitiligo
- Jaundice
- Stigmata of hyperlipidaemia (e.g. xanthomata, corneal arcus in under fifties)

Thyroid

Always examine the thyroid: ?enlargement
General thyroid status

Cardiovascular system

Usual assessment, particularly:

- hypertension (common)
- postural hypotension (overtreated hypertension, autonomic neuropathy, dehydration)
- left ventricular hypertrophy (hypertension)
- systolic murmur (aortic sclerosis, mitral regurgitation—previous myocardial infarct is common)
- peripheral pulses weak or missing (peripheral vascular disease common)
- ankle or sacral oedema (cardiac failure, nephrotic syndrome)

Respiratory system

- Breathlessness—chest infection, cardiac failure (common)
- Asthma or chronic obstructive airways disease: ?on steroids
- Hyperventilation—diabetic ketoacidosis (uncommon)

Abdomen

- Obese (is obesity general or central?)
- Scaphoid (severe weight loss if glucose uncontrolled, or pancreatic cancer)
- Hepatomegaly: alcohol, non-alcoholic fatty liver, haemochromatosis
- Kidneys: tender—pyelonephritis; bruits—renal arterial stenosis
- Bladder tenderness—urinary tract infection
- Epigastric tenderness—severe ketosis
- Genitalia—vulvovaginitis (common) or balanitis from candidiasis

Nervous system (📖 p.292, 306) including eyes (📖 p.294)

- Eyes
  - cataract
  - retinopathy
  - reduced acuity is a late sign of diabetic eye disease
- Hearing
  - deafness hinders education unless recognized
  - deafness can be due to mononeuropathy, infection; rarely congenital rubella, Wolfram's syndrome, etc.
- Cranial nerves
  - stroke
  - mononeuropathy
- Limbs
  - peripheral sensory neuropathy
  - mononeuropathy
  - paresis or other evidence of new or old stroke
- Autonomic neuropathy
  - postural hypotension

Joints and ligaments (📖 p.320)
- Dupuytren's contracture
- Cheiroarthropathy
- Charcot joints
- Arthritis: may make injections difficult or limit dexterity/mobility
- Arthritis: may be on steroid treatment

Feet and legs (📖 p.325)
- Gait: mobility
- Shoes (distorting or distorted)
- Foot hygiene
- Previous surgery or amputation
- Deformities
- Skin: dry, cracked, blisters, blemishes, colour (red, white, purple, blue, black)
- Pressure areas
- Old or current ulcers
- Circulation and pulses, feet hot or cold
- Sensation: monofilament, light touch, pin-prick (Neurotip), position, vibration

When finished
- Record your findings. Negative findings are important—record them
- Feed back to the patient

Information from others
Partners/relatives

Amplification of history if necessary

Information from other health care professionals
- Diagnostic glucose concentrations—if you did not make the diagnosis confirm it before starting lifelong treatment
- Amplification of clinical history

Share findings
- With patient:
  - discuss diagnostic and clinical findings
  - encourage patient to keep copies of this information (see below)
- With relevant health care professionals

Patient folder
Many different versions. The simplest is an envelope folder containing:
- information about help and rescue
- information about diabetes care (GP, clinic, etc.)
- appointment card
- glucose diary if required
- personalized health targets
- copies of laboratory and other test results, including X-ray report
- some centres using hard copies give patients their X-rays to keep
- photocopy of ECG (important)
- relevant information leaflets

Box 2.2 Investigations

- Finger-prick blood:
  - glucose
  - HbA_{1c} (if available)
  - ketones if emergency attender and/or ill/vomiting and glucose >11 mmol/l; or if appears well and glucose >15 mmol/l
- Urine:
  - dipstick glucose, ketones, protein, blood, leucocytes, nitrite
  - if protein dipstick negative—microalbumin-to-creatinine ratio (laboratory or clinic)
- Fasting laboratory venous blood (non-fasting if emergency attender):
  - nothing to eat/drink except plain water for 12 hr pre-test
  - fasting glucose (if diagnosis unproven)
  - fasting cholesterol, HDL, LDL, triglyceride
  - urea and electrolytes
  - creatinine
  - liver function
  - calcium and albumin
  - thyroid function
  - haemoglobin A_{1c}
  - full blood count
  - consider adding C-reactive protein (?infection), urate (?gout)
  - add tissue transglutaminase/anti-mysial/anti-gliadin antibodies in under-twenties
- Chest X-ray if chest signs or symptoms, recent immigrant, Asian
- Foot X-ray if ulcer, possible infection, or injury
- ECG if chest pain, or if age >40 yrs (author's practical suggestion as ECG changes are common at diagnosis and future cardiac events are also common)

This chapter assumes that the person has untreated diabetes. This system can also be used to reassess someone with known diabetes. Full assessment takes at least 30 min. Full dietetic assessment takes another 30 min.

Summary

- Is the patient ill? Always assess for danger signs and treat promptly
- Is the patient high risk—child or pregnant woman?
- Obtain a full history on first encounter. Get to know your patient.
- Detailed examination is important
- It takes up to an hour to assess a new diabetic patient fully. Break this into manageable sessions if necessary
- Every patient needs investigations
- Start the record which will follow the patient for the rest of his/her life
- Share your findings with the patient and with relevant health care professionals

Chapter 3

The aims of diabetes care

Introduction

To enjoy life to the full and stay well

The aim should be for a person with diabetes to enjoy life to the full without their diabetes or its care causing problems now or in the future. This means avoidance of acute glucose emergencies and long-term diabetic tissue damage. It also means as little interference as possible by the process of diabetes care and clinical supervision.

Many people with diabetes simply want to 'get back to normal'. Normality is hard to define. Dictionary definitions include 'ordinary', 'well-adjusted', and 'functioning regularly'. Each person will have their own personal definition. It is devastating to discover that one has a permanent illness which may disable or kill you, which requires uncomfortable and sometimes complex treatment, and which may impact on your job, driving, insurance, and family life. It is misleading and unfair to paint too rosy a picture of life with diabetes, but neither should carers paint too gloomy a future. Help people with diabetes to get back towards their version of normal as soon as possible. If this is not feasible then provide them with sympathetic and practical support through their disappointment and frustration. Help them to build a new 'normality'.

Diabetes education (📖 p.51)

People with diabetes need to understand what diabetes is, what it means for them personally, and what may happen in the future. They need to learn what they themselves can do to reduce the likelihood of glucose problems and tissue complications, and what their diabetes team can do to help them. They should understand how best to use their medication and related technology, how to cope with common difficulties and emergencies, how to seek help, and how to make the most of health resources. Relatives and friends also want to learn and help.

Education is a continuous process, and so there must be opportunities for learning during every interaction with health care staff—and in between. People need revision sessions and opportunities to extend and update their knowledge.

Appropriate accessible care

Appropriate accessible high-standard evidence-based health care

Each person with diabetes should be able to access diabetes care when and where they need it, easily and without barriers. Distant surgeries or clinics, too few diabetes-trained staff, poor public transport, over-busy tired staff, lack of continuity of staff, and lack of expert advice out of hours are some examples of barriers to care. Some can be resolved by increasing resources, and some by additional training.

Staff delivering diabetes care should know about diabetes—in depth. Obvious? Apparently not. Many patients are cared for by health care staff who have had no special training in diabetes care. Nowadays this is not acceptable. Over the past 10 yrs the publication of several large well-planned studies has provided a clear evidence-based blueprint for diabetes care (📖 p.34). Everyone caring for diabetic patients should follow this to the best of their ability and keep up to date. The resources to deliver the highest standards of care are not always available, especially as the frequency of diabetes increases. Therefore we must use what we have efficiently, communicate well within and between primary and secondary care, and avoid duplication or omission. Staff should be supported with good training, updating, and good working conditions.

Each patient is unique

Daisy has lived alone since her husband died. She is 81, walks with a stick, and is blind in one eye. She has peripheral vascular disease and arthritis, and has had several falls. She takes gliclazide for her type 2 diabetes. Her BMI is 24 kg/m^2, BP 165/95, and HbA_{1c} 8.3%.

Malcolm is a successful 32-yr old businessman. He has had diabetes for 5 years which is treated with gliclazide. He works long hours and regards his job as stressful. He enjoys playing football at weekends. His BMI is 24 kg/m^2, BP 165/95, and HbA_{1c} 8.3%.
These are imaginary patients.

Clearly these two patients are very different. One is elderly and frail; the other is young and energetic. One has plenty of time for herself; the other is in a stressful time-consuming job. One finds finger-prick glucose measurements difficult, the other easy. One does not drive and cannot use a bus; the other has a car. Both have elevated BPs and poor glucose balance. So what factors influence the targets we set for Daisy and Malcolm? Think about it.

If it doesn't work for me, it doesn't work

The care plan we produce must be acceptable to the patient and he/she must feel that it will work for them. As with all patients, we need to consider their previous knowledge of their condition and its care, their attitudes, their expectations, their emotional state, their educational level, and factors which may impede understanding.

Physical factors

Factors affecting understanding (e.g. dementia, metabolic disarray), movement and mobility (arthritis, stroke, amputation), sensation (neuropathy), balance (stroke, postural hypotension), concentration (malaise from persistent hyperglycaemia, pain), vision (cataract, retinopathy), and hearing (diabetic deafness) can all impede care, as can comorbidities. For example, do not aim for a BP of 125/75 in someone with postural hypotension.

Practicalities

Modern diabetes care means that the patient must be reviewed more often. He/she needs to be able to get to the surgery or clinic easily. If not, the care should go to the patient. Consider using telephone (landline or mobile), texting, and e-mail (with appropriate confidentiality warning). Many areas have specialist helplines. However, it is often those patients who have most difficulties in hearing or using the phone who cannot get to the surgery, and who have the most medical problems.

It is easier to look after your diabetes if you are financially well off. Meters are not yet available on the NHS and so have to be bought, although some diabetes centres may be able to provide them free. It is easier to enjoy an attractive diabetic diet if you can afford interesting food. Advise low-income patients to check that they have obtained benefits for which they are eligible. Diabetes team members may be able to help advise on economical and healthy food, for example. Now that we are encouraging more frequent check-ups, patients may be worried that they may lose their jobs, those with young families may find it hard to find babysitters, and students may miss school or college. Late evening or weekend surgeries are valued by patients but have to be staffed.

NHS care arrangements are complicated, especially if you have a disability such as amputation, and the planned links between health and social care are welcome. Diabetic patients are often under the care of multiple medical teams. Daisy, for example, sees her GP, the diabetic clinic, the eye clinic, the vascular clinic, the rheumatologist, and the orthopaedic clinic. She has an appointment for care of the elderly about her falls. She sees a chiropodist separately, has a social worker, and her son recently arranged a visit to an osteopath. One health care professional should act as a keyworker for such patients and coordinate care.

Evidence-based diabetes care for adults

There can be few chronic disorders which offer so much scope for preventive health care as diabetes. In this section we discuss the evidence from some recent large studies of diabetes care or subset analyses of studies including diabetic patients. Study acronyms are given, with references at the chapter end. Detailed review is outside the scope of this book (📖 p.48).

There is clear evidence that good diabetes care reduces diabetic tissue damage. Aim for perfect diabetes care for all, tailoring the final decision to suit the patient's situation and wishes. Do not endanger patients in the search for the perfect glucose or perfect BP. However, with care, patients can achieve considerable improvements in both without major physical or emotional side effects. The world of research studies, with frequent discussions with research nurses or doctors, is very different from the busy clinic with too many patients and too few staff. The resourcing of modern diabetes care is a national issue. Focus on the key care issues for each patient and try to deliver them as efficiently and kindly as possible.

Targets

The aim of diabetes care is to return the patient to as close a non-diabetic state as is safe and practical for that particular person. These targets are for adults.

Children also need careful diabetes care, aiming for safe near normalization of parameters, but this has particular risks. They should be cared for by specialist teams.

These targets are stringent, but are supported by the literature and by the relevant specialist societies. They will not be possible in some patients and care is needed in their application. There is increasing evidence that there is no threshold effect for BP or glucose provided that they remain within physiological levels (i.e. providing adequate perfusion and cerebral glucose delivery, respectively). There appears to be no threshold effect for cholesterol either, although research continues. Risk reduction will also be discussed in the chapters on complications of diabetes.

Do not use cardiovascular risk calculators in people with diabetes. Diabetes itself is such a risk that it renders them inappropriate.

Box 3.1 Targets for preventive care in diabetes

- No smoking
- Waist circumference
  - <102 cm in men (<92 cm in Asian men)
  - <88 cm in women (<78 cm in Asian women)
- BMI 18.5–25 kg/m^2
- BP (without postural hypotension)
  - <130/80
  - <125/75 renal disease
- Fasting* lipids
  - Total cholesterol <4 mmol/l or a 25% reduction, whichever is lower
  - LDL cholesterol <2 mmol/l or a 25% reduction, whichever is lower
  - Fasting triglyceride <1.7 mmol/l
- Fasting plasma glucose 4–6 mmol/l (without hypoglycaemia)
- HbA_{1c} 6.0–6.5% (without hypoglycaemia) (📖 p.125)
- No high glucose emergencies
- Urine albumin-to-creatinine ratio normal (📖 p.104)

*Fasting may cause hypoglycaemia in insulin or sulphonylurea-treated patients and is not essential unless triglycerides are raised

Derived from Joint British Societies' Guidelines on the Prevention of Cardiovascular Disease in Clinical Practice: Risk Assessment (JBS2) British Heart Foundation 2006

(Joint British Societies: British Cardiovascular Society, British Hypertension Society, Diabetes UK, Heart UK, Primary Care Cardiovascular Society, The Stroke Association.)

Stop smoking!

- People with diabetes who smoke have at least the same risk of morbidity and mortality as non-diabetics who smoke, and probably greater.
- Diabetics who smoke have about four times the risk of dying from cardiovascular disease (CVD) as those who do not.
- Give smokers support in stopping—stop smoking groups/courses.
- Vigorously discourage young people with diabetes from starting smoking.
- Nicotine may alter the rate of insulin absorption, so monitor glucose after stopping. The insulin dose may need to be adjusted. Nicotine patches can be used by people with diabetes but care should be taken by those with CVD. Avoid patches in those with renal failure.
- Bupropion can also be used in people with diabetes but not in those with renal failure. Monitor BP.

Blood pressure (BP) control (📖 Chapter 14)

For clinical management 📖 p.208.

CVD is the most common cause of death in diabetic patients. Reducing BP greatly reduces the risk of diabetic and cardiovascular events, both fatal and non-fatal, but be constantly aware of the risk of postural hypotension. There is considerable evidence of the benefits of BP lowering.

In UKPDS 38, tight BP control produced a mean BP 144/82 mmHg vs [illegible]4/87 in the less tight control group. The tight control group showed a [illegible]% reduction in diabetes-related endpoints, 32% reduction in deaths due to diabetes, 44% reduction in strokes, and 37% reduction in microvascular endpoints.

Advice about BP targets varies. NICE CG 66 (2008) advocates <130/80 if kidney, eye or cerebrovascular damage and BP 140/80 for others. The Joint British Societies (2005) advocate a resting BP <130/80, and <125/75 if there is any renal impairment. Most patients with diabetes need treatment.

Angiotensin-converting enzyme (ACE) inhibitors (captopril (UKPDS), enalapril (ABCD), fosinopril (FACET, HOT), ramipril (HOPE/MICRO-HOPE)), β-blockers (atenolol (UKPDS)), and diuretic agents bendroflumethiazide (UKPDS), hydrochlorothiazide (not availabe on its own in UK) (Syst-EUR)) are effective and do not produce adverse metabolic effects in diabetic patients. ACE inhibitors appear to have benefits in addition to BP lowering. ACE inhibitors and diuretics are often combined.

Angiotensin receptor blockers (ARBs) reduce CVD endpoints. Losartan reduced cardiovascular events and total mortality vs atenolol (LIFE), and also reduced endstage renal failure vs placebo (RENAAL). Irbesartan reduced endstage renal failure vs amlodipine and placebo (IDNT).

Calcium-channel blockers showed variable results. Felodipine (HOT) and nitrendipine (may not be available in UK) (Syst-EUR) were safe and effective. Amlodipine ± perindopril reduced cardiovascular endpoints more than atenolol ± thiazide and was less diabetogenic in non-diabetics. (ASCOT). ALLHAT showed no difference in cardiovascular endpoints between chlortalidone, amlodipine, lisinopril, and doxazosin, but there was less heart failure on chlortalidone.

Microalbuminuria

Microalbuminuria warns that diabetes has damaged the kidneys and renal failure will follow. The rate of progression to renal failure can be slowed by prompt and vigorous treatment. Risk factors for progression are:

- male sex
- family history
- South Asian or African Caribbean
- smoker
- BP >125/75
- HbA_{1c} >7%
- dyslipidaemia
- retinopathy
- type 1 diabetes onset aged <20 yrs

Trandolapril given to reduce BP to 120/80 reduced development of microalbuminuria vs verapamil (BENEDICT). Enalapril showed a reduction in development of microalbuminuria in normotensive diabetic patients (*Ann Int Med* 1998; **12**:982–8). Ramipril (HOPE and MICRO-HOPE) and losartan (LIFE 2004) are licensed for use in microalbuminuria with or without hypertension. MICRO-HOPE and HOPE demonstrated the benefit of ramipril in reducing deterioration of renal function in diabetic patients with early nephropathy/microalbuminuria, although it was thought that much of this effect was due to BP lowering. The decrease in albuminuria was significantly greater with losartan vs atenolol in the LIFE study. Irbesartan is licensed for use in hypertensive diabetic patients, including those with renal disease, following IRMA-2 in which irbesartan appeared to have an effect upon albumin excretion apart from BP lowering. Valsartan had a similar additional benefit when compared with amlodipine ± other agents as needed to achieve the same BP lowering effect (MARVAL).

Lipid lowering (📖 Chapter 14)

For clinical management see 📖 p.287.

A rigorous low-fat high-fibre weight-normalizing diet reduces lipids. Good glucose control also reduces lipids (DCCT 1995, UKPDS 39). However, lifestyle measures are not enough. The evidence of the benefit of statins is overwhelming, even in patients with "normal" cholesterol levels.

The 5 yr Heart Protection Study (HPS) included 5963 people with diabetes who did not satisfy existing criteria for cholesterol-lowering therapy in 1994. The study compared simvastatin 40 mg with placebo. There was a 22% reduction vs placebo in cardiovascular events in those on simvastatin, with a 33% reduction in those without overt vascular disease at outset and a 27% reduction if LDL-cholesterol <3 mmol/l at the outset. HPS also showed that simvastatin is safe—there was no significant difference in elevation of liver enzyme or of muscle enzyme between the two groups.

CARDS showed a reduction in ACS, coronary revascularization, and stroke, regardless of initial lipids, with atorvastatin vs placebo.

In subgroup analyses of other studies, statins (lovastatin (not available in UK) (AFCAPS/TexCAPS)) and fibrates (gemfibrozil (Helsinki), bezafibrate (SENDCAP)) reduced myocardial infarcts and/or cardiac death in diabetic patients. In studies of patients after myocardial infarction, statins (simvastatin (4S), pravastatin (CARE, LIPID)) reduced cardiac events and death. In DAIS, micronized fenofibrate reduced coronary arterial narrowing in diabetic patients with coronary artery disease vs placebo.

There are fewer studies of lowering triglyceride or raising HDL, although both are risk factors for CVD. Gemfibrozil increased HDL and reduced triglyceride and reduced CVD mortality (*N Engl J Med* 1999; **341**:410–18. Fasting triglycerides should be <1.7 mmol/l.

Box 3.2 Cholesterol lowering

Give simvastatin or atorvastatin to:

- All diabetic patients aged >40 yrs*
- Diabetic patients 18–40 yrs with any of:
  - Retinopathy
  - Nephropathy
  - HbA_{1c} >9%
  - BP >130/80
  - Total cholesterol ≥6 mmol/l
  - Waist circumference
    >102 cm in men (>92 cm in asian men)
    >88 cm in women (>78 cm in asian women)
  - Total Cholesterol > 4 mmol/l
  - Triglyceride >1.7 mmol/l (fasting), >2.0 mmol/l (random)
  - HDL cholesterol <1.0 mmol/l (men), 1.2 mmol/l (women)
  - Family history—premature CVD in first-degree relative

Joint British Societies' *Heart* 2005; **91**(Suppl 5):v1–52

* NICE (2008) advocates statin if CV risk >20% 10yrs (see www.dtu.ox.uk/index.php?maindoc=/riskengine)

**Consider fibrate 📖 p.275

Blood glucose control (📖 Chapters 7–13)

Intensive blood glucose control reduces the development and progression of the complications of diabetes (DCCT, UKPDS).

In DCCT (1993), intensively treated type 1 diabetic patients had a mean blood glucose of 8.6 mmol/l compared with 12.8 mmol/l in the conventionally treated group. Intensive therapy reduced the risk of developing new retinopathy by 76%, and slowed progression by 54% in those with pre-existing retinopathy,. Overall, intensive therapy reduced occurrence of microalbuminuria by 39%, overt proteinuria by 54%, and clinical neuropathy by 54%. The benefit persisted post-trial even though glucose levels rose (DCCT 2000). There was a trend towards reduction of CVD during the original study, and long-term follow-up (DCCT 1995, 2005) showed a significant reduction of 42% in CVD in the intensive therapy group.

In UKPDS (34), intensive treatment with metformin in overweight type 2 patients produced a median HbA_{1c} of 7.4% compared with 8.0% in those treated conventionally. Intensive treatment with metformin reduced any diabetes-related endpoint by 32%. In UKPDS (33), intensive treatment of type 2 patients with sulphonylurea or insulin reduced HbA_{1c} to 7.0% compared with 7.9% with conventional treatment. This reduced any diabetes endpoint by 12%.

ADVANCE (11, 140 patients with Type 2DM) used gilclazide and other drugs to reduce HbA_{1c} to 6.5% vs 7.3% in a standard control group. This intensive glucose control reduced combined major macrovascular and microvascular events by 10%, primarily due to 21% relative reduction in nephropathy. There was no significant difference in mortality (intensive control 8.9% vs standard control 9.6%). This much larger study does not confirm the results of ACCORD, stopped because the very intensive glucose control group (HbA_{1c} < 6.0%) had more deaths (14 /1000/yr vs. 11/1000/yr) then the standard group (HbA_{1c} 7–7.9%) (BMJ 2008; 336: 407).

Intensive blood glucose control increased the frequency of hypoglycaemia, in ADVANCE and DCCT but careful blood glucose monitoring, good access to knowledgeable advice, and appropriate treatment adjustment can reduce this. Quality of life was no different between intensively and conventionally treated patients. Intensive glucose lowering did not appear to have an adverse effect upon cognitive function in DCCT.

The lower HbA_{1c}, the lower is the risk of diabetic tissue damage. The aim for blood glucose is that observed in non-diabetics without any glucose intolerance: a fasting blood glucose between 4 and 6 mmol/l. At other times the glucose should be between 4 and 7 mmol/l. (up to 10 mmol/l after food). HbA_{1c} should be within the normal range for your local laboratory (usually 4.5–6.5%), but only if safe and practical for an individual patient. For a detailed discussion of glucose-lowering agents 📖 Chapters 8 and 9

The main risk is of hypoglycaemia (📖 p.199). Teach all patients on glucose-lowering treatment (whether tablets or insulin) how to recognize and treat hypoglycaemia. Teach them how to adjust their treatment to reduce the risk of further hypoglycaemia. Patients with varied timetables, varied meals, varied exercise, varied emotions, and varied compliance are particularly at risk of hypoglycaemia, as are children and elderly people. Any patient who has had one hypoglycaemic attack is likely to have more. Some patients will be unable to achieve a normal glucose without hypoglycaemia. In this case work together towards the best compromise between safety now and good health long term.

Normalize weight

See 🕮 p.84

Obesity increases insulin resistance, BP, and cardiovascular risk. Weight reduction reduces symptoms of diabetes and reduces the treatment needed to normalize blood glucose, BP, and lipids. Encourage weight loss in people with diabetes (Canadian Task Force 1999).

The aim is a BMI between 18.5 and 25 kg/m^2. Waist circumference provides a better estimate of adiposity and should be <102 cm in men (<92 cm in Asian men); and <88 cm in women (78 cm in Asian women).

In general, the most effective weight reduction strategy combines dietary advice (🕮 Chapter 5), regular exercise (🕮 Chapter 13), and long-term help in changing everyday weight-gaining habits. Very-low-calorie diets are successful. Drugs are methylcellulose, orlistat, which inhibits pancreatic lipase and therefore induces fat malabsorption (and frequent gastrointestinal side effects), and sibutramine and rimonabant, which reduce appetite centrally. All drugs require expert supervision and long-term dietetic support. Bariatric surgery is effective in weight reduction and improving glucose control in obese diabetic patients. A meta-analysis showed that 'diabetes was completely resolved in 76.8% of patients and resolved or improved in 86.0%. Hyperlipidemia improved in 70% or more of patients. Hypertension was resolved in 61.7% of patients and resolved or improved in 78.5%'. Operative mortality was up to 1%. (*JAMA 2004;* **292**:1724–37)

Identification and treatment of tissue damage

The main thrust of diabetes care must be prevention of problems, but in reality much effort is needed to detect and slow progression of diabetic tissue damage. Up to half of patients with type 2 diabetes have obvious tissue damage at the time of diagnosis. Diabetes UK's audit data and regression calculations showed that the onset of coronary heart disease culminating in myocardial infarction is 20 yrs pre-diagnosis, stroke is 12 yrs, nephropathy is 18 yrs, amputation is 7 yrs, and retinopathy is 7 yrs (🕮 p.5) At least half the patients with diabetes on any practice list will have overt tissue damage. Every person with diabetes must be assumed to have hidden tissue damage.

Many diabetic complications have specific treatments and their progress can be slowed by redoubled preventive care (see above and 🕮 Chapters 14 and 15). It is essential to detect any hint of tissue damage early. This means rigorous checks by the patient (reporting visual change, foot problems, etc.) and by health care professionals. Standards for monitoring are described in the relevant chapters. Record negative information (e.g. normal foot pulses, no retinopathy) as well as positive findings. Check tissue damage annually at present (note that there is no evidence to support a 12-month interval as being better than a shorter or longer one). In a perfect world we should probably check more often. But the main difficulty lies in the silence of much severe tissue damage until it is too late to prevent disability.

Delivery of good diabetes care

Annual review

Everyone with diabetes should have a full check by someone trained in the assessment of people with diabetes at least once a year.

Box 3.3 Annual review

- Who is the patient? Age? Child/teenage/adolescent/adult?
- Woman of child-bearing potential?
- How is the person feeling? Any symptoms?
- Life events? Births, deaths, marriages, separations? Moves? Job? Hobbies?
- Emotions. Check for depression or anxiety and manage appropriately if present.
- Driver? If yes, check knowledge of safe driving with diabetes. Told insurance company and DVLA?
- Diet. If unhealthy or overweight, provide appropriate advice and dietetic referral as required. Ideally, everyone with diabetes should see a dietitian annually.
- Exercise? Advise if insufficient.
- Smoker? If yes, help them stop.
- Alcohol? If excessive, help them reduce/stop.
- Hospital attendances or admissions? For diabetes, e.g. hypoglycaemia, high glucose/diabetic ketoacidosis. For non-diabetes reason.
- Symptoms of cardiovascular disease, eye problems, neuropathy, foot problems, sexual dysfunction, other complications.
- Woman. Periods? Planning pregnancy? Contraception?
- Glucose control: HBGM, hypoglycaemia.
- BP (including home monitoring if done).
- Full foot assessment: shape, skin, pulses, sensation. Refer any problems to podiatrist.
- Cardiovascular examination if any hint of cardiac disease.
- Examine other systems if any relevant symptoms.
- Finger-prick or laboratory glucose (± ketone).
- Laboratory HbA_{1c}, cholesterol, HDL, LDL, triglycerides, urea, electrolytes, creatinine, eGFR if relevant, LFT, thyroid function. Full blood count + vitamin B_{12} (if on metformin or otherwise relevant).
- Urine dipstick, laboratory microalbumin-to-creatinine ratio.
- Ensure patient has had visual acuity check and digital photographic retinal screening by a recognized service—and obtain the results.
- Check patient knows what and how to monitor.
- Diabetes education and revision.
- Check patient knows where and how to seek help.
- Any questions?
- Date of next appointment.

Give the patient a copy of the annual review.

Diabetes register: audit and recall system

See 📖 p.500

In order to deliver good diabetes care each unit or practice needs to know who has diabetes in their area of responsibility and what care they have had. This means a register with audit facilities. There should be a recall system for annual review and, optimally, reminders for interim check-ups. Non-attenders have a high rate of complications and should be pursued in a constructive way. There a national diabetes audit programme (www.icservices.nhs.uk/ncasp).

Local support

There should be a local forum for supporting district-wide diabetes care. In many districts this is the Local Diabetes Services Advisory Group. There should be representation from all those involved in receiving, providing, and purchasing diabetes care throughout the district. Such a group can be a major force in communication, education, and improving resources.

Cost-effectiveness

Many health service financial cycles are annual. Diabetic complications take years to become obvious, and so the immediate benefits of intensive management can rarely be demonstrated to a financial manager planning the following year's budget. Both DCCT and UKPDS studied the long-term cost-effectiveness of intensive diabetes care.

DCCT (1996), concluded that intensive rather than conventional therapy for the 120 000 people with type 1 diabetes in the USA would gain 920 000 yrs of sight, 691 000 yrs free from endstage renal disease, 678 000 yrs free from lower-extremity amputation, and 611 000 yrs of life.

In UKPDS 41, intensive management of type 2 diabetic patients 'significantly increased treatment costs but substantially reduced the cost of complications and increased the time free from complications'. They calculated that, with intensive care, the patient would gain 1.14 yrs (confidence interval 0.69–1.61) of event-free time (an event being a diabetic complication, including death). This did not include the non-medical and social benefits such as fitness to work.

National Service Framework for diabetes: summary of standards

Prevention of type 2 diabetes

Standard 1

The NHS will develop, implement, and monitor strategies to reduce the risk of developing type 2 diabetes in the population as a whole and to reduce the inequalities in the risk of developing type 2 diabetes.

Identification of people with diabetes

Standard 2

The NHS will develop, implement, and monitor strategies to identify people who do not know they have diabetes.

Empowering people with diabetes

Standard 3

All children, young people, and adults with diabetes will receive a service which encourages partnership in decision-making, supports them in managing their diabetes, and helps them to adopt and maintain a healthy lifestyle. This will be reflected in an agreed and shared care plan in an appropriate format and language. Where appropriate, parents and carers should be fully engaged in this process.

Clinical care of adults with diabetes

Standard 4

All adults with diabetes will receive high-quality care throughout their lifetime, including support to optimize the control of their blood glucose, blood pressure, and other risk factors for developing the complications of diabetes.

Clinical care of children and young people with diabetes

Standard 5

All children and young people with diabetes will receive consistently high-quality care and they, with their families and others involved in their day-to-day care, will be supported to optimize the control of their blood glucose and their physical, psychological, intellectual, educational, and social development.

Standard 6

All young people with diabetes will experience a smooth transition of care from paediatric diabetes services to adult diabetes services, whether hospital or community-based, either directly or via a young people's clinic. The transition will be organised in partnership with each individual and at an age appropriate to and agreed with them.

Management of diabetic emergencies

Standard 7

The NHS will develop, implement, and monitor agreed protocols for rapid and effective treatment of diabetic emergencies by appropriately trained health care professionals. Protocols will include the management of acute complications and procedures to minimize the risk of recurrence.

Care of people with diabetes during admission to hospital

Standard 8

All children, young people, and adults with diabetes admitted to hospital, for whatever reason, will receive effective care of their diabetes. Wherever possible, they will continue to be involved in decisions concerning the management of their diabetes.

Diabetes and pregnancy

Standard 9

The NHS will develop, implement, and monitor policies that seek to empower and support women with pre-existing diabetes and those who develop diabetes during pregnancy to optimize the outcomes of their pregnancy.

Detection and management of long-term complications

Standard 10

All young people and adults with diabetes will receive regular surveillance for the long-term complications of diabetes.

Standard 11

The NHS will develop, implement and monitor agreed protocols and systems of care to ensure that all people who develop long-term complications of diabetes receive timely, appropriate, and effective investigation and treatment to reduce their risk of disability and premature death.

Standard 12

All people with diabetes requiring multi-agency support will receive integrated health and social care.

http://www.dh.gov.uk/en/Publicationsandstatistics/Publications/PublicationsPolicyAndGuidance/Browsable/DH_4899717

Summary

- The aim should be for a person with diabetes to enjoy life to the full without their diabetes or its care causing problems now or in the future.
- Everyone with diabetes should be taught about their condition and what they and others need to do to ensure optimal care.
- Diabetes care should be appropriate, accessible, high standard, and evidence based.
- Care should be tailored to the individual.
- Diabetes care should be practical.
- Evidence-based care should be used where available.
- Targets for risk reduction are smoking, BP, glucose, cholesterol, weight, and microalbuminuria
- Tissue damage should be detected and treated.
- Every patient should have an annual review.
- Practices and clinics should have a diabetes register with a call and recall system.
- Diabetes services should audit their care.
- Clinical services should make optimal use of resources.
- Care should conform to the NSF standards.

[illegible]

Further reading and references

A detailed analysis of the many diabetes studies is outside the scope of this book.

Suggested further reading

A H Barnett (ed) 2006 *Diabetes; best practice and research compendium.* Amsterdam: Elsevier

References

ABCD *N Engl Med* 1998; **338**:645–52
ADVANCE *N Engl J Med* 2008; **358**; 2560–2572
AFCAPS/TexCAPS *JAMA* 1998; **279**:1615–22
ALLHAT *JAMA* 2002; **288**:2981–97
ASCOT *Lancet* 2005; **366**:895–906
BENEDICT *N Engl J Med* 2004; **351**:1941–51
Canadian Task Force on Preventive Health Care *Can Med Assoc J* 1999; **160**:513–25
CARDS *Lancet* 2004; **364**:685–96
CARE *N Engl J Med* 1996: **335**(14):1001–9
DAIS *Lancet* 2001; **357**:905–10
DCCT *N Engl J Med* 1993, **329**(14):977–86
Am J Cardiol 1995; **75**:894–903
JAMA 1996, **276**, 1409-15
N Engl J Med 2000; **342**:381–9
N Engl J Med 2005; **353**:2643–53
FACET *Diabetes Care* 1998; **21**:597–603
Helsinki *Diabetes Care* 1992, **15**, 820-5.
HOPE/MICRO-HOPE *Lancet* 2000; **355**:253–9
HOT *Lancet* 1998; **351**:1755–62
HPS *Lancet* 2003; **361**:2005–16
IDNT *N Engl J Med* 2001; **345**:851–60
IRMA-2 *N Engl J Med* 2001; **345**: 870–8
Joint British Societies *Heart* 2005; **91**(Suppl V):v1–52
LIPID *N Engl J Med* 1998; **339**:1349–57
LIFE *Lancet* 2002; **359**:995–1003
Lancet 2002; **359**:1004–10
Hypertension 2004; **22**:1805–11
MARVAL *Circulation* 2002; **106**:672–8
NICE (National Institute for Clinical Excellence)
NICE (2008). The management of Type 2 diabetes. www.nice.org.uk/nicemedia/pdf/CG66diabetesfullguideline.pdf National Collaborating Centre for Chronic conditions London. Royal College of physicians. www.nice.org.uk
RENAAL *N Engl J Med* 2001; **345**:861–9
SENDCAP *Diabetes Care* 1998; **21**:641–8
4S *Diabetes Care* 1997; **20**:614–20
Syst–EUR *Arch Int Med*;1998:**158**, 1681–91.

UKPDS http://www.dtu.ox.ac.uk/index.php?maindoc=/ukpds/
UKPDS 33 *Lancet* 1998; **352**:837–53
UKPDS 34 *Lancet* 1998; **352**:854–65
UKPDS 38. *BMJ* 1998; **317**:703–13
UKPDS 39 *BMJ* 1998; **317**:713–20
UKPDS 41 *BMJ* 2000; **320**:1373–8

Chapter 4

Diabetes education

Essential to survival

Diabetes education is essential to patient survival. It is the person who has the condition who determines their own outcome. They need to know:

- How to get help
- What diabetes is
- What it means for them
- How the relevant body systems work
- What to do to stay healthy
- How to treat the diabetes specifically
- What might happen because of the diabetes
- How to avoid problems
- How to manage problems if they occur
- Ways of working out what to do in unexpected situations
- How to include all the above in everyday life in a practical, acceptable way
- How to revise and learn more
- How to get help (duplicated on purpose)

It is particularly important to equip patients with the knowledge to work things out for themselves. Problems may arise which require a logical extension of the instructions given by the doctor or nurse. The situation may deteriorate and the patient has to know when to seek help, and how urgently.

Factors influ[illegible] and application of [illegible]

[illegible] the patient [illegible]

- [illegible] of learning [illegible]
- [illegible]
- [illegible]
- [illegible] diabetes [illegible]
- [illegible]
- [illegible] beliefs
- [illegible] health beliefs [illegible]
- [illegible]
- [illegible] health professionals [illegible]
- Educational background and abilities
- Reading abilities (literacy and numeracy)
- Social factors
- Ethnic and language [illegible] the same [illegible]

[illegible]

At [illegible] diagnosis has [illegible] take the [illegible] overwhelming [illegible] the diabetes teaching and [illegible] the diagnosis [illegible] figures respected, [illegible] managers [illegible] can be a major influence.

[illegible]

The patient's agenda [illegible] want to know [illegible] Patients don't take in [illegible] their concerns [illegible] personal communication [illegible] head [illegible]

Factors influencing learning and application of diabetes education

- Emotions: how the patient feels on the day
- Motivation
- Circumstances of teaching session
- Support from family or friends sharing learning
- Personal experiences of diabetes (e.g. diabetes in a relative or friend, past gestational diabetes)
- Media portrayal of diabetes (television, newspapers, Internet, e.g. entering 'diabetes' into Google™ produced 'Do you have diabetes?… It may lead to kidney damage' as the first item)
- Personal health beliefs
- Personal health beliefs and influences of family and friends
- Anxiety
- Attitudes to health professionals
- Age
- Educational background and abilities
- Reading abilities (if leaflets etc. used)
- Social factors
- Ethnic and language factors—are you both using the same language in the same way?

The impact of friends, family, or 'leaders'

Ask if the patient has a close relative or friend with whom they wish to share the teaching session. Often relatives are more worried about the diabetes than the person who has it. They may harbour misconceptions which subsequently override what you have said. They can also reinforce the diabetes teaching and correct patients' misconceptions. Being allowed to share in the diabetes experience can help relatives overcome feelings of uselessness. 'I want to help but I don't know what to do.' The views of figures respected as religious leaders may influence adherence to advice. For teenagers in particular, the views or behaviour of media stars can be a major influence.

Agendas

The patient's agenda

Teach me what I want to know, when I want to know it. Start with this. People won't take in what you are saying until you have addressed their concerns. 'No question is ever stupid if it has to be a question' (Thomas, personal communication). The patient will not have a tidy curriculum in his/her head. The heart will be pounding and the head will be whirling with confused thoughts and anxieties.

The teacher's agenda

The standard lesson must be tailored to individual need. Patients see many members of the multidisciplinary diabetes team, in both primary and secondary care, as well as other health care professionals not specializing in diabetes care. It is important to educate staff involved in treating diabetic patients elsewhere.

A woman stumbled into a diabetic clinic in tears having been informed by a midwife that she had miscarried because she was injecting her insulin into the subcutaneous tissue of her abdomen. Even people who should have good understanding of human physiology and anatomy may harbour gross misconceptions.

Some patient anxieties

- Is it serious? Am I going to die? Die–abetes!
- Why me?
- Will I get better?
- Am I going to lose my legs like that man in the waiting room?
- Will I go blind?
- Will I lose my job?
- Am I going to lose my driving licence?
- Will I lose my boyfriend?
- What are you going to do to me now?
- Will I need to have injections?
- Will it hurt?
- Will people think I'm a junkie? Will I get addicted to insulin?
- Will I embarrass myself?
- Will I go into a coma?
- Can I eat chocolate?
- Can I go out for a meal?
- Do I have to buy special food?
- Will I have to use complicated machines?
- Something awful will go wrong if I don't do it properly!

'What is diabetes?' may be a long way down the list. Once the shock of diagnosis is over, other questions relating to living with diabetes emerge—what exactly the diagnosis means, what diet and other treatment are needed, how to use the appropriate technology (e.g. finger-prick blood glucose testing, needles, syringes), self-care, the prevention of short- and long-term complications, and how to manage diabetes under different circumstances. Practicalities such as where to get supplies of medication and equipment, clinic/surgery arrangements, and whom to call for help also need to be covered

When and how to teach

The patient's motivation is crucial. Adult learning is usually most enthusiastic when related to solving problems and aiming for specific goals which are not too distant. They have lost some of the childhood joys of discovery. In general, use of the 'teachable moment'—the time when the person formulates the question or needs to know how to resolve a problem—engenders more interest and may lead to better retention of knowledge. However, while one can utilize those teachable moments which occur in front of professionals, one cannot wait until they happen. Some more formalized teaching is needed.

'We can't afford a formal programme'

Structured diabetes education programmes (📖 p.65) have been demonstrated to improve some outcomes and the concept is supported by NICE. However, such programmes may be expensive in terms of finance or staff resource, despite likely long-term savings. The next section provides some practical suggestions for practices and clinics but is not a formal evidence-based programme.

Teaching

There are formal courses on teaching/education at all levels, often available through health care organizations. Surgery or clinic circumstances and surroundings do not always lend themselves to putting the theory into practice. Factors which may help are:

- Use the teachable moment—always answer questions straightaway, and enlarge if appropriate
- Check that the patient can see and hear properly
- Check that the patient can understand your language
- Avoid 'medspeak'. Say 'high blood-glucose level' rather than 'hyperglycaemia', or 'passing lots of water' rather than 'polyuria', or 'fatty tissue under the skin' rather than 'subcutaneous fat'
- Allocate time for teaching
- Use a quiet undisturbed place (divert phones and bleeps)
- Allocate a teaching room with all the leaflets and equipment you need to hand if possible
- Carry your teaching kit with you around the wards or the district
- Involve the patient in the lesson—discussion, question-and-answer format, how is it for you?
- Consider what teaching method you are going to use
- Consider your personal resources—time, knowledge, etc. vs how many patients need to learn.
- One-to-one: more personal and private, but fewer patients seen
- Group: patients bounce ideas of each other, less personal, less private, more time efficient for staff
- Big lecture: more patients can listen, but less will be retained than in sessions where there can be more interaction. Consider mixing patients and health professionals in the audience.
- Discussion: questions and answers; talk, then question and answer.
- Practical demonstration—equipment
- Visual aids: draw a diagram, flip charts, written, moving image, etc.
- Provide leaflets in the right language (discreetly check if the patient can read)
- Provide CDs, DVDs, tapes
- Provide reputable Internet links (e.g. www.diabetes.org.uk)
- Personalize books or handouts by writing in specific comments for the particular patient or encourage the patient to do this him/herself
- Check that you know what the chart, slide, overhead, or book says before you use it
- Check Powerpoint/projection equipment is working and that you know how to use it
- Check understanding. Recheck understanding.

Three-stage programme

- Newly diagnosed—survival kit (Table 4.1)
- Main body of knowledge—the full package
- Revision and update

Survival kit

Table 4.1 The survival kit: vital points to be discussed following diagnosis

The diagnosis	Diabetes:
	is long term but controllable
	has symptoms that will be relieved rapidly
	is not catching
	is not immediately fatal!
Diet	Know what and how much to eat—in simple terms
Treatment	Either tablets or insulin if needed; if insulin, know the basic technology
	Hazard warnings
	Free prescriptions for those on tablets or insulin
Monitoring	Finger-prick blood glucose monitoring (start with urine testing in really nervous patients)
Carry	Diabetes card, and glucose everywhere (unless diet alone)
Drivers	If a driver, tell DVLA and motor insurance company immediately
Implications	Immediate implications for work, family, or leisure activities
Contact	Provide details of whom to contact for help
Concerns	Any questions or concerns
Appointments	With whom, where, when

The details of each of these stages are covered in subsequent chapters. Extend the patient's knowledge in several sessions. Most importantly, in each session give the patient time to talk, listen a lot, and answer the patient's questions. Until you have done this they may not listen to the information which you wish to pass on.

Full package

- What is happening in your body
  - Causes of diabetes
  - Why this person has diabetes
  - How the pancreas works
  - Basic biochemistry of glucose, insulin, and fat
- The implications of diabetes (see sections below)
- Food and drink.
  - What happens to the food you eat
  - What to eat; how much to eat
  - Carbohydrate counting and glycaemic index as appropriate
  - Give more detailed personalized dietary information
  - Achieving and maintaining desirable weight
  - Alcohol
- Exercise.
  - Personalized targets
  - Forms of exercise
  - Glucose control and treatment adjustment
  - Safety (hypoglycaemia, issues around tissue damage)
- Treatment
  - Tablets for glucose control: their name(s), what is the dose, how to take them, how they work, side effects, self-adjustment, what to do if you forget a dose, how to get supplies. Other tablets—same details.
  - Insulin: the name(s), what is the dose, how to inject (ask patient to demonstrate), how insulins work, how injection devices work (ask patient to demonstrate), side effects, injection site problems, self-adjustment, what to do if you forget a dose, how to get supplies, help-lines. Exenatide—same details.
- Finger-prick blood glucose testing
  - How to do it, lancets, finger-pricking devices, strips, meter; how it all works; what to do if it goes wrong
  - Personalized glucose targets
  - Controlling the blood glucose—what to do if it is too low or too high
  - Glucose emergencies—hypoglycaemia, diabetic ketoacidosis
  - Use of more sophisticated monitoring techniques as required
- Can they show you their diabetic card and emergency glucose?
- Sick day rules
- Preventive care
  - Blood pressure—personal target, treatment if appropriate
  - Cholesterol—personal target, treatment if appropriate
  - Glucose and HbA_{1c} personal targets
  - Microalbuminuria
  - Tests—what the doctor/nurse measures (e.g. laboratory tests) and what it means
  - Personal hygiene
- Annual review
  - Weight, abdominal circumference

- Height until fully grown
- HbA_{1c}
- Eye check with digital eye photography in a screening programme
- Foot check, including skin, shape, pulses, sensation
- Blood pressure
- Kidneys: eGFR, microalbumin-to-creatinine ratio (MAC)
- Cholesterol and triglyceride
- Thyroid function in type 1 diabetes
- Coeliac tests if type 1 diabetes <20 years old
- Diabetic complications
  - Eyes
  - Kidneys
  - Nerves
  - Feet
  - Heart
  - Circulation
  - Stroke
  - Skin
- Driving
  - Personal, work-related (LGV, PCV?)
  - Confirm DVLA and insurance company have been told.
  - Safety—hypoglycaemia avoidance; problems from tissue damage, e.g. cannot feel pedals if severe neuropathy
- Work
  - Telling employers and colleagues
  - Safety issues
  - Legal issues
  - Practical issues, e.g. shift work, ability to access food, privacy for injections if desired
- Family
  - Avoiding pregnancy
  - Planning pregnancy—preconception, antenatal care, post-partum care
  - Inheritance of diabetes
  - Sexual dysfunction
- Leisure
  - Practical issues—sports, hobbies
  - Glucose balance and treatment adjustment
  - Safety (hypoglycaemia, issues around tissue damage)
  - Travel
- Smoking—don't
- Street drugs—don't
- Who is who in the diabetes system—primary and secondary care. How the diabetes system works in your district. How to make the best use of this resource
- How to get help—urgent, non-urgent. Where and how to get supplies
- Local and national self-help or support groups
- Useful websites
- How to get help/advice locally
- The next meeting

Revision and update

Skills and knowledge decline rapidly after training, especially if unused. They need updating regularly, perhaps every 6 months. Even the most experienced patient (or diabetes care professional) should have their insulin administration and blood glucose monitoring techniques checked regularly. Information gaps occur. One may discover people who have not informed the DVLA of their insulin-treated diabetes—many years after diagnosis. And why is the diabetes card and glucose always in the other coat?

Misconceptions may persist. Patients and relatives (or friends) may need updating too.

> Jo, an intelligent young woman with insulin-treated diabetes, was recorded as injecting fast-acting Actrapid® three times a day and long-acting Ultratard® (now unavailable) at night. Her blood glucose diary showed gross glucose fluctuations. After several years a doctor discovered that she was taking both Actrapid® and Ultratard® three times a day.
>
> Mavis was losing weight. She often showed urinary ketones. 'My friend's grandfather was diabetic. She said I should never touch starch. Fatal, you see, for a diabetic. Makes sugar. So I'm always very strict. No bread, no biscuits, no potato ever.'
>
> John was admitted to hospital with severe hypoglycaemia. He had collapsed from hypoglycaemia. His neighbour, an ardent first aider, rushed in and diagnosed a 'diabetic coma'. Surrounded by admiring relatives, he injected a large amount of insulin into John's leg.

Speak with one voice

Patients become confused if different staff members provide contradictory advice. The diabetes team should get together and agree a consistent approach to all aspects of diabetes education. This consistency should extend to all involved in patient care—GPs, hospital staff, school teachers. Use the national consensus where possible.

Coordinating diabetes education

The best person to coordinate diabetes education is the diabetes specialist nurse. Every person with diabetes should have access to a nurse with this special training. A chart in the patient's record, preferably the one they themselves hold, can be used to check off items and who has taught them.

Every team member should be able to provide basic diabetes advice—the podiatrist should know about healthy eating, and the dietitian about good foot care. The podiatrist can ask how the blood glucose control is going.

Diabetes education programmes

Diabetes education programmes

Studies of diabetes education have shown reduction in HbA_{1c} in the intervention groups in type 1 and type 2 diabetes, but have not been large or long enough to show that education alone produces major differences in patient outcomes long-term. However, NICE (Technology Appraisal 60, April 2003), stated that 'the Committee was convinced of the importance of patient education in improving glycaemic control and quality of life, while reducing the rate of complications associated with diabetes ... all individuals with diabetes should be offered structured patient education at the time of diagnosis and ongoing patient education as required based on a formal, regular assessment of need, recognising that needs change over time.' The appraisal advised the following.

- The use of established principles of adult education
- A multidisciplinary approach, with teams including, as a minimum, a diabetes specialist nurse (or a practice nurse with experience in diabetes) and a dietitian, with appropriate training provided to educators
- Use of group education sessions
- Provision of educational opportunities that are accessible to the broadest range of people, taking into account culture, ethnicity, disability and geographical issues
- Educational programmes based on a variety of learning techniques, adapted to meet varying needs, and integrated into routine diabetes care over the longer term

Structured patient education in diabetes

http://www.dh.gov.uk/en/Publicationsandstatistics/Publications/PublicationsPolicyAndGuidance/DH_4113195

- Use a structured education programme
- Use trained educators
- Be quality assured
- Be audited

DAFNE (Dose Adjustment For Normal Eating)

Dr Michael Berger developed this programme which teaches patients to adjust their insulin to ordinary eating habits. It does not advocate unhealthy eating. Published benefits include improved glycaemic balance and quality of life. Participants report greater enjoyment of food and flexibility. There may be a reduction in hypoglycaemia. Participants should have had diabetes for at least 6 months, be on multiple insulin injections daily, and be prepared to adjust their insulin according to multiple finger-prick glucose tests daily. Eight self-selected participants attend a 5-day course taught by the multidisciplinary team.

http://www.dafne.uk.com

DESMOND (Diabetes Education and Self-Management for On-going and Newly Diagnosed)

This is a project which assesses educational and psychological factors, and then provides structured education for groups of patients with type 2 diabetes. Participants showed improvements in weight loss, smoking cessation, and beliefs about illness, but not in HbA_{1c}, compared with non-participants (*BMJ* 2008; doi:10.1136/bmj.39474.922025.BE).
www.desmond-project.org.uk

EPP (Expert Patients Programme

'The Expert Patients Programme (EPP) is a NHS-based training programme that provides opportunities to people who live with long-term chronic conditions to develop new skills to manage their condition better on a day-to-day basis.' Up to 16 patients attend six sessions run by a patient trainer looking at different aspects of personal health and wellbeing, and working with health care professionals. Patients reported more self-confidence and control in managing their condition(s) and their lives, healthier eating, and fewer visits to doctors. Most courses are not designed to make a patient an expert in a particular condition.
www.expertpatients.nhs.uk/public/default.aspx

X-pert (Expert Patient Education)

This is a structured education programme for patients with type 2 diabetes developed in the North East.
http://www.xpert-diabetes.org.uk/artman/publish/

Your local diabetes education programme

Check what is available locally. Your local PCT, community diabetes service, Diabetes Centre, diabetologists, and hospital diabetes service may provide an education programme for people with diabetes in your area.

Care planning

Work with the patient to agree his/her plan of care for the year. The education programmes above will help, and care planning training is being developed (for patients and professionals). Patient support organisations can help inform people with diabetes about options. (Example: www.diabetes.nhs.uk/work-areas/year-of-care)

Patient support

Patient support groups

Patients gain much from mutual support,but remember that it is often those most severely affected by a condition who attend meetings most often—which can frighten new and less-affected members. Most areas have local patient support groups and everyone with diabetes can access the national organization Diabetes UK.

Diabetes UK

This is the main UK source of trusted information. It provides support and education for people with diabetes and health care professionals. It was one of the first patient self-help organizations in the world and was founded by a person with diabetes and a doctor specializing in the condition. Diabetes UK provides a wide range of educational resources and patient leaflets in a variety of languages. There is an excellent website for patients and professionals. There are local branches of Diabetes UK in most districts.

Diabetes UK's Careline provides information and support for those with diabetes, but not individual medical advice. It is linked to Language Line to ensure that non-English speakers can be helped.
Tel 0845 120 2960; www.diabetes.org.uk

Pharmaceutical company helplines

NovoNordisk out-of-hours helpline

NovoNordisk has an out-of-hours helpline for users of NovoNordisk insulins from 5.30pm to 11.00pm (working weekdays) and 8.30am to 11.00pm (weekends and public holidays). It is run by NHS diabetes specialist nurses and also uses Language Line for non-English speakers.
Tel 0845 600 5055
http://novonordisk.co.uk/documents/article_page/document/helpline.asp

Sanofi-Aventis Diabetes Information Line:

For people using Sanofi-Aventis insulin or devices.
Tel 0845 606 6887

Eli Lilly Diabetes Careline

For people using Eli Lilly products
Tel 01256 315999

Summary

- Diabetes education is essential to the patient's healthy survival
- Many factors influence whether the patient absorbs what you think you have taught, and whether he/she applies what has been learnt appropriately or at all
- A person with diabetes must understand what diabetes is and how it may affect him./her
- Regard patient education as part of care (like measuring blood pressure)
- The professionals must provide the patient with the knowledge and the tools to monitor his/her condition and to adjust treatment.
- Knowledge should be provided as and when the patient wants it, tailoring the professionals' agenda to the patient's individual needs
- Knowledge should be consistent and teaching should be professional
- Use the three-stage programme: the starter kit, the full package, and the revision and update sessions
- Speak with one voice
- Provide frequent revision sessions and support whenever it is required
- Assess learning needs formally and use a structured education programme, developed either nationally or locally (see NICE guidelines)
- Use the existing literature and professional support
- Tell all patients about Diabetes UK and patient support groups

Chapter 5

Healthy eating and drinking (including management of obesity)

Aims of a healthy diabetic diet

The two parts of the diet are what you eat and how much. A healthy diet provides energy for daily activity and maintains the right body weight for height. It is a lifelong eating plan. It is important that people continue to enjoy their food and that the treatment of their diabetes is adjusted to their usual eating pattern and not vice versa. New patients start enthusiastically and then lapse, so weight may fall and then rise again during the first year.

Box 5.1 Aims of a healthy diabetic diet

- Physically healthy
- Feeling well
- Energy for life and exercise
- Well-balanced diet
- Good day-to-day glucose control
- HbA_{1c} 4.0–6.0% without hypoglycaemia (if safe)
- Total cholesterol <4 mmol/l
- LDL cholesterol <2 mmol/l
- Triglyceride <1.7 mmol/l
- BMI 18.5–25 kg/m^2
- Waist circumference
  - <102 cm in men (<92 cm in Asian men)
  - <88 cm in women (<78 cm in Asian women)
- Alcohol in moderation if desired
- Low salt

Dietitian

Every patient should see a dietitian on diagnosis of diabetes and annually thereafter. The diabetic diet is an integral part of treatment and medical staff must ensure that patients realize this. Patients may wrongly assume that there is no need to worry about the diet if they are taking their diabetes tablets or insulin. All those caring for people with diabetes should be aware of dietary requirements and be able to answer questions about food. Advise patients to keep a week's food diary (using your local format) to help their discussions with the dietitian.

What to eat

A healthy balanced daily diet

- Include:
  - Starchy carbohydrate (CHO) foods such as bread, potato, pasta, rice, cereals spread through the day. They should be high in fibre and not cooked or dressed in fat.
  - Five portions of fruit or vegetables a day (which can include pulses, beans, or fruit juice, but each once a day)
  - Two small portions of meat, fish, or pulses for protein. Remove skin and fat, and do not cook or dress in fat.
  - Three portions of low-fat dairy foods: milk (skimmed/semi-skimmed), cheese (matchbox size), yoghurt (small pot).
  - Alcohol in moderation.
- Exclude:
  - Most sugar and fat. Use low-sugar or low-fat options.
- The recommended daily calorie breakdown is:
  - CHO 55% (45–60%) (sucrose <10% total calories)
  - Fat <30–35%
  - Protein 10–15%
- Calorie content of foods is:
  - Fat 9 kcal/g
  - Protein 4 kcal/g
  - CHO 3.8 kcal/g
  - Alcohol 7 kcal/g
- The standard unit is a kilocalorie. This is expressed as calorie throughout the book as this is common usage. Food also contains water, fibre, and inedible waste such as pips or pith.

Box 5.2 The healthy plate

- One-third protein
- One-third CHO
- One-third salad or vegetables

or

- Half mixed food (e.g. lasagne, meat pie)
- Half salad or vegetables

This advises on proportions of food but not portion size. Big plate—high-calorie diet; small plate—low-calorie diet. But note that there is no specific space for fats and these may be concealed within the protein (fat in meat) and CHO (butter in mashed potato).

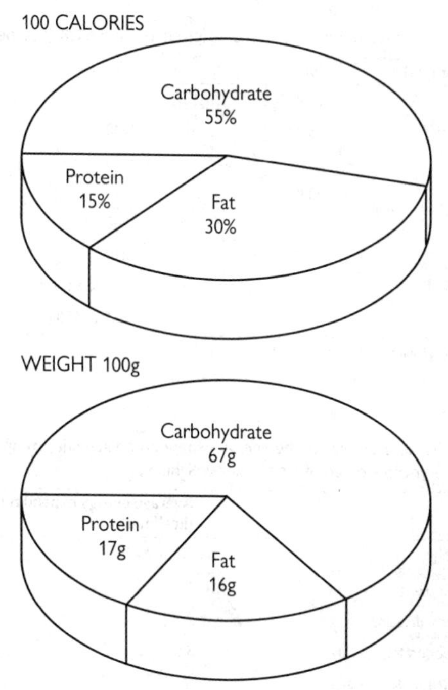

Fig. 5.1 Recommended dietary components by calories and by weight.

Table 5.1 Estimated average requirements for energy in the UK (kcal/per day)

Age range (yrs)	Men	Women
15–18	2755	2110
19–50	2550	1940
51–59	2550	1900
60–64	2380	1900
65–75	2330	1900
75+	2100	1810
Pregnant		+200 last trimester
Lactating		+450 to 570 (1–3 months)

From *Manual of nutrition*, 10th edn TSO 1995 with permission.

Table 5.2 Some examples of the energy expended on activities by an average 25-yr-old woman office worker weighing 62 kg

Activity	Average energy expenditure (kcal/min)
Sitting, eating	1.1
Standing, cooking	2.1
Washing and dressing	2.1
Walking moderately quickly	3.5
Walking up and down stairs	6.5
Office sitting	1.5
Office walking slowly	2.6
Dancing	4.5
Average jogging	6.5

From *Manual of nutrition*, 10th edn TSO 1995 with permission.

Prepared foods are often highly calorific. Fat and sugar make food taste good and act as cheap bulking agents in manufactured prepared foods. Home cooking can also be calorific. Table 5.3 shows an example of a home-cooked family meal—many patients would regard the chicken and dessert portions as small. This might be just one meal for an energetic young man. It would be the food for an entire day for an overweight person on a 1000 calorie diet. 40% of the calories are in the sweet pudding (pastry is high in fat and CHO). Apple alone would be better. There is plenty of fibre in this meal—in the baked beans, cabbage, and apple, and some in potato. The fat in the tomato soup could be reduced; and the chicken could be steamed or casseroled without its skin or added fat.

Table 5.3 Sunday lunch: a 1000 calorie meal

Food	Weight (g)	kcal	Protein (g)	Fat (g)	CHO (g)
Tomato soup	200	110	1.6	6.6	11.8
Roast chicken (meat)	100	148	24.8	5.4	0
Cabbage	200	30	3.4	0	4.6
Baked beans	200	162	9.6	1.2	30.2
Boiled potato	200	152	3.6	0.2	36.0
Apple pie*	100	369	4.3	15.5	56.7
Custard*	30	35	1.2	1.5	5.0
Total	1030	1006	48.5	30.4	144.3
Kcal		1006	193	272	541
Percentage of total kcal		100%	19%	27%	54%

*Made with sugar; full-fat milk in the custard.

Water was drunk with the meal (no calories).

Calculated from figures in the *Manual of nutrition*, 1989.

Food labels

In packaged foods, ingredients are listed by weight, with the first one contributing the biggest proportion to that food by weight.

Table 5.4 Quantities in a complete meal or 100 g snack

Food	A little	A lot
Fat	≤5g	≥20g
Saturated fat	≤1g	≥5g
Sugars	≤5g	≥10g
Fibre	≤0.5g	≥3g
Sodium (1g sodium ≈ 2.5g salt)	≤0.1g	≥0.5g

With thanks to Pat Smith, Dietitian, The Hillingdon Hospital.

What should I eat?

Most patients are concerned to know what they are supposed to eat. Some are prepared to look at their food in detail (see CHO counting), but many are not. The calculations above are rarely necessary. Suggested stages of education are:

- Different types of food (CHO, protein, fat)
- The healthy plate (see above)
- Personal portion sizes (use food diary)
- Personal eating for health, work, exercise, leisure
- CHO counting
- Glycaemic index and glucose load

Carbohydrates (CHOs)—starchy sugary foods

The old rigid division into simple and complex CHOs is not always helpful as many foods and most meals combine more than one sort of CHO.

Sugars

These provide rapidly absorbed CHO. When eaten alone, glucose produces an abrupt rise in blood glucose concentration, starting in minutes and lasting about 2 hr. Normally this stimulates pancreatic insulin release to parallel the blood glucose rise. The insulin or subcutaneous insulin of a diabetic patient may not match the glucose rise. Analogue insulins are designed to mimic natural insulin release (📖 p.164).

- Monosaccharides: glucose, galactose, fructose
- Disaccharides:
  - Sucrose (glucose + fructose) from sugar cane or beet
  - Lactose (glucose + galactose) from milk
  - Maltose (glucose + glucose) from fermenting grain

When sucrose is eaten as part of a meal, the blood glucose rise following that meal is similar to that of a meal of the same caloric value without sucrose. The fat and fibre content of the meal slow glucose absorption. Better compliance may be achieved if patients can have a sweet/pudding during the meal within their total calorie intake.

In insulin-treated patients, exercising vigorously, liver glucose release may not keep up with glucose uptake by muscles. The blood glucose can fall precipitously if the patient does not top up with sugar or glucose (📖 p.264). Thus insulin-treated patients can use sugar-containing foods when exercising. Regular exercise may eventually be fuelled mainly by unrefined CHOs.

Glucose or sucrose ('sugar') is essential in the treatment of hypoglycaemia (📖 p.208). Obvious? Not necessarily. If you tell the patient 'No sugar', he/she may obey you to the letter, fighting off all attempts to treat hypoglycaemia with sugar lumps. Lactose digestion will be slowed by fat in milk products. The fat in chocolate slows digestion/absorption of glucose, sucrose, and lactose. Patients on acarbose, a disaccharidase inhibitor, must use glucose to treat hypoglycaemia. They cannot break down sucrose. Granular sugar substitutes such as sucralose (Splenda®) will not resolve hypoglycaemia! Plain glucose (e.g. glucose tablets) is the best treatment for hypoglycaemia (📖 p.208).

Complex CHOs—starchy foods

More than half of dietary calories should come from starchy CHOs. Each patient will have his/her staples: bread, cereals, corn (maize), legumes (e.g. beans), pasta, potatoes, and rice are the most common. Many of these are made more palatable with fat: bread and butter, cornflakes and milk, pasta with sauce. Some people count beans as protein, but they contain more CHO.

Complex CHOs have to be digested into simple CHOs before absorption. The rate at which this happens varies (📖 p.76, 80).

Fibre

Insoluble fibre (e.g. in wheat bran, vegetables) bulk out food and make it filling. Examples are wholemeal bread, wholemeal pasta, brown rice, potatoes in their jackets, celery, and cabbage. Soluble fibre in beans and pulses slows digestion and absorption of CHO. People with diabetes should eat some beans, lentils, chick peas, or other pulse every day.

More people are used to a high-fibre diet. A patient unfamiliar with this should introduce the new foods slowly to reduce abdominal griping and flatulence.

Box 5.3 Examples of fibre content

White bread	2 g fibre/100g
Baked beans	6 g fibre/100g
Wholewheat bread	7 g fibre/100g
Bran cereal	43 g fibre/100g

Source: USDA database (📖 p.96)

CHO portions and CHO counting

CHO counting was popular for many years, went out of fashion, and is now back, particularly for type 1 diabetes. For many it makes it easier to balance insulin doses with food. The huge range of CHO foods, portion sizes, and presentations available can make this daunting. Patients should start with learning to count the CHO foods they usually eat.

Most books on the subject are American, creating problems for British readers as portions are usually quoted in cups (1 UK cup = 1.25 American cups):
One cup = 16 tablespoons (levelled off for solid foods)
One tablespoon = 3 teaspoons (levelled off for solid foods).

Box 5.4 Example of CHO counting

Chicken sandwich:	
Two slices white bread	2 x 12g
Butter	0
Piece of chicken	0
One medium tomato	5g
One large banana	30g
Total	about 60g CHO 6 x 10g CHO portions

NB this takes no account of calories or fibre

Source USDA database (📖 p.96)

Getting started

A dietitian should advise on the total daily calories to achieve and maintain a healthy weight for that person.

- Total daily diet 2000 kcal/day includes 240–320g CHO, 24–32 10 g portions
- Total daily diet 1000 kcal/day includes 120–160 g CHO, 12–16 10 g portions

Different centres use different 'portions' or 'exchanges'. The latter are familiar to many patients with long-standing diabetes. 10 g CHO is simplest (e.g. small slice of bread, small apple). Packaged food lists CHO content. Patients can use personal observation and detailed records to calculate their insulin dose in units per 10 g CHO portion. Dietitians can provide 10 g CHO portion lists or 'exchanges'. Beware confusion as American books often quote 15 g portions as do some UK centres.

Alternatively, divide 500 by the total daily dose (TDD), i.e. the total of all the insulin injected in 24 hr. Thus if the TDD is 50 units, the insulin-to-CHO ratio is 1 unit insulin to 10 g CHO. For a total daily dose of 25 units of insulin, the insulin-to-CHO ratio would be 1:20 g (📖 p.189).

Patients are often advised to subtract the amount of fibre in the food if over 5g to achieve the final CHO count upon which they base their insulin dose.

Glycaemic index and glycaemic load

The glycaemic index is calculated by performing multiple blood glucose tests in people who have fasted overnight and have eaten the test food on its own. It compares the area under the blood glucose curve after eating a particular food with that after eating an equivalent amount of CHO as glucose. With this technique, an apple has a glycaemic index of 39%, baked beans 40%, brown rice 66%, wholemeal bread 72%, honey 87%, and Lucozade® 98, some cooked potatoes 111%. Glucose is 100%.

The glucose (glycaemic) load uses the amount of CHO to be eaten and its absorption (glycaemic index) to give a figure to indicate the total effect of that food on blood glucose levels:

glucose load = (CHO amount x glycaemic index)/100

Thus the glucose load for a large banana is (30 x 70)/100 = 21. This calculation is not widely used although some patients are doing similar approximations.

The major problem with the use of the glycaemic index, and hence the glucose load, is that foods are rarely eaten on their own. These are some of the factors which alter the rate of CHO absorption.

- Other foods—fats and fibre slow absorption
- Liquids
- Alcohol
- Total quantity of food eaten
- Patient at rest or exercising
- Emotional factors
- Gastric status, e.g. gastroparesis from autonomic neuropathy
- Nausea or vomiting
- Intestinal status, e.g. malabsorption or diarrhoea
- Cardiovascular factors
- Drugs, e.g. acarbose, metformin

Information about the glycaemic index and CHO content of many foods is available at www.glycemicindex.com

Confused?

So are patients. Few patients will be prepared to do the complete complex calculations above. However, a practical working knowledge of the CHO of their usual foods and how fast it is likely to be absorbed can significantly improve their use of insulin and may help tablet-treated patients. The most useful figure is the CHO count, and seeing food as 10 g portions of CHO allows this to be factored into insulin dose calculations.

The CHO foods should be spread out in three meals a day, convenient for the patient. If they are taking insulin, a coffee time and tea time snack may be desirable, and a bedtime snack is usually essential. Insulin may be needed to cover snacks >10 g CHO. Overweight patients not on insulin should avoid snacks.

Fruit and vegetables

We should eat five portions of fruit or vegetables a day. Fruit tastes sweet because it contains sucrose and fructose. The sweeter it tastes (e.g. grapes), the more refined is the CHO it contains. Fruit is an important source of vitamin C. Large amounts of fruit will elevate blood glucose and weight. One portion at a time is best.

Vegetables can be divided into two groups: those which can be eaten in large amounts with little influence on weight or CHO, and those which have to be considered as an energy source. Leafy vegetables such as lettuce and cabbage, big watery containers of small seeds like cucumbers and courgettes, and swollen stalks such as celery can be eaten with impunity. Starchy root vegetables, such as potatoes, and big seeds, e.g. beans, peas, lentils, other pulses, and nuts, contain a lot of CHO to fuel the growing plant after germination. All starchy root vegetables and big seeds need to be considered in the CHO total. Potatoes are not included in the 'five-a-day' totals. Nuts contain a lot of fat.

Fats—greasy oily foods

All fats are fattening! Reduce fat intake. No more than 35% of dietary calories should come from fat. This is a very small amount of visible fat because so much is concealed in other foods, especially manufactured foods. Fat makes food taste good and few people realize how calorific it is. The pat of butter contains as many calories as the slice of bread on which it is spread.

Avoid visible fat. Spread butter thinly; better still, use a polyunsaturated low-fat spread or go without. Eat lower-fat meats such as skinned chicken or turkey. Avoid hard cheese, cream cheeses, and lard or dripping. Avoid cream and use semi-skimmed milk or skimmed milk. Avoid fried foods. Do not use oil-based salad dressings.

Hidden fat can be avoided by self-catering. Do not add fat to cooking unless essential—use low-fat cookery books. Advise patients to read the label on ready-made meals. Warn that 'reduced-fat foods' may still be high in fat (and sugar), e.g. half the calories in lower-fat crisps still come from fat. Meat products (sausages, salami, pork pies, beefburgers) are very high in fat.

Fat slows gastric emptying and hence food absorption.

Saturated, mono-unsaturated, poly-unsaturated, and transfats

- *Saturated* fats are usually found in animal-derived products and increase LDL cholesterol. Intake should be reduced. They are found in dairy and animal fats (e.g. cheese, cream, fat on meat).
- *Mono-unsaturated fats* (e.g. rapeseed oil, olive oil, avocado oil) and poly-unsaturated fats (e.g. sunflower oil, fish oils) have less effect on LDL cholesterol and may enhance HDL. The omega-3 fatty acids found in herring, mackerel, wild salmon, and sardines appear to be cardioprotective. Mono- and poly-unsaturated fats should form a greater proportion of the total fat intake (but should still be limited in weight-reducing diets).
- *Transfats* are found naturally, mainly in animal-derived products. Most are manufactured by hydrogenating vegetable oils to prolong shelf-life and flavour of foods. Many such products become solid at room temperature. Transfats are found in margarines and butter-substitute spreads, dressings, snack foods, biscuits, and some cooking fats. Transfats raise LDL cholesterol, and contain the same amount of calories as other fats. Most are eaten in manufactured biscuits and snacks. Patients should reduce these.

Protein

If 50–60% of the dietary calories are CHO and 30% are fat, that only leaves 10–20% as protein. This is the equivalent of about 150 g (5 oz) of chicken meat in a 1500 calorie diet. Many proteins are closely associated with fat. Skinned white meat, fish, and vegetable protein (e.g. soya) with some low-fat cheese and one or two eggs a week should be the main protein source. Red meat should be lean and grilled or casseroled rather than roasted or fried. Eat one or two portions a week.

Salt

Sodium chloride is linked with hypertension and may worsen fluid retention in oedematous patients. Do not add salt at table and use it sparingly in cooking (unless exercising in hot weather or participating in endurance sports). Avoid too many manufactured foods as these tend to be higher in salt.

Calcium and vitamin D

People with diabetes are more likely to be vitamin D deficient than the general population, even allowing for ethnicity (*Arch Int Med* 2007; **167**:1159–65). Skim milk and other calcium-rich foods should be encouraged, as should safe exposure to the sun. Calcium and vitamin D supplementation may be required in patients who do not drink enough milk and/or those with dark skin, especially if they cover themselves when out of the house.

Iron

Vegetarians and older people are likely to be iron deficient. Encourage red meat (one or two portions weekly) or iron supplements if necessary.

Drinks

Aim for 6–8 cups of fluid a day. Tea and coffee may contain full fat milk, cream, and sugar. Therefore 6–8 cups of tea a day can include a pint of milk and a lot of sugar. Introduce semi-skimmed milk and artificial sweeteners such as aspartame. Better still, use skimmed milk and no sweetener (or even black tea or coffee).

Aerated 'diet' drinks containing artificial sweeteners can be drunk in moderation. Care is needed in reading the labels of some products marked 'sugar-free' which may contain other refined CHOs, e.g. glucose.

Fruit juices may contain a lot of sugars. Read the label. A box of apple juice (262 g) contains 123 kcal, 30 g CHO, 28 g sugars (4 g sucrose, 7g glucose, 15 g fructose) (glycaemic index ~40). Fruit smoothies should be pure fruit. They will also contain some sucrose and will produce a rapid glucose rise as they are easily absorbed. Vegetable juices could be substituted. Other savoury drinks, such as Bovril, can be very salty and should be drunk only occasionally.

Alcohol

Moderation in all things. The recommended amount is 14 units a week for a woman and 21 units a week for a man. A unit is half a pint of beer, lager, or cider, a single pub measure of spirits, or a glass of wine. Therefore 21 units a week is 1.5 pints a night. Alcohol is highly calorific, ranging from 285 kcal/unit for sweet cider to 50 kcal/unit for spirits.

Confusion is generated by the CHO content of alcoholic drinks. Very sweet drinks should be avoided, but otherwise there is no benefit in using low-CHO products as the CHO has been turned to alcohol by further brewing. The total calorie content should be considered if the patient needs to lose weight, but it is better to ignore the CHO contribution of alcoholic drinks.

Alcohol impedes glucose release from liver glycogen stores and may precipitate or worsen hypoglycaemia. It also reduces the growth hormone rise stimulated by hypoglycaemia and therefore lengthens the glucose recovery. People with diabetes should not drink on an empty stomach. A packet of crisps or preferably another lower-fat snack, if available, should be consumed if alcohol is drunk outside mealtimes.

Modified products—'diabetic foods' and sweeteners

'Diabetic foods'

These are sweets, biscuits, and cakes in which glucose and sucrose have been replaced by fructose or sorbitol. There is no evidence that fructose is any better for diabetics than sucrose, and it may be metabolically worse. Sorbitol, the other commonly used sweetener, causes abdominal griping and diarrhoea when consumed in large amounts. It is a polyol compound and, although CHO is not absorbed to the same extent, 15 g of sorbitol should be counted as about 7 g of absorbable CHO. Many of these products contain fat and are highly calorific. Discourage patients from buying them.

Sweeteners

These include Aspartame spartame (Nutrasweet®), saccharin, acesulfame potassium (acesulfame K), cyclamates, and sucralose. There has been concern that aspartame may have adverse effects. The European Food Safety Authority has said that it is safe. The FDA states 'To date, FDA has not determined any consistent pattern of symptoms that can be attributed to the use of aspartame, nor is the agency aware of any recent studies that clearly show safety problems'.

Vary artificial sweeteners so that none is used in excess of advised daily intake.

How much to eat

Eat as much as is necessary to reach and maintain normal weight and fuel current physical activity:

calories in = calories out—weight stays the same.
calories in > Calories out—weight gain
calories in < Calories out—weight loss

Obesity and weight reduction

Obesity is common. Many patients with type 2 diabetes are obese. It is easy to gain weight and hard to lose it. Treat the patient with courtesy and respect. Listen to his/her story.

Recognize patients' difficulties in finding the will-power to lose weight, and their need to have the occasional forbidden food. Discuss the overall goal but set a reasonable interim goal in agreement with the patient. Aim for a loss of 0.5–1 kg per week (1–2 lb per week). Failure to meet the goal is noted and further effort encouraged; praise success, however slight. Success breeds success.

Group support may help, as in Weight Watchers, where there is also a financial incentive. Enlisting a family member to watch the diet and give encouragement may help for some people.

Ask the patient to monitor his/her own progress. Advise weekly weigh-ins, preferably by someone else, at the same time of day and in the same clothes, with the result written on a graph.

There is no easy formula to help people lose weight—the one constant factor of most studies is that continued interest and support is helpful.

Box 5.5 Assessing an overweight patient

- Is the patient worried about his/her weight?
- Does he/she have any weight-related symptoms?
- Will losing weight help this particular patient?
- Is this a good time for him/her to try to lose weight?
- Willingness and motivation to change?
- What is their eating pattern? How does he/she use food?
- Conditions contributing to the obesity
- Medical problems
- Psychological factors
- Medication
- Non-drug treatments
- Previous dietary efforts or weight-reducing treatments or surgery
- Family history, especially of obesity
- Lifestyle, exercise, work, and leisure
- Family and social aspects

Box 5.6 Factors influencing food intake

- Hunger
- Appetite (not the same as hunger)
- Emotion
- Motivation
- Health beliefs
- Previous dietary advice/experience of dieting
- Cultural factors
- Family pressure: 'eat up, clean your plate'
- Outside pressure: friends, health care professionals, other 'advisers'
- Courtesy: don't want to upset their hostess
- Attractiveness or otherwise of food
- Exercise
- Ambient temperature
- Boredom
- Habit (popcorn in the cinema)
- Portion size (self-selected, served at home, served in restaurant, etc.)
- Comfort eating (distress or stress)
- A 'treat'—'naughty but nice'
- Alone or in company
- Because it's there
- To keep up with the insulin or tablets
- To treat a hypoglycaemic episode
- Drugs, e.g. insulin, steroids
- Hormonal conditions, e.g. Cushing's syndrome, polycystic ovary syndrome
- Intracranial and hypothalamic disorders
- Psychiatric illness

Diet diary

Most people do not realize how much they eat. A diet diary (underline the importance of honesty) for a week is helpful guide if the patient wishes to comply. Otherwise take a dietary history

Modify the type of foods eaten

- Reduce fat
- Reduce alcohol
- Reduce manufactured foods and take-aways
- Increase green leafy vegetables; reduce solid starchy vegetables
- Increase large watery fruits or high-fibre crunchy fruits; reduce small sweet fruits or starchy fruits.
- Avoid sauces or dressings unless low calorie

Reduce the quantities eaten

Obese people often choose larger portions than slim people. Use a small spoon and a small plate. Eating out often presents larger portions. Ask for a smaller helping, or leave some. Eat more slowly so that the food lasts.

When is the food eaten?

Eat at mealtimes and not in between. Enjoy the food. Avoid habit eating, e.g. while watching television, while driving (dangerous, illegal), while working at a desk, while serving behind the counter, while chatting. This food is chewed but not savoured. Substitute calorie-free chewing gum or a minimum calorie drink.

Why do people eat?

Overweight people need to eat very little to survive. Appetite can overcome satiety—we can be completely full of meat and vegetables but still fancy a piece of chocolate gateau. Food is a great comforter. It is an excuse for a social or family gathering. It is an expression of welcome, a thank you present, a sign that you care, a religious symbol. It is sometimes used as a weapon, especially by children. Eating may simply be something to do with your hands. Find out why your patient is eating the foods he/she eats and suggest substitution of another activity or lower-calorie foods as appropriate.

Where is the food eaten and with whom?

Eating alone allows unwitnessed greed. Eating with a bad influence can encourage dietary sinning. No one actually likes being good all the time. What food is available at work? Could a packed lunch be taken?

Home-cooked meals may prove difficult if the cook is not the person with diabetes and does not understand dietary requirements. Wives usually change their diet to suit their husband's diabetic diet. A husband rarely changes his diet if his wife has diabetes.

Read the label

Most foods now have detailed content and calorie lists. However, few packs weigh exactly 100 g. And what is a gram? Many British cooks still think in pounds and ounces. 100 g is 3.5 oz. One ounce is about 30 g.

Increase exercise

Advise at least 30 min of moderate intensity physical activity on at least 5 days a week (📖 p.262). Continue this regardless of weight lost. Any exercise is better than none—just walking round the garden, for example. Glucose-lowering treatment may need to be reduced to avoid hypoglycaemia and patients should be warned about this.

Weight-reducing drugs

NICE CG43 states that 'Drug treatment should be considered for patients who have not reached their target weight loss or have reached a plateau on dietary, activity and behavioural changes alone'. Weight-reducing drugs should be prescribed only as part of a weight-reducing plan which includes psychological support, dietetic support for healthy eating, and exercise—and a plan for post-drug care. Do not prescribe more than one weight-reducing drug at a time.

The drugs available act either within the gastrointestinal tract or centrally acting drugs. Those acting within the gut are orlistat and methylcellulose. The latter is a high-fibre bulking agent aiming to induce satiety and is rarely used. Centrally acting drugs are sibutramine and rimonabant. Both have multiple cautions and contraindications, and worrying side effects and should be used with caution in diabetic patients. Similar drugs used in the past (dexfenfluramine, fenfluramine, and phentermine) have been linked with valvular heart disease and the risk of pulmonary hypertension.

Orlistat

Mechanism of action of orlistat

Inhibition of lipase which reduces absorption of fat.

Beneficial effects of orlistat

Weight loss when used with a low-fat weight-reducing diet.

Indications for orlistat

Criterion for use in diabetic patients is a BMI of 28.0 kg/m^2

Contraindications and cautions for orlistat

- Patients who refuse to reduce their fat intake should not be prescribed orlistat (avoid)
- Chronic malabsorption (avoid)
- Cholestasis (avoid)
- Breastfeeding (avoid)
- Pregnancy (caution)
- Gastrointestinal problems or diarrhoea for any reason (caution)
- Known faecal continence problems or anal problems (caution)

Dosage of orlistat

- 120 mg orally immediately before, during, or up to 1 hr after each main meal (up to a maximum of 360 mg daily). Gradual increase advised.
- Therapy should be continued beyond 3 months only if the person has lost weight since starting drug treatment.

Side effects of orlistat

Gastrointestinal side effects are common and may lead the patient to stop taking orlistat. They are usually due to excessive fat intake. As the fat is not absorbed, it passes through the bowel causing oily diarrhoea and rectal leakage or incontinence. Specifically warn patients of this risk.

- Gastrointestinal: rectal oil leak, oily diarrhoea, faecal urgency, faecal incontinence, flatulence, abdominal distension, abdominal pain; rarely rectal bleeding; very rarely diverticulitis, cholelithiasis, hepatitis
- Impaired absorption of fat-soluble vitamins (if supplement needed take at least 2 hr after orlistat or at bedtime, whichever is the longest)
- Tooth and gum problems
- Respiratory and urinary tract infections
- Tiredness
- Anxiety
- Headache
- Menstrual problems
- Hypoglycaemia
- Very rarely, skin problems and blisters
- Withdrawal: weight may rise

Sibutramine

Use this drug cautiously in diabetic patients—most will have a reason for caution or a contraindication.

Mechanism of action of sibutramine

Sibutramine inhibits the re-uptake of noradrenaline and serotonin.

Beneficial effects of sibutramine

Reduced appetite and weight loss when used with a weight-reducing diet.

Indications for sibutramine

Criterion for use in diabetic patients is BMI $\geq$27.0 kg/m^2. Sibutramine should not be prescribed unless there are adequate arrangements for monitoring weight loss, pulse, and blood pressure.

Cautions for sibutramine

- Already on drugs which may cause bleeding
- Predisposition to bleeding
- Sleep apnoea syndrome
- Epilepsy
- Ocular hypertension/glaucoma (now or past, or risk of)
- Family history of motor or vocal tics
- Past depression
- Hepatic impairment (avoid if severe)
- Renal impairment (avoid if severe)

Contraindications for sibutramine

- Aged <18 or >65 yrs
- Pregnancy
- Breastfeeding

- Cardiovascular problems including:
  - coronary artery disease
  - cardiac failure
  - arrhythmias
  - tachycardia
  - peripheral vascular disease
  - uncontrolled hypertension
- Cerebrovascular disease
- Psychiatric illness including eating disorders
- Drug or alcohol abuse (now or past)
- Tourette syndrome
- Prostatic hypertrophy
- Endocrine problems:
  - hyperthyroidism
  - phaeochromocytoma
- Interactions. Avoid in these patients taking:
  - warfarin—risk of bleeding
  - non-steroidal anti-inflammatory drugs—risk of bleeding
  - all antidepressants—risk of central nervous system toxicity

Dosage and monitoring of sibutramine

- Initially 10mg daily in the morning:
  - increase to 15 mg daily if weight loss <2 kg after 4 weeks
  - discontinue if weight loss <2 kg after 4 weeks at higher dose
- Maximum period of treatment 1 yr
- Therapy should be continued beyond 3 months only if the person has lost weight since starting drug treatment
- Monitor blood pressure and pulse rate at weeks 2, 4, 6, 8, 10, 12, 16, 20, 24, and then at least every 3 months thereafter
- Monitor for pulmonary hypertension
- Discontinue if:
  - blood pressure >145/90 mmHg
  - systolic or diastolic pressure raised by more than 10 mmHg
  - pulse rate raised by 10 bpm at two consecutive visits
  - weight loss after 3 months <5% of initial body weight
  - weight loss stabilizes at <5% of initial body weight
  - individuals regain 3 kg or more after previous weight loss
- Treatment should be continued only if weight loss is associated with other clinical benefits

Side effects of sibutramine

- Hypersensitivity reactions including angioedema and anaphylaxis, rash, urticaria, Henoch–Schönlein purpura
- Bleeding: thrombocytopenia, cutaneous bleeding disorders
- General: insomnia, light-headedness
- Gastrointestinal: dry mouth, taste disturbance, nausea, vomiting, constipation, diarrhoea, gastrointestinal bleeding, haemorrhoid problems
- Cardiovascular: tachycardia, palpitation, arrhythmias, hypertension, flushing
- Neurological/psychological: headache, anxiety, depression, seizures, memory disturbance, paraesthesia

- Genitourinary: menstrual problems, sexual dysfunction, urinary retention
- Renal: interstitial nephritis, glomerulonephritis
- Skin: sweating, alopecia, hypersensitivity reactions
- Eyes: blurred vision, very rarely angle-closure glaucoma
- Withdrawal: weight may rise, rarely headache and increased appetite

Rimonabant

Mechanism of action of rimonabant

Rimonabant is a cannabinoid receptor antagonist developed by blocking the pathway thought to be responsible for the 'munchies' observed in people abusing cannabis.

Indications for rimonabant

Criterion for use in diabetic patients is BMI ≥ 27.0 kg/m^2.

Beneficial effects of rimonabant

Weight loss when used with a weight-reducing diet.

Cautions for rimonabant

- Age <18 or >75 yrs
- Epilepsy
- Hepatic impairment (avoid if severe)
- Plasma concentration of rimonabant increased by ketoconazole

Contraindications for rimonabant

- Pregnancy
- Breastfeeding
- Severe renal or hepatic impairment
- Depression and any other psychiatric illness

Dosage of rimonabant

- 20 mg daily before breakfast
- Warn patient of risk of depression; if present, stop it immediately and seek medical advice
- Rimonabant is not licensed for use for >2 yrs

Side effects of rimonabant

- Gastrointestinal: anorexia, dry mouth, nausea, vomiting, diarrhoea, hiccoughs
- Psychiatric: depression (10%) may come on very suddenly in patients with no previous evidence of depression, mood changes, anxiety, nervousness, irritability, anger, sleep disorders, memory impairment, impaired attention; rarely hallucinations
- Neurological: hypo-aesthesia, sciatica
- Musculoskeletal: tendonitis, muscle cramp
- Skin: itching, sweating
- General: dizziness, hot flush, asthenia, influenza-like symptoms
- Withdrawal: weight gain

Comment

The author no longer uses this drug because of concerns about depression.

Bariatric surgery

Surgery to reduce gastric capacity is successful in long-term weight reduction in carefully selected patients and is a NICE-approved therapy.

Bariatric surgery is recommended as a treatment option for people with diabetes and obesity if all the following criteria are fulfilled.

- They have a BMI between 35 and 40 kg/m^2
- All appropriate non-surgical measures have been tried, but have failed to achieve or maintain adequate clinically beneficial weight loss for at least 6 months
- The person has been receiving or will receive intensive management in a specialist obesity service
- The person is generally fit for anaesthesia and surgery
- The person commits to the need for long-term follow-up.

(CG43 NICE Guideline 2006)

Many obese patients are not fit for surgery and/or have not shown commitment to long term therapy.

Different diets

Vegetarians often find a healthy diet easy. They may well be following it anyway. Vegans can obtain protein from vegetable sources (such as quorn, pulses, nuts) but may become deficient in vitamin B_{12}, requiring replacement therapy. Lacto-vegetarians should use lower-fat dairy products.

Be sensitive to religious dietary requirements (📖 p.415). Limitations on meats are rarely a problem in working out the diabetic diet, but some traditional ways of cooking may use a lot of fat (e.g. ghee). Brown rice or wholemeal flour can be substituted for lower-fibre products (but remember that to eat white rice may reflect higher status). Rural diets of peoples in South Asia and Africa are high in fibre and low in sugar, but urban diets in those countries or in emigrants to the West may not be. Unless the person who actually cooks the patient's food sees the dietitian or diabetes team it is unlikely that dietary advice will succeed (📖 p.86).

Fast days or periods of denial occur in many religions, both Eastern and Western. Ramadan places particular demands on insulin-treated patients. Most religious leaders will exempt a diabetic person from this religious observance, but the patient may feel participation to be essential for spiritual well-being. Sometimes meals are eaten during the hours of darkness, and attention should be given to long-lasting CHO with plenty of fibre in the last meal before dawn. Insulin doses must be adjusted to cope with the long period without food. (📖 p.418)

Never underestimate the strength of a person's belief in the rightness of his/her usual diet. Many hours of explanation may be needed to convince the patient that the new diabetic diet is better for them.

Eating out and abroad

People with diabetes need not avoid other people's cooking. The occasional non-diet meal can be included. However, if they eat out often, care is needed. A reasonable meal could be a starter of melon or consommé, a main course of grilled fish or steak, or skinless chicken, with baked or boiled potatoes and vegetables or salad, followed by fruit. Avoid sauces and roast dishes, limit alcohol, and limit the sweet trolley.

When abroad, identify the local staple CHO. The patient should ensure regular clean meals. He/she can enjoy trying local foods. Some homework beforehand may make CHO counting easier.

Emergency foods

Everyone taking insulin injections or other glucose-lowering medication, should carry glucose to treat hypoglycaemia and keep a store of emergency food to substitute for a missed meal. It should be durable, conveniently packaged, and easy to carry around. The wide range of muesli and high-fibre bars contain some starchy CHO and some sucrose mixed with fibre, but watch the fat content. They fit in a pocket, handbag, or workbox and keep for months. Small boxes of fruit juice, nuts and raisins, and packs of savoury snacks are useful.

Eating disorders in diabetes

There is debate as to whether eating disorders are more common in people with diabetes than in non-diabetics. The constant emphasis on food and diet in diabetes may encourage unusual eating behaviours, whether or not they can be formally defined as eating disorders. Eating problems associated with diabetes range from restriction of CHO or omitting meals to reduce the blood glucose to a more sinister severe CHO restriction to reduce the insulin dose and reduce weight. Some anorexic patients deliberately induce insulin deficiency and hyperglycaemia to lose weight. They tend to be admitted in biochemical chaos and ketoacidosis. Laxative abuse and insulin deficiency cause dangerous hypokalaemia. Anorexia nervosa may alternate with bulimia. Bulimia produces gross fluctuations in glucose balance as the overeating may need large insulin doses, but the self-induced vomiting then precipitates hypoglycaemia. Such patients should be referred to a specialist diabetes service and be seen in conjunction with psychiatric and psychological support. Abnormal eating patterns may persist for many years before being detected, and some people with diabetes never again have a normal attitude to food (📖 p.454).

Summary

- A diet is what you eat. Teach patients about the types of food and the amounts of food to eat.
- A healthy diet should be high in CHO, high in fibre, low in sugar, low in fat, and low in salt, with alcohol in moderation.
- Weight reduction is the most important part of treatment for the obese type 2 patient.
- All patients should achieve normal weight for their height.
- Try to strike a balance between practicality and theory. Use common sense and do not forget that patients are people.
- Adapt the treatment to the patient, not the patient to the treatment.

Further information

NICE Clinical guideline CG 43
The USDA National Nutrient Database for Standard Reference http://www.nal.usda.gov/fnic/foodcomp/search/ gives full nutritional information for a wide range of foods including CHO values by weight or portion size
Glycaemic index www.glycemicindex.com
Virtual supermarket tour for patients: www.storetour.co.uk/Store.aspx
Patient leaflets for healthy eating:
British Dietetic Association. www.bda.uk.com/latest-food-facts.php
Diabetes UK www.diabetes.org.uk

Chapter 6

Urine testing

Introduction

Urine has been studied for thousands of years. Nowadays, patients may feel embarassed about providing a sample and often fail to comply, or do not follow instructions. Provide discreet facilities and clear explanations, especially about 24 hr collections which are inconvenient, often incomplete, and or inaccurately timed. Beware the shy patient who repeatedly fails to provide urine for testing—they may have hidden nephropathy.

Uses of urine testing

- Annual review for protein (micro- or macroalbuminuria)
- Patients with micro- or macroalbuminuria—to confirm this and monitor
- Symptoms of urinary tract infection
- Unwell diabetic patient with no obvious cause
- Hyperglycaemia: ?ketones, ?infection
- Unstable glucose control: ?ketones, ?infection
- Impaired renal function for cells, casts, blood, protein, and infection
- Patient glucose self-monitoring (unusual nowadays)
- But NOT to diagnose diabetes

Unexpected glycosuria in a non-diabetic should be followed by blood tests (📖 p.8) but cannot be used to diagnose diabetes. Non-diabetic patients with a low renal threshold will have glycosuria. Because of the variation in renal threshold, absence of glycosuria does not exclude diabetes. Post-prandial testing is more likely to detect diabetes than fasting samples. Up to 15% of pregnant women show glycosuria, but most of these do not have diabetes.

Home urine glucose monitoring can be used for some patients, as can urine ketone assessment at times of hyperglycaemia.

Practical points

- Teach all patients how to do a clean midstream urine suitable for microbiological testing.
- Always use this method for spot urine samples, whether done at home or in the clinic.
- Encourage them to do an early morning sample at home on the day of clinic.
- Keep all samples until the end of clinic.
- Send off those requiring microbiological testing at the end as this avoids the need for repeat urine samples.
- Give patients a urine sample bottle for next time as they leave.
- Ask all female patients of child-bearing age if they are menstruating.
- Keep urine pregnancy testing kits in clinic.

Urine glucose monitoring

The person testing the urine must:
- understand why they are doing the test
- be capable of following instructions
- follow the instructions
- not be colour blind
- not suffer visual impairment
- not have impeding upper-limb disabilities

Home urine glucose monitoring is not precise and can be misleading. It will not detect hypoglycaemia and the variability of renal threshold, from person to person and over time, makes results hard to interpret. Urine glucose testing can be a first step to learning about self-monitoring, or be the only means of self-monitoring in needle-phobic patients or in those whose renal threshold allows consistency.

Ideally, urine glucose monitoring should be used only after urinalyses during an oral glucose tolerance test or blood glucose series have demonstrated the renal threshold. The threshold is usually about 10 mmol/l. Urine glucose monitoring is too imprecise for insulin-treated patients. Do not use it as the sole means of testing in any patients capable and willing to measure finger-prick blood glucose. Some physicians advocate urine testing for well-controlled type 2 patients and blood testing for type 1 patients. While there may be less rapid fluctuations in blood glucose concentration in type 2 diabetes, it is helpful for patients to have an accurate knowledge of their blood glucose status. Some patients like to use both blood and urine testing.

When to test for glycosuria

To monitor the overnight blood glucose balance, test the first urine passed on rising in the morning. For a fasting pre-breakfast test, empty the bladder on rising, and then test a specimen voided 30–60 min later, but before eating. Remind patients that the concentration of glucose in the urine depends upon the height of the blood glucose above the renal threshold during the period since last voiding (often many hours) and the volumes of fluid passed. Many patients think that the urine glucose now reflects the blood glucose now. The results should be written down, with an indication of the period covered.

Urine vs blood glucose testing

In the UK it is now unusual to monitor glucose control using urine testing.

For

- No needles, no finger-pricks
- No risk of infection to the tested and minimal risk of infection to testers.
- Simple equipment—just a bottle of strips—which is easy to use

Against

- The method is dependent upon renal threshold which varies from person to person and over time in one individual
- Needs a lavatory or other appropriate place
- It is retrospective
- If there is no glucose in the urine the patient does not know whether his/her blood glucose is normal, or whether he/she is hypoglycaemic—hence the old advice to keep a trace of glucose in the urine (which, in practice, meant keeping the blood glucose >10 mmol/l, hardly normoglycaemia).
- Aspirin and vitamin C interfere with urine glucose testing, giving false-negative results.

Urine ketones

Ketones are a product of fat breakdown. Their presence in urine is a sign of insulin deficiency. However, anything which causes major fat breakdown, such as a strict weight-reducing diet, produces ketonuria, as can alcohol excess. Some patients have been alarmed by the teaching that ketonuria always means impending coma.

Ketone testing strips are available in bottles and individually foil-wrapped. The latter are most suitable for patient use as they keep well and most patients need them infrequently. The strips measure acetone, but the predominant ketone in diabetic ketoacidosis is β-hydroxybutyrate which can now be measured by finger-prick testing (📖 p.126). Urine ketones levels above ++ require immediate action (?DKA). Type 1 patients with any ketonuria require review of their clinical condition (?developing DKA) and insulin treatment unless they are well and are deliberately reducing calorie intake to lose weight.

When to test for ketones

New patients

Always test newly diagnosed diabetic patients for ketones. If present in large amounts they indicate the need for insulin treatment.

Ill insulin-treated patients

❶May have relative insulin deficiency and should be encouraged to test for ketones. This is especially important if they are vomiting or are short of breath. Such patients who present to their doctor must have a urine or blood ketone test and require emergency admission.

Very high blood glucose

❶ Type 1 patients should test for ketones if their blood glucose concentration is >15 mmol/l, even if they are otherwise well.

Urine vs blood ketone testing

For

- Widely available
- Cheap
- Combined with other tests on a single familiar strip

Against

- Must wait for patient to urinate
- Cannot be used in anuric patients
- Need lavatory or suitable place
- Measures acetone
- False positives—levodopa (e.g. sinemet), valproic acid, vitamin C, phenazopyrazine

Urine protein

Which test?

Laboratories may measure total protein or albumin in the urine. Albumin assay costs more, but should be use in microalbumin tests, ideally as a ratio with urinary creatinine. Check your local laboratory practice and normal ranges. There are a variety of point-of-care strips which test albumin or albumin-to-creatinine ratio (ACR). Renal physicians check total protein in patients with macroproteinaemia to monitor progression.

Everyone loses some albumin in their urine—in fit adults the loss ranges from 2.5 to 11 mg per 24 hrs. Albumin excretion rate varies during 24 hrs depending on, for example, posture and exertion. Albumin excretion above 25 mg per 24 hrs is not only a marker for the development of diabetic nephropathy but also, in type 2 diabetes, for early mortality (mostly from cardiovascular causes). Therefore efforts are being made to detect small, early increases in albuminuria (microalbuminuria). Albustix© will detect 300 mg/l albumin in urine, but this is not sensitive enough for early detection. More sensitive point-of-care strips are available to test for microalbuminuria or microalbumin-to-creatinine ratio. Laboratories will measure albumin, protein, ACR, or protein-to-creatinine ratio (PCR).

Which sample for protein testing?

- ***Timed overnight urinary ACR***. Gold standard but rather impractical. During a normal night at rest less than 30 μg albumin should be passed per minute. Can use PCR.
- ***Overnight urine collection*** The albumin concentration should be below 20 mg/l. Less precise than timed samples, bigger volumes, unpopular with patients and laboratories. Can use PCR.
- ***Early morning urine ACR***. Sample from first urine passed on waking. Normal <3.5 mg/mmol in women and <2.5mg/mmol in men. Can use PCR.
- ***Urine ACR on sample passed in clinic***. Normal taken as <3.5 mg/mmol in women and <2.5mg/mmol in men, but less reproducible because of exercise and posture. Can use PCR.

False positives

- Cetrimide (e.g. Savlon®)
- Chlorhexidine (e.g. Hibitane®)
- Concentrated urine

When to test for albumin

All newly diagnosed patients

Should have an urine test for protein or albumin. If this is negative, micro-albumin should be measured.

All patients

Should have their urine albumin checked annually using a microalbumin technique. If they already have proteinuria detectable using protein or albumin test strip there is no need for the more sensitive test.

Patients with microalbuminuria

If microalbuminuria is confirmed on two further tests during the next month prescribe ACE inhibitor treatment. Repeat tests at least annually after intervention to monitor progress. (📖 p.302)

Overt proteinuria

Some units are now using spot ACR or PCR to monitor overt proteinuria rather than performing 24 hr urine collections which are unpopular with patients and laboratories and are often incomplete. PCR has been shown to be a good indicator of 24 hr protein excretion. PCR may be used in preference to ACR in known chronic kidney disease.

Multiple test analysis

Urinary tract infections (UTIs) are common in men and women with diabetes. Some clinics use multiple dipstick urine checks at every clinic visit. This often detects unsuspected UTIs.

Test for UTIs

- Check blood, protein, nitrite, and leucocytes in:
  - patients with symptoms of UTI
  - pregnant diabetic women every visit (risk of premature labour with UTI)
  - patients with renal disease every visit
  - unwell patients
  - patients with high glucose or erratic glucose control
- False positives:
  - failure to close bottle of strips between tests
  - contamination during urination.

Summary

- Remember that patients may find providing urine samples embarrassing
- Patients may not follow instructions for collection, or may not provide the sample at all. Beware repeat lack of samples and hence hidden early nephropathy.
- Beware false negatives and false positives in all forms of urine testing.
- Urine glucose testing of post-prandial samples can be used to detect diabetes but laboratory venous glucose is required for diagnosis
- Urine glucose testing can be used to monitor glycaemic balance but is less reliable than blood glucose testing.
- Urine ketone (acetone) testing should be used to detect the need for insulin therapy in newly diagnosed patients. It may indicate the need for increased insulin dosage in those who are ill or markedly hyperglycaemic. Finger-prick blood ketone (β-hydroxybutyrate) testing is better.
- Urine albumin testing includes albumin-to-creatinine ratio (ACR) to detect microalbuminuria, or tests for albuminuria. Urine microalbumin testing detects patients at risk of worsening nephropathy at a stage when intervention may slow the rate of progression. It also warns of increased risk of cardiovascular mortality in type 2 patients. Spot ACR generally correlates with 24 hr urinary protein excretion and can be used in patients who find 24 hr collection difficult.
- Protein:creatinine ratio (PCR) is used to monitor patients with known chronic kidney disease
- General multiple test dipstick urinalysis can detect urinary tract infections which are common in men and women with diabetes.

Further reading

NICE (2008). Management of type 2 diabetes. Inherited Clinical Guideline 66. www.nice.org.uk
The Renal Association. www.renal.org

Chapter 7

Blood glucose and ketone testing

Blood glucose

Blood glucose assessment includes capillary blood glucose monitoring from finger-prick samples, laboratory estimation of venous plasma (or whole blood) glucose, or retrospective measures using glycosylated proteins (fructosamine and HbA_{1c}).

Blood glucose results from separate but simultaneously taken samples in the same person may vary for the following reasons.

- Whether arterial, venous, or capillary sample
- Whether whole blood or plasma used in assay
- Fasting or post-prandial
- The level of blood glucose (more variation at higher readings)
- Patient's central and peripheral temperature
- The state of the patient's circulation
- Laboratory or hand-held meter assay
- Which meter is used

Laboratory venous plasma glucose is the international gold standard (WHO). On fasting samples, capillary whole-blood glucose is usually lower than or similar to venous plasma glucose. On 2 hr post-prandial samples capillary whole-blood glucose is higher than venous glucose. (*Diabet Med* 2003; **20**:953–6) Because this is a complex topic with no clear answer, in this book it is assumed that, for practical purposes, venous plasma glucose and capillary glucose targets are approximately the same.

Blood glucose targets

Whenever possible the target should be to have a glucose level within the non-diabetic range, provided that this is safe and practical for that individual.

Table 7.1 Blood glucose targets (laboratory or capillary)

Situation	**Blood glucose target**	
	Before food	**2 hrs after food**
Most people	4–6 mmol/l	4–8 mmol/l
❶Hypoglycaemia prone or poor warnings of hypoglycaemia	6–8 mmol/l	8–10 mmol/l
Pregnant women	4–6 mmol/l	4–6.9 mmol/l
	❶Beware hypoglycaemia	

Blood glucose laboratory estimation

This is the gold standard against which other methods are compared. When taking venous blood, record the time. Same-day analysis is best, but if this is not possible, the sample can be kept in a 4°C refrigerator. Record the results, tell the patient, and act as outlined below. Temper these guidelines with your knowledge of the individual patient. (Table 7.1)

Box 7.1 Results of laboratory venous plasma glucose test

< 3.9 mmol/l
Telephone patients on glucose-lowering medication to make sure that they are not still hypoglycaemic. Did you or the patient realize that they were hypoglycaemic at the time? If not, warn the patient that they have hypoglycaemic unawareness. And you need to sharpen your clinical observation. Reduce glucose-lowering treatment unless it was a one-off low with a one-off explanation.

4.0–6.9 mmol/l
Within normal limits; no action need be taken

7.0–10.9 mmol/l
OK if post-prandial. Too high before food. Discuss eating less or increasing glucose-lowering treatment.

11.0–19.9 mmol/l
Too high. Review diet, self-adjustment of treatment, exercise. Increase treatment if necessary.

20 mmol/l or more
Much too high. Many patients tolerate blood glucose levels like this much of the time. Others will be symptomatic or ill. Telephone the patient that day and check that they are alright. If the level is ≥30 mmol/l the patient should be seen by a doctor that day. They may need insulin and most need hospital admission (p.226).

Capillary blood glucose testing

Capillary blood glucose testing

This is a more direct and precise way of monitoring blood glucose concentration than urine testing. Urine testing should not be used by professionals in hospitals or surgeries to monitor glycaemia in known diabetes. The Medicines and Healthcare Products Regulatory Agency (MHRA) (www.mrha.gov.uk) tests meters and highlights problems. Visit the website regularly.

Diabetes UK's position is 'that people with diabetes should have access to home blood glucose monitoring based on individual clinical need, informed consent and not on ability to pay. Home monitoring is essential in the context of diabetes education for self-management in order to enable the person to make appropriate treatment or lifestyle choices'.

Home finger-prick blood glucose monitoring (HBGM) is expensive and thus causes concern for those with financial responsibilities for health care who may put pressure on prescribers to reduce glucose test strip prescriptions. HBGM is a waste of time, pain, and money without appropriate patient education about what results mean and what to do about them.

Who can use capillary glucose testing?

Professionals

For rapid bedside measurement of blood glucose. If the test is performed properly, the results are nearly as accurate as those obtained in the laboratory. If the user and the meter participate in a quality assurance scheme and the user has regular retraining, the results can be used for most diabetes management. All hospitals and clinics using this technique should participate in a quality assurance scheme. Record the results on a hospital-wide chart (Figure 7.1 📖 p.115). Finger-prick glucose tests should not be done on cold or 'shut-down' hands. Problems may arise when inexperienced personnel are asked to test blood glucose without any training. Every finger-prick glucose-testing problem investigated in one busy district general hospital was found to be due to user error.

People with diabetes or their relatives or carers

HBGM has taken the guesswork out of life with diabetes. Patients no longer have to rely on urine tests and symptoms to manage their diabetes. HBGM allows patients to adjust their treatment and eating, and to monitor their own condition. It should not be a ritual just to produce numbers for the doctor.

The person testing the blood must:

- understand why they are doing the test
- understand when the test is or is not appropriate
- learn how to obtain an appropriate blood sample
- be aware of health and safety issues of blood testing and safe disposal of sharps
- be aware of normal and abnormal results—and what to do about them
- have had a formal training session with the device and be able to demonstrate its use
- be aware of potential technical problems and what to do about them

The Hillingdon Hospital **NHS**
NHS Trust

Blood Glucose Monitoring

Name:

Blood glucose (mmol/1) **Comment** *e.g. treatment*

Below 4 = hypoglycaemia, give glucose, tell doctor
Above 20 = very high, tell doctor

Times	Pre b'fast		Pre lunch		Pre dinner		Pre bed		
Date ▽									

HIL028

Fig. 7.1 An example of a hospital blood glucose monitoring chart.

- know how to seek help
- take part in a quality assurance system (e.g. using manufacturer's test samples)
- not be colour blind unless using a meter
- not suffer visual impairment unless using a talking meter
- not have severe impeding upper-limb disabilities.

A patient produced her home glucose-testing diary. Every day for a month her glucose was 9.6 mmol/l. When asked to demonstrate the test she pricked her finger, ignored the blood, and looked at the meter, which was set on memory and showed the result of 9.6 produced when the diabetic nurse had originally demonstrated blood glucose testing.

How to do a finger-prick blood glucose test

Like all laboratory techniques performed outside the laboratory, finger-prick blood glucose measurement is a waste of time unless it is done properly. Important factors are as follows.

- ***The finger*** should be warm, clean, and dry. Wash with water and then dry. Do not use alcohol swabs, which may interfere with the test. Sticky fingers give falsely high blood glucose levels. The sides of the finger are less sensitive than the tip. The ear lobe can be used.
- ***Making the hole*** Finger-pricking lancets are for single use only. Spring-loaded devices are less painful. Many devices have platforms to press on to the finger. Platforms of different thickness allow deeper or shallower finger-prick. In hospitals or clinics use individually spring-loaded lancets for each patient to avoid transmission of blood-borne infection which is a risk with devices with platforms. One meter (Ascensia Esprit 2™) has a built-in finger-pricker. A laser light device (Lasette™) uses a laser to make a small hole in the skin (www.nutech-international.com). It may be less painful that a lancet, but UK experience is limited.
- ***The blood drop*** should be allowed to form naturally. If necessary blood may be 'milked' up from the base of the finger. Squeezing the finger tip may dilute the blood with serum and may make the finger sore. Drop the blood onto the strip without smearing. Some systems wick up the blood from the end of the strip.
- ***The electrode strips*** must be in date and dry. Never handle the pad onto which the blood will be dropped—your sticky fingers might influence the result.
- ***Read the result*** A properly used meter is best. Visually read strips are rarely used nowadays. Each bottle of strips has a colour chart against which to match the colour changes of the strips in that bottle. (The dyes in each batch may change slightly, so strips must not be matched against a bottle from a different batch.) The person reading the result must have normal colour vision. People with diabetic retinopathy, especially those who have had laser treatment, may not have normal colour vision.

People may not always understand instructions.

One elderly couple tried to make words out of the numbers on the meter.
A nurse read a meter upside-down— 07 instead of LO.
Warning messages may be misinterpreted—a nurse said a patient had ketones in her blood. When asked how she had measured this, she said 'Came up on the meter'. What the biosensor actually indicated was 'Check ketones'! Optium Xceed™ does measure ketones but only if a specific ketone strip is used.

Record the result

Many patients do not record their results. While a one-off test may be of use at the time it was done, without a record neither the patient nor their carer can assess overall glucose balance and the need or otherwise for intervention. There may be other problems.

A teenage patient produced a tidy glucose diary with lots of tests for the past month. Unfortunately I had seen her making-up the results in the waiting room!

There is a human tendency to under-read or to fail to record unpalatable results. A few patients make up their results to please their doctor. A sophisticated faker may be detected only by repeated marked disparity between the glycosylated haemoglobin and home-recorded glucose levels. With modern meters with memories it possible to review, with the patient, what the results actually were. Many patients prefer using software to download the results onto a computer. Clinics can also do this.

Acting on the result

It is no use noting an abnormal result and doing nothing about it. In one district general hospital audit, only one in four markedly abnormal blood glucose results recorded by nursing staff was acted upon. Patients frequently record high or low results for weeks without taking action.

Protecting staff

There is an obvious risk of infection with blood-borne diseases and staff must take care. Use disposable gloves to protect from blood contamination. Use finger-prickers which retract the needle into a safety cover.

Strips and meters

Nowadays, most people use meters but these are not currently available at NHS expense. Keep them clean, handle them gently, follow the instructions, and calibrate new packs of strips. Ask the company trainer to visit the surgery, clinic, or ward each year to update staff. Use the test solutions provided and share in any quality assurance scheme for meters. Many patients buy meters off the shelf. Check that they are using them properly; some are easier to use than others. Some download to computers.

The MIMS (Monthly Index of Medical Specialties) website has an up-to-date list of meters, strips, finger-prickers and lancets.
http://www.healthcarerepublic.com/mims/Tables/28928/

HBGM in insulin-treated diabetes

It is essential that these patients learn how about HBGM—how to use it for insulin dose adjustment and for safety checks.

HBGM in non-insulin-treated type 2 diabetes

The benefits (or otherwise) of HBGM are difficult to study. More motivated patients are more likely to wish to test and to use the results. It can be hard to separate the effects of education from the effects of testing. For some reason, while insulin-treated patients are encouraged to use test results to adjust their treatment, tablet-treated patients are not. Provided that patients are aware of the dosage range of their medication, the adjustment rules for each tablet, the interval (usually weeks) required to assess effect before further change, and safety issues, there is no reason why they should not self-adjust tablets according to blood results.

A recent study (*Br Med J* 2007; **335**:132–9) selected non-testing, non-insulin-treated type 2 diabetic patients and randomized them to intensive or non-intensive HBGM with educational packages vs a non-testing control group. Only 15% of 8457 patients were entered into the study and so its generalizability is limited. HbA_{1c} fell slightly, but not significantly, in the HBGM groups but there was no difference between intensive and non-intensive testers. The study excluded those already testing, who might have been those for whom there was value in HBGM. Similar studies are ongoing (*Br Med J* 2007; **335**:105)

A practical approach seems to be to use HBGM for patients who are willing and capable of using it for safety and treatment monitoring. It should not be continued for patients are not using HBGM, despite prescription, or are not finding the results helpful.

When to test

Test whenever you want to know the blood glucose. Tell patients that HBGM allows them to check their glucose at any time, virtually anywhere, to ensure that they are safe and comfortable, and that any changes in treatment, eating, or exercise can be made on a day-to-day basis. On most occasions when you see someone with diabetes, measure his/her finger-prick blood glucose. HbA_{1c} provides good long-term information about glycaemia but an HbA_{1c} of 7.0% can be achieved by oscillating between 1 and 20 mmol/l. Also, some patients may be having unrecognized problems with accurate measurement (or simply not checking). If this is the case, HBGM is unlikely to helpful. A small but significant number of insulin-treated patients will be hypoglycaemic while talking with you. Use local HBGM guidelines if available.

Consider the difference between HBGM to assess overall glucose control (HbA_{1c} is usually better for this), and testing during times when glucose changes may be expected (e.g. illness, new treatment, etc.).

Insulin-treated patients

Should test before each meal and before bed until their blood glucose levels are stable. Patients using short-acting insulin pens or pumps should continue to test four times a day for optimum flexibility in insulin dosage adjustment and glucose control. If the number of tests is being reduced, the one that should always remain is the pre-bedtime test to ensure that patients go to bed with a safe glucose concentration.

Non-insulin-treated patients

Can test two to four times a day when treatment has just started or if their treatment regimen has been changed (to see if the new treatment is working and to check for hypoglycaemia). The most important test in type 2 diabetes is the pre-breakfast, fasting test as this is a useful indicator of overall glucose balance. It should be 4–6 mmol/l. These patients can learn how to adjust their tablets according to blood glucose levels. Patients with good fasting glucose but high HbA_{1c} should test post-prandially. There is usually no need to continue routine testing if the HbA_{1c} is within target for that patient unless the patient wishes. However, patients who find it helpful, e.g. those who are on repaglinide or nateglinide and adjust their treatment for meals and exercise, should continue to test.

Illness, pregnancy, or exercise

More frequent finger-prick glucose tests may be needed in illness or pregnancy, or when undergoing new, hazardous, or vigorous exercise.

Post-prandial tests

Post-prandial hyperglycaemia contributes considerably to overall glycaemia. Test results 1–2 hrs after a meal should be between 4 and 8 mmol/l without hypoglycaemia at other times.

Night-time tests

If under intensive control, e.g. when pregnant, waking hypoglycaemia after reduction in overnight insulin, waking high glucose (to check if nocturnal hypoglycaemia).

Safety checks

Drivers, especially PCV and LGV drivers, on glucose-lowering treatment which could cause hypoglycaemia, and others involved in hazardous activities should test regularly to avoid hypoglycaemia.

Continuous blood glucose monitoring

Transcutaneous glucose monitoring

Glucowatch G2 Biographer™ (www.glucowatch.com). This system draws glucose through the skin into gel discs from which the electrode measures the glucose. This allows readings up to every 10 min for 13 hrs. The device has to be calibrated with capillary glucose readings and has a long stabilization period. Adverse skin reactions are common. Patient feed-back has been variable. Computer analytical software is available.

Continuous glucose monitoring system

CGMS® System Gold™ and Guardian® REAL-Time Continuous Glucose Monitoring System™. (www.minimed.com). A needle sensor records up to 288 multiple interstitial fluid glucose levels a day, and can be used for 3 days. Patients wear a recording device. Patients have to calibrate the system with four finger-prick glucose readings a day. The Guardian system uses wireless technology. Both have analytical computer software. The systems and the single-use sensors are expensive.

Indications suggested by the manufacturers:

- Raised HbA_{1c}
- Hypoglycaemic episodes and unawareness
- Hyperglycaemic episodes
- Diabetic ketoacidosis
- Unexplained blood glucose excursions
- Gastroparesis
- Gestational diabetes, preconception, pregnancy, and nursing
- Evaluation of therapeutic changes to medication regimen
- Evaluation of behavioural modifications affecting glycaemic control
- Patients undergoing erythropoietin therapy because $HbA1_C$ may be unreliable.

Table 7.2 Suggested indications for HBGM

Which patients?	Frequency of testing
What is my glucose? (all patients)	Any time
Illness (all patients)	4–6 times daily until well
Unusual circumstances/exertion (all patients)	Any time
Planned exercise (all patients*)	pre/post-exercise until stable
Unstable glucose (all patients)	2–4 times daily
Change in treatment (all patients)	2–4 times daily
Pre-pregnancy	4–6 times daily
Pregnancy (type 1/2, gestational diabetes)	4–6 times daily
Insulin pump patients	4–6 times daily
Type 1 or 2 diabetes (basal-bolus insulin)	4 times daily
Type 1 or 2 diabetes (twice daily insulin)	2 (vary times) to 4 times daily
Type 2 on basal insulin	Fasting daily; post-prandial 1–7 times a week
Type 2 on sulphonylureas (initial/change dose)	Fasting + a post-prandial daily until stable, then weekly
Type 2 on glitazones (initial/change dose)	Fasting + a post-prandial daily until stable, then weekly
Type 2 on diet or metformin alone*	Not routinely unless patient wishes or as above; use HbA_{1c} every 2–6 months

Table 7.3 Indications for finger-prick capillary glucose monitoring in hospital/clinic/practice

Situation	Frequency of testing
Hospital	
ITU/HDU/resuscitation area	Hourly
In theatre and recovery area	Hourly
Very ill patient anywhere	Hourly
Insulin—sliding scale	Hourly
Acute ward	6 hourly (pre-meals, pre-bed)
Nocturnal hypoglycaemia?	2 a.m.
Not ill but awaiting care package	As for Table 7.2
Clinic/practice	
Annual check	
Each visit	

Factors affecting capillary glucose results

Different meters may be affected in different ways by the patient's age, condition, or treatment. Check that the meter you are using is right for the job—especially in a neonatal or maternity unit.

Box 7.2 Factors affecting capillary glucose results*

- Variation in haematocrit—neonates, pregnancy
- Peripheral shut-down, e.g. hypotension, dehydration, shock, peripheral vascular disease
- Over-squeezing finger (dilutes with tissue fluids)
- Water on finger
- Glucose on finger
- Oedema of finger
- Dialysis treatments: some peritoneal dialysis fluids may contain maltose which interferes with some strips
- Variations in oxygenation, e.g. intensive oxygen therapy
- Non-glucose reducing substances, e.g. ascorbic acid infusions
- Jaundice
- Hypertriglyceridaemia
- Total parenteral nutrition

***See MRHA website www.mrha.gov.uk**

Glycosylated haemoglobin

Glucose binds with many proteins—glycosylation. Glycosylated haemoglobin A_{1c} (HbA_{1c}) is used to monitor glucose balance because it is a marker for the risk of diabetic tissue damage—the higher the HbA_{1c}, the greater is the risk. HbA_{1c} is related to glycaemia over the life of the red cell, which is about 120 days.

- Glucose in the preceding:
  - 30 days contributes to ~50% of the HbA_{1c}
  - 30–90 days contributes to ~40% of the HbA_{1c}
  - >90 days contributes to ~10% of the HbA_{1c}
- In general:
  - mean plasma glucose <10 mmol/l ≈ HbA_{1c} ≤7%
  - mean plasma glucose >15mmol/l ≈ HbA_{1c} ≥10%
  - HbA_{1c} does not correlate so well with individual HBGM testing time points, especially those before lunch. Type 1 diabetic patients with near-normal fasting glucose can still have a raised HbA_{1c} (*Diabetes Care 2002;* **25**:275–8).

HbA_{1c} is expressed as percentage of total haemoglobin. There are several different methods for measuring glycosylated haemoglobin. The current UK standard is **HbA_{1c} DCCT aligned**. This refers to the reference methods used in the Diabetes Control and Complications Trial (*New Engl J Med* 1993; **329**:977–86). However, this method includes a mixture of glycated haemoglobins. The International Federation of Clinical Chemists (IFCC) agreed a more precise method measuring a single molecular species of HbA_{1c}.

An international consensus statement (*Diabetologia* 2007; **50**:2042–3) agreed that:

- HbA_{1c} test results should be standardized worldwide
- The IFCC reference system should be used
- HbA_{1c} should be reported worldwide in IFCC units (mmol/mol) and derived National Glycohemoglobin Standardization Program (NGSP) units (%) using an IFCC–NGSP master equation
- An HbA_{1c}-derived average glucose (ADAG) will also be reported to make it easier for patients to understand HbA_{1c}. A study detailing this is due to report.

HbA_{1c} looks at the past, and reflects mean blood glucose concentration, but not sufficiently to rename the HbA_{1c} test the 'mean glucose test' as some have suggested. A finger-prick blood glucose relates to 'now', and fluctuates during the day.

Check glycosylated haemoglobin twice a year in stable patients, and preferably on every visit more than 2 months since the last test. Patients can attend the laboratory for a blood test 1–2 weeks before clinic so that the result is available for discussion. Some units estimate this in blood-spots on filter paper or little finger-prick collector bottles sent in by the patient a week or two in advance. There are several near-patient testing systems for HbA_{1c}.

Non-glucose factors influencing HbA_{1c}

- Rapid turnover of red cells
- Anaemia
- Variant haemoglobins
- Frequent blood transfusions (e.g. in thalassaemia major)
- Erythropoietin therapy

Some centres use fructosamine which measures glycosylation of several plasma proteins, especially albumin. Therefore it reflects glucose balance 1 or 2 weeks before the sample is taken. Fructosamine is affected by anything which influences plasma protein levels and should be corrected for plasma protein level. It is not regarded as such a reliable test as HbA_{1c} but is quicker and cheaper to measure, and does reflect a shorter time span. Fructosamine should be used in some of the situations listed above (e.g. thalassaemia). Seek laboratory advice.

HbA_{1c} targets

HbA_{1c} in a person with diabetes should be same as that for a non-diabetic person provided that treatment does not induce hypoglycaemia. The higher the HbA_{1c} the greater is the risk of diabetic tissue damage.

Table 7.4 HbA_{1c} targets (DCCT aligned)

Treatment	HbA_{1c} target (lab non-diabetic range 4.0–6.0%)
Diet alone	4.0–6.0%
Metformin alone	4.0–6.0%
Oral agents which can cause hypoglycaemia	6.0–6.5% if safe and practical
Insulin	6.0–6.5% if safe and practical
	6.5–7.4% if hypoglycaemia prone

Table 7.5 HbA_{1c} DCCT aligned vs. IFCC units

DCCT aligned(%)	IFCC (mmol/mol)
4.0	20
5.0	31
6.0	42
7.0	53
8.0	64
9.0	75
10.0	86

Blood ketone testing

Management of hyperglycaemia and DKA has been revolutionized by finger-prick capillary ketone testing (MediSense Optium Xceed™ diabetes monitoring system). This measures β-hydroxybutyrate, the main ketone in ketoacidosis, the urine test measuring acetone (📖 p.102). Blood ketone measurement is a better predictor of DKA than urine ketones (*Diabetes Metab* 2007; **33**:135–9). Blood ketones can be used in A&E departments to identify which hyperglycaemic patients have DKA or compensated DKA (*Diabet Med* 2005; **22**:221–4). Ketones rise in fasting, insulin-deficiency and alcohol excess.

Table 7.6 Indications for finger-prick blood ketone testing

Situation	Frequency of testing
Patients/carers	
Vomiting, insulin-treated	Daily. If ketones present, 6 hourly until gone
Ill, insulin-treated	Daily. If ketones present, 6 hourly until gone
Glucose >15 mmol/l	Once. If ketones present, 6 hourly until gone
Insulin pump patients	Should have a pack of strips to use as above
Patients with frequent DKA	Provide strips to use as above
Healthcare professionals	
Vomiting, insulin-treated	Once
Ill, glucose >11 mmol/l	Once
All emergency attenders	
Glucose >11 mmol/l	Once
'Well', glucose >15 mmol/l	Once
Ketones ≥1 mmol/l	6 hourly until <1 mmol/l
Ketones ≥3 mmol/l	❶ ?DKA. Admit 2 hourly until <1 mmol/l
Ketones ≥6 mmol/l	❶Risk of death. Admit HDU/ITU

Table 7.7 Act on finger-prick blood ketone results

Ketones (mmol/l)	Action
<1 mmol/l	Good glucose balance + nutrition
1–2.9 mmol/l	Risk of DKA. Increase insulin, check nutrition
≥3 mmol/l	❗ DKA. Extra insulin preferably IM. 999 to A&E Admit. IV fluids, IV insulin sliding scale

Summary

- Hyperglycaemia is one manifestation of diabetes, which is a multisystem disorder.
- Laboratory venous glucose is the only criterion for formal diagnosis of diabetes. Laboratory glucose levels should be checked from time to time in patients in whom other glycaemic monitoring techniques are in use.
- For everyday use, finger-prick blood glucose monitoring provides instant assessment of blood glucose concentration any time, anywhere. It can be used by professionals and patients or their carers.
- Finger-prick blood glucose testing is a laboratory method carried out away from the laboratory. The results are only of use if the test is performed accurately, according to instructions.
- Pay attention to each stage of the testing technique, whether performed by doctor, nurse, or patient.
- Use all meters and sensors according to instructions: the result is only as good as the user's technique. There is a wide range to choose from.
- Anyone with diabetes can use finger-prick blood glucose measurement provided that they can understand what they are doing and why, and are properly taught with regular revision sessions.
- Finger-prick blood glucose testing is more useful than urine glucose testing.
- Blood glucose levels should be 4–6 mmol/l before meals and 4–8 mmol/l afterwards (without hypoglycaemia). Targets should be tailored to individuals.
- HbA_{1c} provides a longer-term view of glycaemia. The higher the HbA_{1c} the greater is the risk of diabetic tissue damage. HbA_{1c} should be within the non-diabetic range for that laboratory, avoiding hypoglycaemia (e.g. 4.0–6.0%).
- Finger-prick blood ketone measurement allows prompt recognition of ketosis and can be used to help manage DKA
- Patients at risk of DKA should have a pack of ketone strips and the relevant meter at home.

Non-insulin medications

Treat each patient according to his or her individual condition.
Always check drug information in a current edition of the British National Formulary (BNF) www.bnf.org before prescribing any medications described in this book. Be alert for warnings from the MHRA (www.mhra.gov.uk). To review the Summary of Product Characteristics (SPC) and Patient Information Leaflet (PIL), see www.emc.medicines.org.uk

Introduction

This is a difficult chapter to keep up to date as new agents are being introduced for the treatment of type 2 diabetes. These new agents have yet to find their place in patient care. Concerns are being raised about potential risks of some drugs. Readers are strongly advised to check local prescribing policy and discuss any questions with a local consultant diabetologist.

When to use non-insulin medication

Hypoglycaemic drugs are used in type 2 diabetes. Immediate insulin treatment is essential in type 1 diabetes. Adding metformin to insulin may improve glucose control in type 1 patients, especially if they are overweight. Oral hypoglycaemic agents work only if the patient is producing insulin. By the time diabetes has been diagnosed about half the insulin production has failed in most patients, and about 4% is lost every year thereafter. Many patients with type 2 diabetes will need insulin (usually added to metformin ± sulphonylurea).

Provide education about diabetes and lifestyle advice for all patients—healthy eating, regular exercise, not smoking, alcohol in moderation. Previous advice was to try diet and exercise in all before adding glucose-lowering medication. Most patients find it hard to keep to a new diet. Each month of high glucose increases the risk of tissue damage.

Practical suggestions for patients with type 2 diabetes are as follows.

- Glucose levels ≥20 mmol/l:
  - diet and glucose-lowering medication at diagnosis
  - adjust according to glucose level
  - reduce or stop if hypoglycaemic symptoms, glucose <4 mmol/l, or HbA_{1c} below target range (📖 p.125)
- Glucose levels ≥11 mmol/l and patient symptomatic, or has infections or diabetic complications:
  - add glucose-lowering medication at diagnosis
  - reduce or stop it if patients succeed in dietary measures (or if glucose falls as infection resolves)
- Glucose <11 mmol/l or asymptomatic, uncomplicated patient:
  - start with diet and exercise alone
  - if, after 2 months, HbA_{1c} is not within patient's target range (📖 p.125) start oral hypoglycaemic tablets while continuing diet/exercise advice
  - at any time, if glucose ≥11 mmol/l and patients become symptomatic, glucose rises, or infections, complications, or problems appear, start glucose-lowering medication

In 2007 NICE reviewed usage of oral hypoglycaemic drugs in the UK in 2005–2006. £147 million was spent on some 16 million prescriptions, of which 53% were for metformin, 35% for sulphonylureas, 9% for glitazones, 1% each for meglitinides and acarbose, and 2% for metformin with rosiglitazone, Studies of adherence to glucose-lowering medication have shown that up to half the patients do not take it as prescribed. Check concordance before increasing the dose.

Patient education

- These tablets work only if you are making or taking insulin. They help control the blood sugar levels.
- These tablets are not insulin. They help control your glucose in other ways.
- They must be taken in the dose prescribed, at the right time every day.
- If the dose is to be adjusted to finger-prick glucose levels, explain how to do this and what the target glucose range is.
- They are a long-term treatment, not a short course.
- Warn about hypoglycaemia if relevant.
- Double-check for contraindications, including previous intolerance or hypersensitivity.
- Warn about relevant side effects and the need to report these to staff.
- Warn about interacting medications—there are a lot (most just require more frequent HBGM).

Non-insulin glucose-lowering medications

- Biguanide: metformin
- Sulphonylureas: glibenclamide, gliclazide, glimepiride, glipizide, gliquidone, tolbutamide
- Thiazolidinediones: rosiglitazone, pioglitazone)
- Meglitinides (prandial glucose regulators): repaglinide, nateglinide
- Incretin-effect enhancers: exenatide injections, sitagliptin
- α-Glucosidase inhibitor: acarbose

Which drug?

Set individual targets for blood glucose or HbA_{1c},taking the patient's overall clinical state, mental state, and personal circumstances into consideration. Strict glucose balance may not be appropriate in an elderly person living alone, for example.

Start with metformin, especially in overweight patients. In patients for whom metformin is inappropriate or not tolerated use generic sulphonylureas. In those in whom it would be helpful to adjust tablet dose to food or exercise use meglitinides. Consider glitazones in patients in whom metformin is inappropriate or not tolerated (but check safety concerns).

Metformin and glibenclamide (and glipizide in fewer patients) were used in UKPDS (📖 p.39). Giclazide (modified release) was the sulphonylurea used (with additional agents as required) in ADVANCE (📖 p.40). Giclazide is the commonest sulphonylurea used in the UK.

If glycaemic targets are not met, check that the patient understands how to take the medication, and is actually taking it, and then increase the dose according to licensed guidance, rechecking HbA_{1c} every 2 months until the target is achieved and stable.

Combined therapy

If patients on sulphonylureas or metformin fail to achieve acceptable blood glucose levels, add the other agent. The combination of a sulphonylurea and metformin produces significant glucose lowering and may stave off insulin therapy. Some doctors give small doses of each together early in treatment because each potentiates the effect of the other. Glitazones may be added to either, or can be used for triple therapy.

In UKPDS 34: 'When metformin was prescribed in the trial in both non-overweight and overweight patients already treated with sulphonylurea there was a significant increase in the risk of diabetes-related death and all-cause mortality.' The authors point out that the patients on sulphonylurea were older, more hyperglycaemic, and followed up for 5 yrs less. They concluded: 'The epidemiological analysis did not corroborate an association of diabetes-related deaths with combined sulphonylurea and metformin therapy although the confidence intervals were wide.' The National Institute for Clinical Excellence (NICE), in its guidance on rosiglitazone states 'Patients with inadequate blood glucose control on oral monotherapy (metformin or sulphonylurea) should first be offered metformin and sulphonylurea combination therapy, unless there are contraindications or tolerability problems.'

Check the patient every 2 months until glycaemic targets are met.

Combined preparations are metformin and rosiglitazone, and metformin and pioglitazone

Right drug, right patient

- ***Overweight*** Metformin, glitazones, incretin-effect enhancers
- ***Very symptomatic*** Sulphonylureas, then add others
- ***Need short-acting preparation*** Meglitinides, tolbutamide, gliquidone
- ***Need flexible dose for variable meals*** Meglitinides
- ***Drives for a living, dangerous job or leisure activity*** Metformin, consider incretin-effect enhancer (but not approved by DVLA yet)
- ***Gastrointestinal problems*** Sulphonylureas (but see below)
- ***Problems remembering medication*** Once-daily preparations (e.g. modified release), combined preparations
- ***Hypoglycaemia*** Metformin, incretin-effect enhancer
- ***Fasting hypoglycaemia on sulphonylureas*** Metformin, glitazones, meglitinides, incretin-effect enhancer

High-risk patients

This list is not exhaustive.

- ***Problems learning about, recognizing, or treating hypoglycaemia*** Any patient like this should be given metformin if possible. Add incretin-effect enhancers if needed. Use other agents with care to avoid hypoglycaemia.
- ***Old age*** Start on a very small dose and increase it cautiously. Start with metformin. Tolbutamide or glipizide are short-acting and perhaps safer. Gliclazide may also be used but is longer-acting. Emphasize the need for regular meals.
- ***Cardiac disease*** Metformin may cause lactic acidosis in severe cardiac failure or hypotension. Glitazones contraindicated. β-Blockers can reduce symptoms of hypoglycaemia. Diuretics reduce the glucose-lowering effect. ACE inhibitors may cause hypoglycaemia. Use insulin in patients with acute myocardial infarction (📖 p.279).
- ***Renal disease*** All glucose-lowering agents are potentially hazardous in patients with reduced creatinine clearance. Gliclazide and gliquidone are the best options, but insulin will probably be needed. Metformin is contraindicated in severe renal impairment.
- ***Hepatic disease*** The liver is involved in the metabolism and/or excretion of all sulphonylureas, so these are usually avoided. Glitazones can worsen liver function (although some diabetologists have been using them in patients with fatty liver–non-alcoholic steatohepatitis (NASH)). Metformin is contraindicated as lactic acid accumulation can occur in hepatic decompensation. Alcohol excess can predispose to lactic acidosis. This means that patients with severe hepatic disease should be treated with insulin (in an alcoholic, for example, this can be very difficult).

- ***Gastrointestinal disease*** Any condition which could seriously impair absorption of oral medication is an indication for insulin therapy. Metformin and incretin-effect enhancers have gastrointestinal side effects. Avoid acarbose in patients with gastrointestinal disease. Cimetidine interacts with both metformin and sulphonylureas.
- ***Arthritis*** Anti-inflammatory drugs, including aspirin, can also potentiate the hypoglycaemic effect of sulphonylureas.
- ***Anticoagulant treatment*** May displace sulphonylureas from protein binding and potentiate their action, and vice versa.
- ***Allergy to sulphonamides*** Precludes the use of sulphonylureas.
- ***Porphyria*** Do not give sulphonylureas.
- ***Galactose intolerance*** Avoid all tablets which contain lactose.

Metformin

Suggested mechanisms of action

- Reduces appetite
- Reduces glucose absorption from the gut
- Enhances glucose uptake and utilization by tissues
- Acts mainly on glucose rise after a meal
- Reduces gluconeogenesis and hence liver glucose release
- Does not enhance pancreatic insulin production

Beneficial effects

- Lowers the blood glucose towards normal but is unlikely to cause hypoglycaemia
- Prevents/delays onset of diabetes in patients with impaired glucose tolerance (evidence-based but unlicensed use)
- May reduce weight
- In polycystic ovary syndrome (unlicensed use unless patient also diabetic) may improve ovulation and hirsutism—but probably will not
- May improve NASH
- Possible lipid-lowering effect

Indications

- Uncontrolled glucose in type 2 diabetes alone or in combination.
- Consider metformin as the initial treatment for any type 2 diabetic patient, but particularly:
  - *obese patients* because metformin may reduce appetite and may be less likely to cause weight gain than sulphonylureas
  - *vocational drivers* of large goods vehicles, passenger-carrying vehicles, and trains should be started on metformin because of the minimal risk of hypoglycaemia
  - *those who operate hazardous machinery, or others in whom hypoglycaemia would be especially dangerous*
  - *older patients*: consider metformin because of the reduced risk of hypoglycaemia, but beware the risk of lactic acidosis in those with cardiac, renal, or hepatic disease
  - *Polycystic ovary disease with diabetes* (used but not licensed for polycystic ovary disease without diabetes)
  - Metformin may also be added to the usual insulin treatment in type 1 diabetic patients whose glucose is high, especially if they are overweight

Contraindications

- Type 1 diabetes unless on insulin; diabetic ketoacidosis
- Pregnancy: not licensed for use in pregnancy but has been used to stimulate ovulation in polycystic ovarian disease, and in pregnancy in some countries (not UK) (📖 p.373)
- Breastfeeding (excreted in breast milk)
- Kidney disease: creatinine >130 micromol (NICE) or eGFR <60 ml/min (manufacturers' SPCs) to reduce risk of lactic acidosis
- Conditions risking acidosis, e.g. low blood pressure, hypoxia, shock, dehydration, severe cardiac or respiratory disease
- Alcohol excess or alcoholism
- Liver dysfunction
- Radiological investigations using injected contrast media which could cause kidney dysfunction—stop the metformin before the procedure and restart 48 hrs later after checking renal function
- Gastrointestinal disease, e.g. ulcerative colitis, where it could precipitate or worsen symptoms
- Warfarin dose may need to be adjusted
- Cimetidine reduces renal clearance of metformin

Dosage

Standard release (generic metformin or Glucophage)

- 500 mg or 850 mg tablets
- Start gradually to reduce likelihood of gastrointestinal side effects.
- Gastrointestinal side effects may settle if a low dose is continued for a few weeks
- Prescribe metformin 500 mg daily with breakfast, increased by 500 mg every 10–15 days according to HBGM
- Usual dosage range is 500–1700 mg/day in divided doses *after meals*.
- Some physicians prescribe up to 3000 mg daily, suggesting that this may enhance the weight-reducing effect even though glucose balance is normal. (maximum licensed dose 2000mg).

Modified-release (Glucophage SR)

- 500 mg daily, increased every 10–15 days
- Maximum 2 g once daily with evening meal, or 1 g twice daily
- Change to standard release if target glucose not reached.
- May have reduced side effects

Tests

- Before starting check renal function.
- On treatment check:
  - vitamin B12 and folate levels annually in patients on ≥1500 mg/day
  - plasma creatinine or eGFR annually in patients without renal impairment, and at least 6-monthly in those with impairment. If creatinine rises, stop metformin and discuss the patient's treatment with a diabetologist.

Side effects

- Poor appetite
- Nausea and vomiting
- Diarrhoea (which may be severe)
- Abdominal discomfort, cramp or pain
- Unpleasant or metallic taste
- ❗Lactic acidosis (in alcohol excess, or elderly with renal impairment, hypotension, or hypoxia); requires immediate admission, often to ITU/HDU. Stop metformin and avoid in future
- Decreased vitamin B12 absorption (up to 30% of patients on high-dose or long-term treatment (*Arch Intern Med.* 2006; 166:1975–9)
- Decreased folate absorption
- Skin: erythema, pruritus, and urticaria
- Liver: hepatitis

Box 8.1 Information for patients on metformin

Your diabetes tablets are called metformin.
Take............mg (... tablet) with or after breakfast;
Take............mg (... tablet) with or after lunch;
Take............mg (... tablet) with or after main evening meal.

Metformin will help your diabetes diet to control your blood glucose level. It will only help you to lose weight if you stick to a weight-reducing diet.

The tablets will work only if you take them regularly as prescribed!

If you are too unwell to take your tablets for any reason contact your doctor or diabetes nurse immediately.

If you cannot eat, or are vomiting, do not take your tablets but contact your doctor or diabetes nurse immediately.

Occasionally metformin can cause stomach and bowel upsets,but these are often temporary and less likely if treatment is started gradually. Never exceed your alcohol limit (ask your doctor what this should be)—excess alcohol could make you very ill. Large doses of metformin may cause anaemia by reducing vitamin B_{12} and folate absorption. If you take 1500 g or more a day have an annual blood count and B_{12} and folate check. Patients with severe kidney trouble should not take metformin. Ensure that your doctor checks your kidney function regularly.

Over the years your diabetes may slowly progress. As your pancreas 'wears out' the tablets may become less effective. Some people may need insulin injections eventually. You may also need insulin temporarily if you are ill or have an operation.

Although your diabetes does not need insulin treatment at present you must take just as much care of yourself in general as someone on insulin injections. There is no such thing as mild diabetes. Your doctor will help you to stay well.

Carry a diabetes card with you.

Sulphonylureas

Mechanisms of action

- Enhancement of glucose-stimulated insulin release
- Possible formation of new α- and β-cells
- Increased insulin binding and receptor density in peripheral tissues.

Beneficial actions

- Reduces glucose and improves HbA_{1c}
- Recent long-term outcome data for glibenclamide. (UKPDS 📖 p.39). and gliclazide modified-release (ADVANCE 📖 p.40)

The drugs, their dosage and approximate duration of action are shown in Table 8.1. Start with a small dose. Adjust the dose of sulphonylurea every 2 weeks according to HBGM.

Table 8.1 Dosage for sulphonylureas

Name	Dosage range per 24 hrs	Dosage frequency
Chlorpropamide	100–500mg	Once daily
Glibenclamide* (Daonil®)	5–15mg	Once daily
Gliclazide* (Diamicron®)	40–320 mg	Once/twice daily
Gliclazide m/r (Diamicron 30 MR®)	30–120 mg	Once daily
Glimepiride (Amaryl®)	1–6 mg	Once daily
Glipizide* (Glibenese®)	2.5–20 mg	Once/twice daily
Gliquidone (Glurenorm®, Minodiab®)	15–180 mg	Once to three times daily
Tolbutamide	500–2000 mg	Once to three times daily

*Generic version available

UK brand names shown-names vary world-wide

Indications

Uncontrolled glucose in type 2 diabetes—alone or in combination. The SPCs exclude children but sulphonylureas are being used in the under-18s as the frequency of type 2 diabetes increases in these young people. Sulphonylureas are used to treat monogenic diabetes (MODY) associated with HNF1–α (📖 p.15)

Which sulphonylurea?

The one you are used to.

- *Gliclazide* is widely used. It may reduce platelet stickiness which could reduce the risk of vascular complications, but glucose-lowering itself can have effects on platelets. Gliclazide also seems less likely to produce sudden hypoglycaemia than glibenclamide. There is good long-term efficacy and safety evidence.
- *Glibenclamide* is widely used worldwide, although less so in the UK. The glucose-lowering effect may last >24 hrs, especially in renal impairment. Glibenclamide may cause profound or prolonged hypoglycaemia even at a dose of 2.5 mg. It is the most common cause of hypoglycaemia due to oral agents. One in three patients taking glibenclamide experiences hypoglycaemia.
- *Tolbutamide* and *gliquidone* are both short-acting and can be linked to meals to allow some patients flexibility in dosage—small meal, small dose; big meal, big dose. Tolbutamide treatment was linked to cardiac events in a 1970s study, but these conclusions have been questioned since.
- *Chlorpropamide* is rarely used nowadays.

Contraindications and cautions

- Type 1 diabetes or diabetic ketoacidosis
- Pregnancy
- Breastfeeding
- Allergy to sulphonamides
- During surgery (📖 p.471)
- Serious infections
- Caution in renal dysfunction
- Caution in hepatic dysfunction
- Some drug interactions with sulphonylureas are outlined in Table 8.2
- Manufacturers state that these drugs should not be used in children, but as type 2 diabetes becomes more commoner in the under-18s, sulphonylureas are being used in this age group.
- Porphyria

Table 8.2 Possible drug interactions with sulphonylureas

	Lower blood glucose	Raise blood glucose
General	Alcohol (+flushing)	
Antimicrobials	Chloramphenicol Co-trimoxazole Miconazole Fluconazole Sulphonamides Ciprofloxacin Norfloxacin Ritonavir	Rifampicin
Cardiovascular	β-Blockers (+ reduce hypo warning) ACE inhibitors Fibrates	Diazoxide Loop diuretics Thiazides (risk of low sodium with chlorpropamide) (Nifedipine)
Anticoagulant	Warfarin	
Gastrointestinal	H2 antagonists	Aprepitant
Endocrine/metabolic	Octreotide Lanreotide Testosterone	Corticosteroids Oestrogens Progestogens Contraceptives
Joints	Aspirin Phenylbutazone NSAIDs Sulphinpyrazone Azapropazone Leflunomide	
Psychotropic	MAOIs	Lithium Phenobarbitone Tricyclics (+postural hypotension) Phenothiazines

This list changes—see the British National Formulary for an up-to-date list.

Tests

Before starting and on treatment check:

- Renal function
- Liver function

Side effects

- Hypoglycaemia
- Allergic rashes
- Gastrointestinal disturbances (usually mild) such as anorexia, nausea and vomiting, altered bowel habit
- Reduction in platelets and white cells, or aplastic anaemia (rare)
- Alcohol flushing (especially with chlorpropamide)
- Weight gain
- Hepatic dysfunction
- Hyponatraemia (especially with chlorpropamide)

Box 8.2 Information for patients on sulphonylurea tablets

Your diabetes tablets are called ....

They belong to a family of medicines called sulphonylureas.

Take..........mg (............tablet(s)) before breakfast;

Take..........mg (............tablet(s)) before main evening meal.

The tablets will help your diabetic diet to control your blood glucose level.

The tablets will work only if you take them regularly as prescribed!

If you are too unwell to take your tablets for any reason contact your doctor or diabetes nurse immediately.

If you cannot eat, or are vomiting, do not take your tablets but contact your doctor or diabetes nurse immediately.

Side effects are usually mild and infrequent, and include stomach or bowel upset and headache. Flushing may occur with alcohol. Allergic rashes, jaundice, and blood problems occur rarely.

These tablets work by reducing the blood glucose. Sometimes the blood glucose may fall too low (i.e. below 4 mmol/l). This is called hypoglycaemia and may happen if you are taking too big a dose, eat too little, or exercise more than you expect. If you feel muddled, slow-thinking, tingly, unduly emotional or cross, sweaty, or shaky, or notice your heart thumping fast, eat some glucose, then have a big snack. Contact your doctor or diabetes nurse. You may need to reduce your dose of tablets.

Over the years your diabetes may slowly progress. As your pancreas 'wears out' the tablets may become less effective. Some people may need insulin injections eventually. You may also need insulin temporarily if you are ill or have an operation.

Although your diabetes does not need insulin treatment at present you must take just as much care of yourself in general as someone on insulin injections. There is no such thing as mild diabetes. Your doctor will help you to stay well.

Always carry a diabetes card and some glucose with you.

Meglitinides (prandial glucose regulators)

[illegible]

- Severe hepatic impairment

[illegible]

Meglitinides (prandial glucose regulators)

Mechanism of action

Also known as prandial glucose regulators
Stimulate insulin release from pancreas by acting on pancreatic β-cell receptors

Beneficial effects

- Glucose-lowering
- Rapid absorption from gut and rapid action and duration
- Reduced likelihood of hypoglycaemia especially overnight

Indications

- Uncontrolled glucose in type 2 diabetes
- Repaglinide—alone or combined with metformin
- Nateglinide only combined with metformin

Contraindications

- Pregnancy
- Breastfeeding
- <18 yrs of age
- >75 yrs of age
- Debilitated or malnourished patients
- Severe renal impairment
- Severe hepatic impairment
- During surgery—stop that morning, restart with normal eating.

Interactions

Repaglinide may interact with gemfibrozil, causing severe hypoglycaemia. Avoid the combination. Repaglinide may also interact with ciclosporin, clarithromycin, itraconazole, trimethoprim, octreotide, lanreotide, and rifampicin. See Table 8.2—many interactions are similar.

Interactions for nateglinide include fluconazole, gemfibrozil, rifampicin, ACE inhibitors, and drugs which inhibit cytochrome P450

Dosage

Repaglinide (UK-Prandin®)

- Start with 500 mcg within 30 min before main meals
- If transferring from another glucose-lowering drug, start with 1 mg of repaglinide before each main meal; adjust the dose every 1–2 weeks according to HBGM
- Maximum single dose, 4 mg.
- Maximum total dose in 24 hrs, 16 mg

Nateglinide (UK-Starlix®)

- Start with 60 mg, within 30 min before breakfast, lunch, and evening meal
- Adjust the dose every 1–2 weeks according to HBGM
- Maximum dose 180 mg three times daily

Tests

Before starting and on treatment check:

- Renal function
- Liver function

Side-effects

- Hypoglycaemia can occur (glucose will stimulate further insulin release so continue monitoring; further glucose and food as necessary for 6 hrs)
- Gastrointestinal: nausea and vomiting, abdominal pain, altered bowel habit
- Rash, pruritus, urticaria
- Vasculitis
- Visual disturbance
- Transient elevation in liver enzymes; it would seem prudent to stop the drug if liver enzymes rise >3 x ULN.

Thiazolidinediones (glitazones)

Mechanisms of action

These drugs are peroxisome-proliferator-activated receptor-gamma (PPAR-γ) agonists and thus reduce the body's resistance to insulin action. PPAR-γ has multiple effects on the body, including influencing production of osteoblasts in the bone marrow.

There has been increasing concern about the non-glucose effects of glitazones, e.g. glitazones increase fracture risk in women. A meta-analysis suggested that rosiglitazone was associated with an increased risk of myocardial infarction (*New Engl J Med* 2007; **356**:2457–71), and further studies are awaited. The CVD effects of pioglitazone vs placebo were studied in PROactive. Pioglitazone did not reduce first CVD endpoints but did reduce second endpoints (total mortality, myocardial infarct, stroke) (*Lancet* 2005; **366**:1279–89). Both glitazones increase the risk of heart failure, especially when combined with insulin. Following review in December 2007, 'the European Medicines Agency has advised that the benefits of both rosiglitazone and pioglitazone in the treatment of type 2 diabetes continue to outweigh their risks. However, the prescribing information will be updated to include a warning that, in patients with ischaemic heart disease (i.e. that caused by a reduced blood supply to the heart), rosiglitazone should be used only after careful evaluation of every patient's individual risk. In addition, the combination of rosiglitazone and insulin should be used only in exceptional cases and under close supervision' (www.mhra.gov.uk).

Beneficial effects

- Reduction in glucose and HbA_{1c}
- Reduction in combined cardiovascular endpoints (but also linked with cardiac problems—see above)

Indications

- Uncontrolled type 2 diabetes only
- Alone if metformin is inappropriate, especially if patient is overweight
- With metformin if sulphonylureas inappropriate
- With a sulphonylurea if metformin inappropriate
- With both metformin and a sulphonylurea as triple therapy
- Pioglitazone only—with insulin in metformin-inappropriate patients (with care)

Contraindications

The SPC lists some of these as cautions, but while concerns have been raised about glitazones, especially rosiglitazone, it would seem prudent to avoid starting the drug in these situations unless benefit would exceed risk.

- Pregnancy—avoid
- Breastfeeding—avoid
- Ischaemic heart disease—avoid for rosiglitazone, care with pioglitazone
- Cardiac failure past or present—avoid
- Hepatic impairment, raised liver enzymes
- Severe renal impairment—risk of fluid retention
- Macular oedema
- Surgery—stop that morning
- Rosiglitazone—do not use with insulin
- Osteoporosis
- Interact with sulphonylureas, meglitinides, NSAIDs, paclitaxel, gemfibrozil, rifampicin, and other inducers or inhibitors of cytochrome P450 2C8 (e.g. gemfibrozil, cerivastatin, repaglinide, carbamazepine, cyclophosphamide, omeprazole, phenytoin, trimethoprim, warfarin).

Dosage

- Rosiglitazone (UK-Avandia®) 4 mg once daily, increasing to 8 mg daily after
  8 weeks if necessary.
- Pioglitazone (UK-Actos®) 15–30 mg once daily, increasing to 45 mg once daily if necessary
- Combination preparations with metformin are available

Tests

- Before starting check:
  - weight
  - cardiac function (for risk of failure or ischaemic event)
  - liver function
  - full blood count
  - renal function (avoid if eGFR <10 ml/min/1.73 m^2)
  - lipids
  - calcium
- On treatment check
  - liver function every 2 months (stop if ALT >3 x ULN). Warn patients to report symptoms such as jaundice, abdominal pain, nausea, vomiting, dark urine
  - lipids regularly

Side effects

- Hypoglycaemia
- Oedema, especially when used with insulin
- Myocardial infarction (under debate at present)
- Cardiac failure (especially when combined with insulin)
- Fractures
- Hyperlipidaemia (increased LDL and HDL cholesterol)
- Anaemia (thought to be due to haemodilution)
- Weight gain
- Headache
- Gastrointestinal symptoms
- Abnormal vision—macular oedema
- Arthralgia
- Dizziness
- Fatigue
- Lactic acidosis
- Women with polycystic ovary syndrome may ovulate as insulin resistance is reduced—risk of pregnancy, and the drug is contraindicated in pregnancy
- Hepatic dysfunction: troglitazone, the first thiazolidinedione on the UK market, was withdrawn because of reports of liver damage; rosiglitazone and pioglitazone may cause hepatic dysfunction and should be stopped if liver enzymes are >3 x ULN.

Incretin-effect enhancers

Exenatide injections (UK-Byetta®)

Mechanisms of action

- Injectable incretin peptide mimetic, i.e. a glucagon-like polypeptide-1 (GLP-1) agonist. Acts like GLP-1 to enhance glucose-dependent insulin secretion by the pancreatic β cells
- Reduces glucagon production
- Slows gastric emptying

Beneficial effects

The position of exenatide in the care of type 2 diabetes has yet to be defined.

- Improves glycaemic control when added to metformin ± sulphonylurea
- When used alone is unlikely to cause hypoglycaemia
- Weight loss—particularly suitable for seriously overweight patients otherwise requiring insulin

Indications

- Combined with metformin ± sulphonylureas—not alone
- In patients with type 2 diabetes whose glucose is not controlled on maximally tolerated doses of metformin ± sulphonylureas

Contraindications

- Pregnancy
- Breastfeeding
- <18 yrs old
- Caution in >75-yr-olds
- Severe renal impairment (eGFR <30 ml/min/1.73 m^2)
- Gastrointestinal disease
- Caution in underweight patients
- Interactions—warfarin, statins

Dosage

- By SC injection 60 min *before* morning and evening meal
- Initially 5 mcg twice daily increasing after 1 month to 10 mcg twice daily if necessary
- Maximum dose 10 mcg twice daily
- The injection is given with a pre-filled pen, similar to an insulin pen. See Chapter 9 (📖 p.186) for injection sites, techniques. etc.
- Do not give drugs whose action depends on gastric emptying within 1 hr of exenatide injections.

Side effects

- Hypoglycaemia is increased in patients on sulphonylureas
- Nausea and vomiting occur in about half the patients but usually settle with time. If severe they may cause dehydration.
- Gastrointestinal symptoms: anorexia, dyspepsia, reflux, abdominal pain, abdominal distension, diarrhoea, constipation, flatulence, burping
- Weight loss

- Slowed gastric emptying may delay absorption of other drugs—this may affect lipid levels.
- Feeling jittery or dizzy
- Headache
- Sweating
- Anaphylaxis
- Rash, urticaria, pruritus, angioneurotic oedema

Sitagliptin (UK-Januvia®)

Mechanism of action

- An oral dipeptidyl peptidase 4 inhibitor. Inhibits clearance of the incretin GLP-1, thus increasing the amount available to stimulate glucose-stimulated insulin secretion
- Reduces glucagon release
- May slow gastric emptying

Beneficial effects

The position of sitagliptin in the care of type 2 diabetes has yet to be defined.

- Improves glycaemic control when added to metformin or glitazone
- Used alone is unlikely to cause hypoglycaemia

Indications

- Combined with metformin or glitazone.
- Type 2 diabetic patients whose glucose is not controlled on metformin or glitazone alone.

Contraindications

- Type 1 diabetes
- Pregnancy
- Breastfeeding
- <18 yrs of age
- Renal impairment (eGFR < 50 ml/min/1.73 m^2) (drug excreted in urine)

Dosage

100 mg once daily by mouth.

Side effects

- Nausea, anorexia, abdominal pain, altered bowel habit
- Weight loss
- Nasopharyngitis
- Upper respiratory tract infection
- Headache
- Oedema (with glitazone)

Vildagliptin (UK-Galvus®)

(New drug. see SPC)

Acarbose

Mechanism of action

Acarbose (UK-Glucobay®) is an α-glucosidase inhibitor which reduces the rate of sucrose digestion in the small intestine so that less glucose is absorbed after a carbohydrate meal.

Beneficial effects

- Glucose-lowering
- Encourages reduced intake of sucrose
- Used alone dose not cause hypoglycaemia

Indications

- Alone or in combination in type 2 diabetic patients in whom glucose is not controlled.
- Patients must adhere to a low sugar (sucrose) diet.

Contraindications

- Pregnancy
- Breastfeeding
- <18 yrs of age
- Gastrointestinal disorders, e.g. intestinal obstruction, inflammatory bowel disease, colonic ulceration, hernias, any chronic gastrointestinal problem
- Malabsorption
- Patients prone to flatulence or in whom increased flatulence would be problematic
- Liver impairment
- Renal impairment
- Interactions—pancreatic enzymes, neomycin, colestyramine, digoxin
- May interfere with absorption of other drugs

Dosage

- Dose is 50 mg initially, increased to twice a day either chewed with the first mouthful of the meal, or before food with a drink of water. Increase gradually to 50 mg three times a day. The dose can be increased after 6–8 weeks to 100 mg three times daily if necessary. Gradual increase is best.
- Maximum dose 200 mg three times daily. Larger doses should be used with care (see SPC).
- ❶Warn patients about drugs which may cause hypoglycaemia (e.g. sulphonylureas), that they may become hypoglycaemic, and that hypoglycaemia must be treated with glucose and not sucrose because the latter will not be digested.

Side effects

- Side effects often preclude long-term use
- Gastrointestinal side effects are common. Most patients experience flatulence—also bloating, flatulence, diarrhoea, and nausea. Because acarbose interferes with carbohydrate metabolism, fermentation is increased. Symptoms are worse if patients eat sugar
- Liver—elevated liver enzymes, jaundice, hepatitis
- Skin rashes

Monitoring non-insulin therapy

Patient knowledge

- Does the patient know what and how much he/she is taking?
- When should he/she take the medication?
- What is it for?
- What should he/she do if he/she becomes ill?
- What precautions should he/she take?
- Is he/she aware of potential side effects?
- Is the patient on sulphonylureas aware of the risk and symptoms of hypoglycaemia?

Diabetes card? Carrying glucose?

Ask the patient to show it to you.

Hypoglycaemia

Always ask if patients have experienced this.

Blood glucose balance

Check this every 2 months until stable and then every 6 months. If the blood glucose is persistently above targets for that patient check adherence to diet, exercise, and medication, and increase or augment hypoglycaemic therapy. If the glucose remains uncontrolled despite maximal oral therapy in an appropriate combination, the patient needs insulin.

❶Do not delay insulin injections in a mistaken attempt to be kind. Diabetic tissue damage is not kind!

Clinical state

- Apart from usual tissue damage monitoring, have any conditions arisen which make it inadvisable to continue oral hypoglycaemics?
- Is there any evidence of side effects of treatment?
- Does the medication need changing?
- Check weight in all before and during treatment
- Check cardiac function before starting glitazones or metformin, and during treatment

Laboratory monitoring

Continue usual diabetes monitoring. These tests are for specific reasons with all or some hypoglycaemic drugs.

- Before starting hypoglycaemic drugs check the following in everyone unless specified:
  - HbA_{1c}
  - urea and electrolytes
  - creatinine (eGFR)
  - liver function
  - full blood count (metformin, glitazones, sulphonylureas)
  - lipids (glitazones)
  - calcium (glitazones)
- During treatment:
  - HbA_{1c}
  - urea and electrolytes
  - creatinine (eGFR)
  - liver function (or at least ALT)
  - lipids (glitazones)
  - full blood count (glitazones, metformin $\geq$ 1500 mg daily)
  - vitamin B_{12} + folate (annually in metformin $\geq$1500 mg daily)
  - calcium (glitazones)

Take home message

Write down the dose the patient should be taking and when. Remind the patient or rewrite it each visit. Make sure he/she has a copy of the sick day/missed medication rules (see below).

Sick days and missed medication

If the patient misses a tablet he/she should not take double next time! Discuss each case individually. If the error is realized within 2 hrs of the correct time take the missed dose immediately. In someone on once-daily breakfast-time therapy, the missed dose could be taken within 4 hrs of the correct time.

If the patient has a vomiting illness or severe diarrhoea not only will he be unable to keep his tablets down (or fail to absorb them), but the illness is likely to push his blood glucose concentration up. The patient must contact his doctor immediately. Monitor the blood glucose carefully and use insulin to control it. Diabetic patients on non-insulin glucose-lowering treatment who have illnesses severe enough to require hospital admission (e.g. cardiovascular diseases, infections, surgical emergencies) should be changed to insulin treatment until their condition has stabilized and they are eating normally. Some may require long-term insulin.

Keep a particularly careful eye on the blood glucose levels of elderly patients, as vague confusion may indicate hypoglycaemia. Non-specific symptoms can be accompanied by gross metabolic derangement and high glucose levels.

Summary

- Always check the British National Formulary before prescribing medications. Even the drugs are very familiar, review them when the new edition arrives as information changes.
- Check BNF and MHRA web sites regularly for updates and warnings.
- Non-insulin hypoglycaemics should be used early if dietary control fails or is unlikely to work.
- Non-insulin hypoglycaemics work only if the patient is making some of their own insulin.
- Non-insulin hypoglycaemics work only if the patient takes them!
- Eventually many patients taking oral hypoglycaemic agents will need insulin
- Use the drug you are most familiar with, but consider the patient and his/her needs
- Non-insulin hypoglycaemic drugs can cause hypoglycaemia. Be alert for this as the symptoms may be less clear cut than in insulin-treated patients.
- Use insulin if severe illness occurs.
- Patient education about therapy is as important as in insulin treatment.
- Tablet-treated diabetes is not mild. It can maim, blind, or kill.

References and further reading

British National Formulary (BNF) http://www.bnf.org
SPCs and PILs (Electronic Medicines Compendium
http://www.emc.medicines.org.uk/
Medicines and Healthcare Products Regulatory Agency (MHRA)
http://www.mrha.gov.uk
Monthly Index of Medical Specialties (eMIMS) http://www.emims.net
NICE is revising the diabetes guidelines www.nice.org.uk
UKPDS 34 *Lancet* 1998; **352**:854–65.
ADVANCE New Engl J Med 2008; 358:2560-72

Chapter 9
Insulin treatments

Treat each patient according to his/her individual condition. Always check drug information in a current edition of British National Formulary (BNF) www.bnf.org before prescribing any medications described in this book. Be alert for warnings from the MHRA (www.mhra.gov.uk). To review the Summary of Product Characteristics (SPC) and Patient Information Leaflet (PIL) see www.emc.medicines.org.uk

'I won't have to inject insulin, will I?'

For many people, having diabetes means insulin injections. They think that these injections will start on their first visit to the diabetic clinic. Sometimes this unexpressed anxiety can impede communication. This may be an unfounded fear, but unfortunately some people do need insulin, and, at present, most patients give this by injection.

Who needs insulin?

- All with type 1 diabetes—such patients will die without insulin treatment
- Type 2 patients with hyperglycaemia uncontrolled on non-insulin treatments
- Patients with acute onset of severe symptoms

Intense thirst and polyuria can be devastating. Insulin cures these symptoms by reliably reducing the blood glucose towards normal. Thus all such patients should be considered for insulin therapy, at least initially, to make them feel better. If the symptoms have arisen within weeks, or have progressed rapidly, it is likely that the patient requires long-term insulin therapy. If these symptoms are combined with ketosis and weight loss insulin is mandatory (Table 9.1).

Ketone producers

In someone with diabetes whose blood glucose concentration is ≥10 mmol/l, moderate to high ketonuria, or blood ketone levels >1 mmol/l suggests the need for insulin therapy unless they are on strict weight-reducing or 'Atkins style' diet. (Lower ketone levels do not definitely exclude the need for insulin.)

Insulin treatment is life-saving in acute diabetic ketoacidosis. Any patient who has had an episode of proven diabetic ketoacidosis in the past is likely to need lifelong insulin treatment. Rarely, patients subsequently produce enough of their own insulin to return to oral hypoglycaemic therapy. This decision should be made by a consultant diabetologist. However, patients should be encouraged to test their blood glucose particularly assiduously during intercurrent illness or stress. They should keep insulin in the refrigerator for immediate use if the blood glucose concentration rises to avert a further episode of ketoacidosis.

Table 9.1 Target blood glucose concentrations in people with type 1 diabetes

	Target finger-prick whole blood glucose level (mmol/l)
Before meals	4.0–6.0 mmol/l
2 hrs after meals	4.0–8.0 mmol/l (10.0 mmol/l if hypoglycaemia prone)
Before bed	6.0–8.0 mmol/l*
HbA_{1c}†	6.0–6.4% without hypoglycaemia 6.5–7.4% if hypoglycaemia prone

Set targets according to each individual's age, general health, and circumstances. For example, strict glucose balance is not always appropriate in a very elderly person living alone. Take care to avoid hypoglycaemia and always reduce the blood glucose gradually.

*This is to reduce the risk of nocturnal hypoglycaemia and assumes that bedtime is 4–6 hrs after the last meal. Patients on insulin should always have a bedtime snack.

†This will vary according to the laboratory's ULN. In DCCT(📖 p.124) the mean $HbA1_c$ of the intensively treated group, which showed a dramatic reduction in tissue damage, was 7%. However, most insulin-treated patients will have hypoglycaemia at levels within the non-diabetic population normal range, and 6–7.4% is usually safer.

People who have lost weight unintentionally

Marked weight loss (e.g. >3 kg) in anyone with newly diagnosed diabetes, especially those who have lost weight despite eating well, may indicate the need for insulin treatment.

Ill people

Insulin should be given to all new or established patients with acute myocardial infarction.

People with diabetes who have an infection, an accident, or a surgical illness often need insulin until the additional illness is under control. The necessity of insulin treatment should be assessed in all diabetic patients urgently admitted to hospital.

Children and young people

The majority of people whose diabetes develops at <30 yrs of age have type 1 diabetes with an absolute insulin requirement. Type 2 diabetes is increasing in this age group, but the decision not to use insulin should be taken very carefully by a consultant diabetologist or paediatric diabetologist.

Pregnant women

It is usual to give insulin to pregnant women with diabetes who cannot control their blood glucose by diet alone (📖 p.373).

Patients who are hyperglycaemic despite non-insulin hypoglycaemic drugs

Patients whose post-prandial blood glucose tests are usually ≥10 mmol/l, fasting ≥6 mmol/l, or who have a persistently raised haemoglobin $A1_c$ should be assessed as likely to benefit from insulin treatment. In obese people or those who eat a lot of sugar it may be possible to improve matters by re-evaluation of the diet.

Many patients who have declined insulin for years are astonished at how much better they feel on insulin and wish they had agreed to have it years before.

Patients with complicated diabetes

Insulin may help patients with severe painful diabetic neuropathy, even if their glycaemic balance approximates to normal on oral therapy. The rationale is that aggressive normalization of the blood glucose with insulin may relieve the symptoms. Patients with other tissue damage may benefit.

Patients with severe hypertriglyceridaemia (i.e. ≥10 mmol/l) and diabetes are usually treated with insulin to achieve normoglycaemia and normotriglyceridaemia. A very low fat diet and carefully balanced carbohydrate intake are needed, and lipid-lowering drugs may also be required (📖 p.288).

Insulin species

There are many insulin preparations on the market (Table 9.2).

Human insulin is made from bacteria using recombinant DNA technology. Novo Nordisk use *Saccharomyces cerevisae*, and Eli Lilly and Sanofi Aventis use *Escherichia coli*. The human insulin is then modified to produce analogue insulins (e.g. insulin lispro, aspart, or glulisine) which do not form hexamers, thus speeding absorption. Porcine and beef insulins are produced from animal pancreas. Animal insulins are more antigenic than human insulin, but antibodies can be formed to all insulins.

When human insulin was introduced there was concern that its use might be associated with reduced warning of hypoglycaemia. Several careful studies have shown that this is not so. Highly purified insulin is less antigenic than older insulins, and so small dose changes may have a larger glucose-lowering effect than that of an older insulin in a long-term user. An aim of near normoglycaemia means an increased risk of hypoglycaemia with fewer warning symptoms. As human insulin was introduced the old dilute insulins were withdrawn. Concentrated U100 insulin requires more precision in drawing up than older insulins. It seems likely that all these factors played a role in the development of hypoglycaemia in people with long-standing insulin-treated diabetes coincidentally changed to human insulin. In addition, long duration of diabetes may be associated with reduction in warning symptoms of hypoglycaemia.

However, the issue highlighted the need to consider the effects of recent care improvements on patients' daily lives, and on the incidence of hypoglycaemia. If individual patients believe that they have experienced problems on human insulin, prescribe animal insulins if that is the patient's preference.

Whenever any patient's insulin is changed, whatever the make or species, they must be warned that they may experience unexpected hypoglycaemia and perhaps with different warning symptoms

Problems with injectable insulin

At the time of writing inhaled insulin is not available for new prescription. Refer these patients to a diabetologist.

- Bleeding disorders such as thrombocytopaenia. Caution: risk of bleeding at injection site
- Major skin diseases affecting potential injection sites
- Severe needle-phobia (always refer such patients to a clinical psychologist)
- Hypersensitivity to insulin or preservatives
- Hypersensitivity to syringe or pen components
- Religious or ethical objections, e.g. to animal insulin or recombinant DNA technology (📖 p.416)
- Inability to inject insulin oneself (family or nurses can do it)

Side effects of injectable insulin

Many of these effects relate to the rapid reduction of hyperglycaemia. It is best to decrease glucose gradually to reduce sudden changes in osmolality.

- Hypoglycaemia
- Injection site problems - bruising, bleeding, irritation, erythema
- Hypersensitivity reactions - local or generalised, itching, urticaria, including, rarely, anaphylaxis.
- Injection site infections
- Insulin lipohypertrophy (common) or lipoatrophy (uncommon) (📖 p. 186)
- Oedema - "insulin oedema" is uncommon but well-recognized and lasts days or weeks usually. Exclude cardiac or renal causes.
- Blurred vision as glucose falls - usually days or weeks - common. Ensure patient has had a full eye check including fundoscopy or digital retinal photography. Advise them not to buy expensive spectacles but use over-the-counter ones until the vision stabilises.
- Rapid worsening of neuropathy which may be painful. This relates to rapid reduction of hyperglycaemia and gradually resolves but may take months to improve. Overall progression of neuropathy is reduced by improved glucose balance.
- Rapid worsening of retinopathy (as above). Overall near-normalization of blood glucose reduces the likelihood of deterioration in retinopathy but a few patients whose glucose is very high initially do show worsening at first.

Prescribing insulin

Prescribing errors are common. Many doctors are not taught how to prescribe insulin—they should be! The prescription should include the following.

- Full name of insulin(s) (e.g. Novomix 30, not just Novomix)
- Prescribe vial/cartridge and/or the pen or injection device to be used
- The amount of each dose
- Write 'units' in full (otherwise the U may be seen as an 0 causing hypoglycaemia). Thus 10 units, not 10 U.
- Time of each injection
- Start date
- Route—usually SC
- Self-administering yes/no if in hospital (📖 p.478)
- Name and signature of prescriber and date prescribed
- Then check it. Show the patient (they are usually more familiar with their insulin regimen than you are)

Table 9.2 Insulin preparations available in the UK

Preparation	Manu-facturer	Spe-cies	Form	Onset (approx.)	Peak activity (approx.)	Duration of action (approx.)
Neutral insulin injection						
Actrapid®	Novo Nordisk	Human	V	<30 min	1.5–3.5h	7–8h
Apidra® (insulin glulisine)	Sanofi Aventis	Human	V,P,C_5, C_2	10–20 min	55 min	1.5–4 h
Humalog® (insulin lispro*)	Lilly	Human	V,P,$C_{3,4}$	15 min	1.5 h	2–5 h
Humulin S®	Lilly	Human	V,P,$C_{3,4}$	30 min–1h	1–6 h	6–12 h
Hypurin Bovine Neutral®	Wockhardt	Bovine	V,C_3	30 min–1h	1.5–4.5 h	6–8 h
Hypurin Porcine Neutral®	Wockhardt	Porcine	V,C_3	30 min–1h	1.5–4.5 h	6–8 h
Insuman Rapid®	Sanofi Aventis	Human	P,C_5	<30 min	1–4 h	7–9 h
NovoRapid® (insulin aspart)	Novo Nordisk	Human	V,P,C_1	10–20 min	1–3 h	3–5 h

V, vial; P, preloaded pen; C, cartridge; C_1, compatible with NovoPen 3; C_2, compatible with OptiClik; C_3, compatible with Autopen Classic; C_4, compatible with HumaPen Ergo/HumaPen Luxura; C_5, compatible with OptiPen Pro 1 and Autopen 24; D, InnoLet delivery device

Pen needles: Microfine, NovoFine, Penfine, and Unifine are compatible with all preloaded and reusable pens.

*Insulin lispro, human insulin analogue

Reproduced from MIMS *Monthly Index of Medical Specialities* with permission. This table is updated monthly; please see the current issue for up-to-date information. http://www.healthcarerepublic.com/mims/Tables/28933/insulin-preparations/

Table 9.2 (*Continued*) Insulin preparations available in the UK

Preparation	Manufacturer	Species	Form	Onset (approx.)	Peak activity (approx.)	Duration of action (approx.)
Biphasic insulin injection†						
Humalog Mix25®	Lilly	Human	P,$C_{3,4}$	15 min	2 h	22 h
Humalog Mix50®	Lilly	Human	P,$C_{3,4}$	15 min	2 h	22 h
Humulin M3®	Lilly	Human	V,P,$C_{3,4}$	30 min–1 h	1–12 h	22 h
Hypurin Porcine 30/70®	Wockhardt	Porcine	V,C_3	<2 h	4–12 h	24 h
Insuman Comb 15®	Sanofi Aventis	Human	V,P,C_5	30 min–1 h	2–4 h	11–20 h
Insuman Comb 25®	Sanofi Aventis	Human	V,P,C_5	30 min–1 h	2–4 h	12–19 h
Insuman Comb 50®	Sanofi Aventis	Human	V,P,C_5	<30 min	1.5–4 h	12–16 h
Mixtard 30®	Novo Nordisk	Human	V,D,C_1	<30 min	2–8 h	24 h
NovoMix 30®	Novo Nordisk	Human	P,C_1	<10–20 min	1–4 h	24 h

†Speed of onset is proportional to amount of soluble insulin

Table 9.2 (*Continued*) Insulin preparations available in the UK

Preparation	Manufacturer	Species	Form	Onset (approx.)	Peak activity (approx.)	Duration of action (approx.)
Isophane insulin injection						
Humulin I®	Lilly	Human	V,P,$C_{3,4}$	30 min–1 h	1–8 h	22 h
Hypurin Bovine Isophane®	Wockhardt	Bovine	V,C_3	<2 h	6–12 h	18–24 h
Hypurin Porcine Isophane®	Wockhardt	Porcine	V,C_3	<2 h	6–12 h	18–24 h
Insulatard®	Novo Nordisk	Human	V,D,C_1	<1.5 h	4–12 h	24 h
Insuman Basal®	Sanofi Aventis	Human	V,P,C_5	<1 h	3–4 h	11–20 h
Insulin–zinc suspension (mixed)						
Hypurin Bovine Lente®	Wockhardt	Bovine	V	2 h	8–12 h	30 h
Protamine–zinc–insulin injection						
Hypurin Bovine® PZI	Wockhardt	Bovine	V	4–6 h	10–20 h	24–36 h
Long-acting insulin analogues						
Lantus® (insulin glargine)	Sanofi Aventis	Human	V,P,C_5, C_2	2.5 h	–	24 h
Levemir® (insulin detemir)	Novo Nordisk	Human	P,C_1, D	2.5 h	–	24 h

Concentration of insulin

All insulin in the UK is provided as 100 units per millilitre (U100). Other countries may not conform to this system and patients should be very careful if they obtain their insulin abroad. A few insulin-resistant patients use U500 insulin (1 unit ≈ 5 units of U100).

Duration and peak action of different insulins

Keep up-to-date about available insulins as manufacturers introduce new insulins and remove others from the market. Warn patients if their usual insulin will no longer be available and discuss other options with them. Ensure that they are taught how to use their new insulin. Changing insulin type is worrying for patients.

Very-short-acting insulins (Analogues)

The insulin made by the normal human pancreas is a clear colourless fluid which, when released into the bloodstream via the portal vein, produces an effect upon the blood glucose within minutes.

These insulins are modified so that they do not form hexamers which take time to separate. Active insulin is available straightaway. They are absorbed and start working within 15 min of injection and clear in 2–5 hrs. Very rapidly acting insulins can (and indeed must) be injected either immediately before eating, or during or immediately after food. Better glucose balance is achieved if the insulin is injected immediately before food. However, if one is uncertain what food will be provided (e.g. in a restaurant) insulin can be injected as the meal finishes.

Insulin lispro (Humalog®), insulin aspart (NovoRapid®), and insulin glulisine (Apidra®) can be used in basal-bolus insulin patterns, or mixed with intermediate-acting insulins in twice-daily regimens. Because insulin levels peak with the glucose absorption from food they produce an insulin effect similar to that of the normal pancreas. Because the insulin more closely matches the food, proper use of such insulins reduces the frequency of hypoglycaemia. However, hypoglycaemia can occur, and it may come on quickly and be severe. The insulin may 'run out' before the next injection and meal. Thus there can be post-prandial normoglycaemia or hypoglycaemia, but pre-prandial hyperglycaemia.

Very-short-acting insulins are increasingly popular with patients as they allow more flexibility of lifestyle and enable more scope for fine-tuning glucose than older insulins. Some patients use ultra-short-acting insulins for some meals and short-acting insulins for others. This produces a very complex pattern and is only suitable for patients who are very knowledgeable and careful about diabetes self-care.

Short-acting insulin

All short-acting insulins are clear and colourless. They include Actrapid®, Humulin S® (Humulin R® in USA), Insuman Rapid®, Hypurin Porcine®, or Bovine Neutral and pork Actrapid®. The main difference between insulin in the non-diabetic person and insulin in the diabetic person is its route of delivery into the bloodstream and the lack of fine control. There is a tendency to forget that the effect of human insulin released by the pancreas in direct response to circulating blood glucose concentrations cannot be the same as the effect of subcutaneous insulin absorbed regardless of the blood glucose concentration. Even continuous intravenous insulin infusion cannot mimic the finely tuned glycaemia-appropriate response of the normal pancreas.

Intermediate-acting and long-acting insulins

These cloudy insulin suspensions are modified to reduce their solubility and hence to prolong their absorption from the insulin injection site. There are several methods of modifying insulins.

Isophane (NPH) insulin is produced by adding protamine and a small amount of zinc at the body's normal pH. This produces insulins which last for about 12 hrs. Examples of isophane (NPH) insulins are Humulin I®, Insuman Basal®, Hypurin Bovine®, Porcine Isophane®, and Insulatard®. Short-acting insulin can be mixed with isophane insulins and the mixture will remain stable. This is the basis of the fixed proportion mixtures, or of mixtures made by patients themselves.

Zinc is used to precipitate insulin crystals, hence the insulin–zinc suspensions. Insulin is absorbed slowly into the bloodstream from these crystals in the injection site. Current versions include insulin–zinc suspension, protamine–zinc–insulin, and Hypurin Bovine Lente®. Mixtures of these insulins with short-acting insulin are not stable.

Current long-acting analogue insulins are insulin glargine and detimir. Detimir and glargine are clear and colourless.

Combination or pre-mixed insulins

These are stable mixtures containing varying proportions of short-acting insulin and isophane (NPH) insulin. These mixtures are inflexible—if the dose is increased, both the short-acting and the isophane insulin dose is increased. However, they have gained in popularity because of their simplicity and their avoidance of drawing-up errors (📖 p.184). They include NovoMix 30®, Mixtard 30® or 50, Humulin M3®, Humalog Mix 25® and Mix 50®, Insuman Comb® 15, 25, and 50, Hypurin Porcine 30/70®, and Pork Mixtard 30®.

Insulin in the user's hands

Tell patients how to look after their insulin. If it is not looked after properly, it may not work properly and have increased antigenicity.

Checklist for patients

- Learn the name of your insulins and the devices you use to inject them.
- Do you have the right insulin(s) for you? Check before you leave the pharmacist every time you get a new prescription.
- If you have different insulins, have you labelled them clearly to reduce errors (e.g. sticker on pen, different coloured pens).
- Protect all insulin from light and vibration.
- Storage of insulin: 2–8°C in a fridge, away from the freezing compartment.
- Insulin pen/vial in use: keep out of the fridge. If first use, keep at room temperature for 1–2 hrs before injection. Stable at 2–25°C. Avoid heating or freezing. Discard if unused after 28 days.
- Is it within its use-by date?
- Is it within its expiry date?
- Is the bung dirty? If yes, clean thoroughly with alcohol wipe.
- Is the bung damaged? If yes, do not use.
- Does clear insulin look clear or cloudy? If cloudy, do not use.
- Has your insulin been shaken so that it is frothy? If so, wait until foam settles.

Preparing insulin for injection

- Keep your current pen/vial out of the fridge. Cold insulin stings more.
- Check that you have the correct insulin for that dose and time of day.
- If you use a cloudy insulin rotate the pen/vial gently 20 times between your hands. Do not shake as it will foam. Do not shake or rotate clear insulin.
- Expel any air bubbles (if using a syringe do not work the plunger up and down too vigorously or microscopic particles will shear off the syringe into the insulin, causing the plunger to 'stick').
- Expel insulin from pen ('safety test') before use, following individual manufacturer's instructions. Usually 2 units are expelled before use, more if it is first use of that pen.
- Use a new needle each time. Take if off after the injection and dispose of it safely.

Contamination may occur with the introduction of cloudy insulin into the clear bottle by the uneducated self-mixer who has forgotten that one should draw up the clear insulin first (📖 p.184). Another form of contamination is to leave short-acting insulin and zinc suspension insulins in the syringe for more than a few seconds before injection. The short-acting insulin will gradually be converted to slower-acting insulin.

Modified insulins—the longer-acting insulins—should be mixed gently by rotating the bottle between both hands before drawing up the dose, or the amount of insulin complex injected may vary. Overzealous mixing can make the insulin foam and this causes frustrating delay in clearing air bubbles and measuring the right dose.

Obviously, the patient or their carer should give the right insulin for that person for that occasion. Mistakes happen all too easily.

Insulin injection equipment

Syringe and needle

All patients should know how to use a syringe and needle and be provided with some of these for emergencies, even if they use pens or pumps.

There are several U100 insulin syringes on the market: 1 ml (100 units of insulin), 0.5 ml (50 units), and 0.3 ml (30 units). Most have a fine integral needle. They are manufactured for single use only. Potential problems include sticking with some cloudy insulins. The fine needles bend easily. Very rarely, if inserted up the hilt and bent, they can snap.

Insulin pens

These devices have an insulin cartridge instead of ink and a double-ended needle instead of a nib. This pierces the bung of the insulin cartridge ready for use. The insulin dose is dialled up or clicked in at the other end of the pen or on the side. A plunger pushes the bottom of the cartridge down, ejecting the chosen dose of insulin through the needle.

Each device has a slightly different action. The pen does the same job as a syringe and needle without the need to draw up the insulin dose from a bottle. This improves accuracy, but only if the patient dials up the right dose in the first place. Insulin pens are also much more portable than a full syringe and needle, and can be carried in a pocket or bag without the insulin in the cartridge 'going off'.

Choose the best pen for each user. Different pens have different features, including the way in which the insulin dose is selected, whether this is counted or dialled up, the ease of operation, delivery of the dose (by a twisting motion, depressing a plunger, or by a slider), knowing whether the insulin has gone in, knowing how much insulin is left, and knowing when to change the cartridge. Most devices are quite robust. There are chunky pens which are easy to grip, pens with concealed needles, and one which delivers 0.5 units of insulin. Unless the insulin dose is large, it is better to be able to make 1 unit changes in dose. It is essential to teach the patient how to prime the pen, load an insulin cartridge, and expel air from the needle before each injection. Patients are usually advised to hold the pen vertically, needle up, and waste a few units of insulin before each injection to clear the needle of air—'safety check'. If there is air in the needle or cartridge this may remain undetected and cause dosage errors. The patient must always read the instructions and practice with a diabetes specialist nurse or other person trained in pen use.

Table 9.3 Examples of Insulin pens

Name of pen	Smallest dose	Maximum dose	Insulins to be used in pen (3 ml cartridges)
Autopen 24®	1 2	21 42	Sanofi-Aventis Sanofi-Aventis
Autopen classic®	1 2	21 42	Eli Lilly and CP Eli Lilly and CP
Humapen ergo®	1	60	Eli Lilly Humulin/Humalog
Humapen luxura®	1	60	Eli Lilly Humulin/Humalog
Humapen luxura HD®	0.5	30	Eli Lilly Humulin/Humalog
Injex needle-free system®	5	30	Any 10ml insulin vial
Novopen Junior®	0.5	35	NovoNordisk Penfills
Novopen 3 Demi®	0.5	35	NovoNordisk Penfills
Novopen 3 Classic® or Fun	1	70	NovoNordisk Penfills
Optipen Pro®	1	60	Sanofi-Aventis Insuman
SQ-pen Needle-free injector	1	50	Any insulin 10ml vial or 3 ml cartridge

All the pen names are registered trademarks.

Insulins and pen injectors are updated from time to time. Check the Monthly Index of Medical Specialities MIMS: http://www.healthcarerepublic.com/home/

There is now a range of pre-loaded disposable insulin pens. The patient screws on a pen-needle, dials up the dose, and injects the insulin. Loading errors are abolished as the insulin is already in the pen. These pens can be used by patients of all ages, including some elderly people (or their families) who might otherwise need supervision by the district nurse. Some pens cannot deliver a dose smaller than 2 units, which may be difficult for patients on small doses. Pre-loaded disposable pens currently available on prescription include Apidra® ,Humalog ®, Humulin S®, Insuman Rapid®, NovoRapid®, Insuman® and Hypurin Mixtures®, Novomix30®, Humulin I®, Insuman Basal®, Lantus®, and Levimir®. A wider pre-filled device with a dial-up dose (Innolet®) may be easier for people with dexterity problems; it contains Insulatard® or Mixtard 30®.

Magnifiers are available for people with poor vision. All patients on insulin should be considered for insulin pen therapy—it is usually more accurate, convenient, comfortable, and practical. However, it is the patient who must choose the method he/she prefers.

Continuous subcutaneous insulin infusion pumps

Continuous subcutaneous insulin infusion (CSII) uses continuously infused short-acting or very-short-acting insulin (the latter usually provides more predictable glucose lowering) to provide background (basal) insulin and bolus insulin for meals or high glucose correction. Insulin is loaded into a special vial within the pump which then pumps it via fine tubing to an indwelling Teflon or metal cannula inserted subcutaneously. The cannula is left *in situ* for a several days. The tubing can be disconnected to allow showers etc., and some pumps are waterproof. The pump is worn on a belt or in a pocket or clothing, and the patient adjusts the infusion rates with the buttons (like programming a mobile phone). Mealtime boluses can be started at the press of a button and may be short or long. Some pumps calculate doses based on glucose levels transmitted by continuous glucose-monitoring devices or entered, along with carbohydrate counts, by the patient. These 'wizards' depend on the insulin sensitivity calculations previously entered by patient or professional, and the insulin doses delivered may not, in fact, be appropriate for the situation.

CSII should be started and managed by trained specialist diabetes teams (diabetologist, diabetes nurse and dietitian) only. The method can be used in adults and children (including babies).

Who should have an insulin pump?

Patients using CSII (or their carers) should:

- be willing and able to learn and prepared for a lot of 'homework'
- be persistent, and able and willing to problem-solve
- be emotionally stable (CSII is *not* the solution to psychologically driven brittle diabetes)
- be using basal–bolus insulin regimens already
- be checking finger-prick blood glucose at least four times every day
- be using carbohydrate counting to adjust insulin doses
- be able to calculate insulin doses to correct high blood glucose
- have and use a mobile phone (i.e. be capable of managing the electronic device)
- have good hygiene habits
- be prepared to have a cannula permanently *in situ*.

NICE (Technology Appraisal TA151 2008 states that CSII is recommended as a possible treatment for type 1 patients >12 yrs if attempts to reach target HbA_{1c} levels with multiple daily injections result in the person having disabling hypoglycaemia; or HbA_{1c} levels have remained $\geq$ 8.5% with multiple daily injections despite the person and / or their carer carefully trying to manage their diabetes. In the UK the diabetologist will have to obtain permission from the primary care trust for funding for CSII.

How does the patient manage his/her insulin doses?

Insulin pump users will:

- have one or more basal insulin rates, e.g. 0.5 units /hr)
- have an insulin-to-carbohydrate ratio, e.g. 1 unit of insulin to 10 g carbohydrate
- have a correction calculation, e.g. 1 unit of insulin for every 2 mmol glucose above their target glucose (e.g. 7 mmol/l)
- use such corrections programmed into their pump (which can be changed)
- use blood glucose results from SC glucose sensors sent to their pump in pre-programmed correction calculations.

Problems with insulin pumps and what to do

Pump patients should have had a thorough education in potential problems and how to manage them. All the pump companies provide 24 hr helplines for equipment problems. Back-up for other problems should be provided by the specialist team managing the patient, although this cannot always be a 24 hr service.

A&E staff and on-call medical teams faced with a pump patient should note the following points.

- If a pump patient arrives, contact the specialist diabetes team immediately (follow local guidelines but phone the diabetologist at home if necessary).
- Hyperglycaemia: these patients have no long-acting insulin depot. If their insulin supply fails (e.g. air in the line, kinked cannula) they will become ketoacidotic within hours, and some patients have died.
    - Glucose ≥11 mmol/l, urine, or blood ketones present but otherwise well, normotensive, not shocked: inject SC insulin, e.g. 6–10 units (or double the patient's usual correction dose), immediately. Ask patient to use intermittent SC insulin according to finger-prick blood glucose level, including long-acting insulin if appropriate, until they can replace the infusion set and insulin reservoir, and check pump function.
    - Glucose ≥11 mmol/l, ill, vomiting, hypotensive, ketones present: manage as for DKA. Inject 10 units of insulin IM or IV. Start IV insulin infusion as soon as possible (📖 p.241)
- Hypoglycaemia: pump runaways are very rare with today's sophisticated insulin pumps but are still a possibility. Pump 'wizards' may calculate an overdose if wrongly programmed. If the pump appears to be malfunctioning, disconnect it and revert to intermittent insulin with syringe or pen. Contact the pump company helpline immediately.
    - Glucose <4 mmol/l, patient able to self-treat: give oral glucose as usual (📖 p.208). Once patient is recovered (i.e. blood glucose ≥6 mmol/l and 45 min after ingesting oral glucose) ascertain why they became hypoglycaemic. If hypoglycaemia is unexplained, ask them to ensure that pump is working properly and not overdosing. If any doubt, continue intermittent SC insulin and contact pump company helpline.

- Glucose <4 mmol/l, patient to ill or confused to self-treat: give IV glucose or SC/IM glucagon (📖 p.209). Disconnect the pump infusion line from the cannula—it can usually be pulled off the button stuck onto the skin. If profound hypoglycaemia and you cannot disconnect the tubing from the cannula, pull out the abdominal cannula. Insert IV cannula and infuse glucose. Once glucose has risen, ensure that the patient has intermittent insulin injection treatment or IV sliding scale, depending on their clinical state and according to blood glucose measurements. ❗Danger: patient may go from hypoglycaemia to DKA without their pump.
- Infusion site infection. Ask patient to remove cannula (or do so yourself). Send cannula to microbiology if feasible. Give anti-staphylococcal antibiotics. Ensure patient's personal and pump hygiene, especially site preparation, are checked. Until infection cleared use intermittent subcutaneous insulin injections or IV sliding scale depending on clinical condition. Toxic shock syndrome or necrotizing fasciitis are rare complications.
- Keep the pump with the patient—they cost over £1000. Turn it off if you can or simply allow it to continue to pump into a polythene bag (e.g. a blood sample bag). It will produce only a drop of fluid. If malfunction is suspected, it is important to contact the pump company helpline. Pumps can be interrogated electronically by the company to detect errors provided that the battery is still working, so time is of the essence.

Other methods of insulin delivery

Continuous intravenous insulin infusion (insulin sliding scale)—inpatients only

This can be used to control glucose in any diabetic patient in hospital who is hyperglycaemic, ill, or nil by mouth. It does not provide good control for patients who are eating unless additional units are added at mealtimes.

Implantable insulin infusion devices

There are several implantable insulin pumps with an insulin reservoir which can be filled through the skin. The insulin is pumped either directly into a vein or intraperitoneally. At present they are mainly used as a last resort in people in whom no other method has succeeded in preventing frequent diabetic ketoacidosis. When reliable implantable glucose sensors are widely available there will be further exciting possibilities with implantable system, the aim being to have a fully automated system which measures the glucose, calculates the insulin dose, and gives it. This is not far off now.

Insulin jet injectors

These 'guns' drive insulin spray through the skin. They may help people with needle phobia, but can leave lumps, bruises, or sore areas at the injection site and insulin may ooze out afterwards. Needle-phobic patients are usually better with devices which hide the needle from view.

SQ-pen®

SQ-X devices use a powerful spring to push a plunger which forcibly ejects a jet of insulin through the skin.

The Hillingdon Hospital

Insulin Sliding Scale

(ADDRESSOGRAPH LABEL)

Human Actrapid Insulin

50 units in 50ml 0.9% Sodium Chloride intravenous infusion

Blood glucose mmol/l	Date Dose (units/hour)	Date Dose (units/hour)	Date Dose (units/hour)	Date Dose (units/hour)	Date Dose (units/hour)
0.0-3.9 call doctor	**0**				
4.0-5.9	**0.5**				
6.0-7.9	**1.0**				
8.0-9.9	**1.5**				
10.0-11.9	**2.0**				
12.0-13.9	**2.5**				
14.0-16.9	**3.0**				
17.0-19.9	**4.0**				
20.0-24.9	**5.0**				
over 25 call doctor	**6.0**				
	Signature	Signature	Signature	Signature	Signature

- Dosage suggestion for adults only. Reduce dose for children.
- Adjust insulin dose according to blood glucose response.
- Infuse glucose IV simultaneously if blood glucose below 12mmol/l.
- Seek help early if problems (your consultant or Diabetes Team).

Please attach to back of drug chart

HIL 145

Fig. 9.1 Example of an insulin sliding scale.

Disposal of sharps and syringes

All needles, lancets, and syringes are pre-packed and sterilized by the manufacturers. They are made for single use only.

It is each professional's and patient's personal responsibility to ensure that used sharps and used syringes are properly disposed of. Every patient should have a needle clipper (B-D Safeclip® and others) and use it (Figure 9.2). The clipped and thus unusable syringes can then be put in a sharps box to be returned to the chemist, hospital, or surgery for formal disposal. In the UK it is the local council's responsibility to provide safe sharps disposal arrangements. Arrangements can be found on council websites or by telephoning waste management. There is a risk of needle-stick injuries when clipping needles, emptying finger-pricking devices, and handling lancets. Needles and lancets should never be resheathed. Lancets should withdraw the needle out of harm's way.

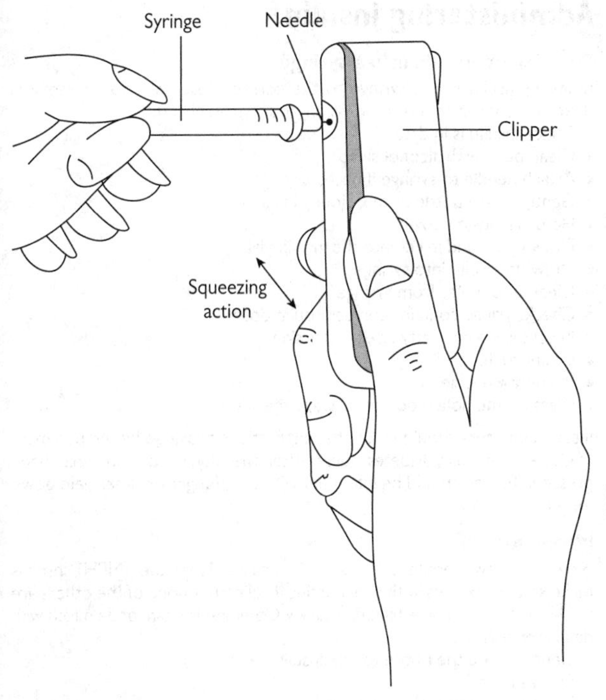

Fig. 9.2 Needle clippers in use.

Administering insulin

Drawing up insulin into a syringe

Drawing insulin into a syringe to the correct dose with no air requires dexterity, concentration, good vision, and a steady hand.

- Check insulin is in date
- Clean bung with alcohol swab
- Attach needle to syringe if necessary
- Gently rotate bottle to mix cloudy insulins
- Hold vial upside down
- Draw up air and inject into the insulin vial
- Draw up insulin into syringe
- Clear air bubbles from syringe
- Check syringe contains correct insulin dose
- Inject insulin into fatty layer under skin
- Count to 10
- Withdraw needle
- Press on the hole—do not massage the site.

Insulin pen users should follow the instructions provided by the pen manufacturer and their diabetes nurse. After the plunger or slider has been pressed, the pen should be left *in situ* with the plunger or slider held down for a count of 10.

Mixing insulin

Nowadays few people self-mix their insulins. Isophane (NPH) insulins make stable mixtures with short-acting insulins, but none of the others are stable and should be injected immediately. Other insulins cannot be mixed with detimir or glargine.

- Gently rotate the bottle to mix insulin
- Draw up air
- Inject air into cloudy insulin bottle
- Put cloudy insulin down
- Draw up air
- Inject air into clear insulin bottle.
- Draw up clear insulin
- Express air bubbles and check you have drawn up correct dose of clear insulin
- Draw up correct dose of cloudy insulin
- Inject

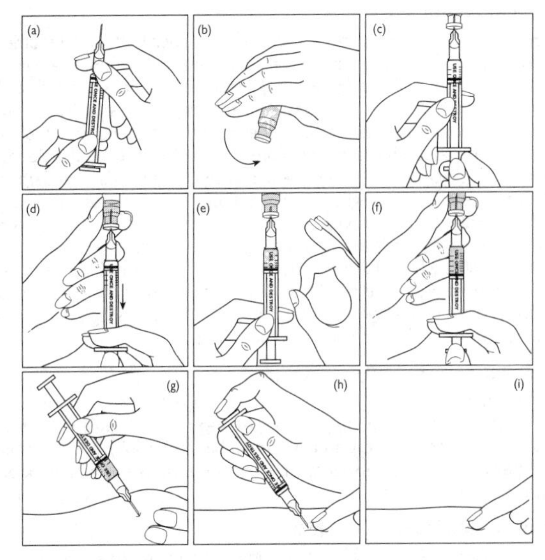

(a) Attach needle to syringe if necessary
(b) Gently rotate bottle to mix insulin
(c) Draw up air and inject into the insulin bottle
(d) Draw up insulin
(e) Clear air bubbles
(f) Check syringe contains correct insulin dose
(g) Inject insulin into fatty layer under skin
(h) Withdraw needle
(i) Press on the hole

Fig. 9.3 Drawing up and injecting insulin.

Injecting insulin

Insulin is injected subcutaneously into bare skin. Injecting through clothes risks infection. A shallow injection may produce a painful intradermal blister with unpredictable insulin absorption. A deep injection which penetrates intramuscularly will lead to rapid insulin absorption and may cause severe hypoglycaemia. The patient should take a thick pinch of skin and subcutaneous tissue and insert the needle at an angle of 45°. An angle of 90° can be used if there is enough subcutaneous fat. The insulin is then injected, the needle left *in situ* for a count of 10, and then withdrawn. Some patients press a clean tissue, cotton-wool swab, or finger over the hole for a few moments.

If the skin is dirty it should be washed and dried. Skin cleansing with alcohol or surgical spirit is not usually necessary, and may causing stinging during injection, and skin hardening if used regularly. Bruising occurs occasionally, as does a tiny trickle of blood. Patients need to be reassured that this is most unlikely to mean that the insulin has been injected intravenously. Some doctors advocate withdrawing the plunger before injection to ensure that a vein has not been entered, but many no longer consider this useful.

Insulin injection sites

The most commonly used sites are the thighs, upper buttocks, abdomen, and upper arms. A few patients use their calves and forearms. Rotate sites to avoid over-use and insulin fat hypertrophy. Insulin absorption varies with each injection site. It is most rapid from the abdomen, then the arms, thighs, and buttocks. Therefore a multi-site rotation scheme can cause variability in blood glucose balance, although this may be more of a problem in some people than others. It may be better to use, say, the abdomen during the day and thighs at night, or to use the left and right side of a particular site for a week or two and then change. Patients who are prepared to monitor this closely with blood glucose testing can work out which site is most appropriate for which circumstance.

Patients will all have favourite sites, usually those which are easy to reach, and there will be areas which gradually become numb through repeated use. Occasionally one discovers small black holes in a patient's leg or abdomen into which he/she has been putting insulin for years!

Insulin fat hypertrophy or atrophy

Insulin has a direct effect on fat cells and often causes hypertrophy at over-used injection sites. These unsightly bulges also cause variability in insulin absorption. The commonest area is paraumbilical. Atrophy due to insulin antibodies is rarely seen nowadays. Encourage patients the whole extent of each available injection site.

When should insulin be injected?

Insulin should be injected before meals in most patients. Analogue insulins can be injected immediately before or after eating. Other insulins take 10–30 min to be absorbed. Insulin is given after meals more often than we realize—patients forget, or they have never understood when to give it, or the district nurse is late. If eating is very erratic (e.g. a person with dementia) it may be safer for carers to give very-short-acting insulin once the meal has definitely been eaten, and just give a little longer-acting insulin once a day to prevent decompensation.

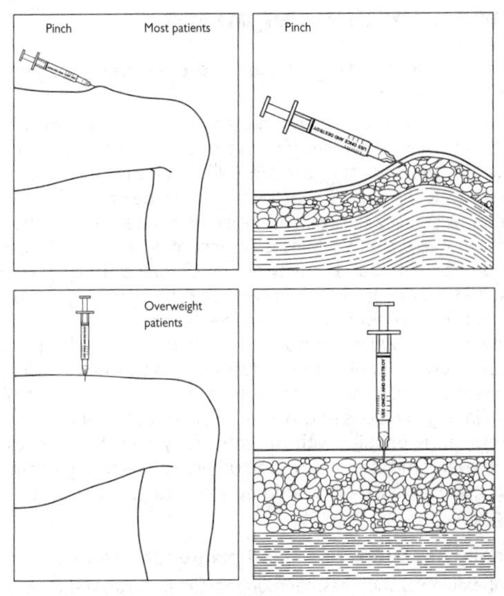

Fig. 9.4 Different methods of injecting insulin.

Factors affecting insulin absorption

These are myriad and tend to be forgotten when the patient and diabetes adviser are poring over the blood glucose diary.

- Type of insulin
- Location of injection site
- Amount of subcutaneous fat at injection site
- Depth of injection
- Size of insulin depot
- Temperature of injection site and patient overall
- Exercising underlying muscle (e.g. thigh or arms)
- Hypotensive shock (never give subcutaneous insulin in this situation)
- Vasoconstrictor compounds/medication (e.g. nicotine)
- Vasodilator medication (e.g. nitrates)

The amount of insulin cleared from an injection site within 24 hrs can vary from 20% to 100% from person to person and within the same person. With such considerable variability in insulin absorption added to the effects of food, exercise, and emotion, the mystery is not why the blood glucose balance is so variable, but why it is possible to control it at all!

Common insulin regimens

Thrice-daily short-acting insulin and once-daily longer-acting insulin: basal–bolus

This provides sophisticated and flexible insulin treatment which can often allow a very varied lifestyle. Use background (basal) insulin overnight (e.g. detimir, glargine, isophane (NPH), or zinc suspension insulin) and give short-acting or very-short-acting insulin before each meal (bolus). Sometimes twice-daily background insulin is needed. Adjust the dose of short-acting or very-short-acting insulin according to blood glucose at that time, food to be eaten, and activity planned. Using carbohydrate counting to adjust the insulin dose more precisely can improve glucose control. The insulin is usually given with a pen injector (📖 p.175). Properly used, this regimen can produce normoglycaemia. However, to do so requires a sophisticated use of insulin dose adjustment and careful observation by the patient of their glucose responses to insulin, food, and activity. A basal–bolus insulin regimen does not, in itself, produce better glucose control.

This regimen is popular with patients. Many find that they can move meals and even omit them. However, others still need regular mealtimes and snacks, and all must eat a bedtime snack to guard against nocturnal hypoglycaemia

Twice-daily injections of a fixed-proportion mixture

This inflexible regimen has been unpopular, popular, and is now unpopular again. Patients find it simple and convenient and drawing-up errors are minimized. There was a wide range of mixtures but manufacturers have withdrawn many of them. Current options are given on 📖 p.167. It is probably the easiest regimen to start with and can be converted to a more flexible pattern if required. However, many diabetologists feel patients should start with basal–bolus straight away. Most patients on mixtures use insulin pens.

Twice-daily self-mixed short-acting and longer-acting insulin

This has largely been superseded by the basal–bolus regimen. The usual insulins are a short-acting types such as Actrapid® or Humulin S® and an isophane such as Insulatard® g.e. or Humulin I®. This regimen gives four points at which the insulin dose can be adjusted. It is essential that the patient understands this—many do not. It is very prone to dosage error. Full use of this regimen is possible only with knowledgeable home blood glucose monitoring.

Box 9.1 Calculating short-acting insulin doses

Basal–bolus insulin or CSII

Intensive glucose control is usually started and monitored by DSNs, dietitians, and diabetologists. It is effective but complex and time-consuming. ❶There is a risk of misunderstanding and of hypoglycaemia.

These calculations provide an approximation which must be checked by the patient against what actually happens to his/her HBGM. There are other ways of calculating these ratios. Patients starting on insulin pumps or unfamiliar regimens usually reduce the total daily dose (TDD) by 25% before using it in the calculations below to avoid hypoglycaemia.

Add up TDD of all insulin	= TDD
Insulin-to-carbohydrate (CHO) ratio	
CHO g covered by 1 unit of insulin	= 500/TDD
Correction dose	
Glucose fall for 1 unit of insulin	= 100/TDD
Example	
John takes:	
10 units analogue insulin with each meal	= 30 units
20 units long-acting insulin at bedtime	= 20 units
TDD	= 50 units
John's insulin-to-CHO ratio:	
500/TDD = 500/50 = 10g CHO	=1 unit per 10 g CHO
John's correction dose:	
100/TDD = 100/50 = 2 mmol glucose	=1 unit insulin per 2 mmol glucose
John's meal contains 60 g CHO	= 6 units insulin
His pre-meal glucose is 13 mmol/l	
His target is 7 mmol/l	
13 – 7 = 6 mmol/l excess glucose	
@ 2 mmol fall per unit	= 3 units insulin
Total short-acting insulin for that meal	= 9 units insulin

Staff should atterd training on using this system before teaching patients e.g. DAFNE 📖 p.64. Also 📖 p.79.

Once-daily long-acting insulin ± short-acting insulin

This regimen is used in type 2 patients uncontrolled on oral agents. It may be sufficient to improve glycaemic balance without mealtime insulin. It rarely produces good glucose control unless the patient is making some of their own insulin. Other situations in which it can be useful are when a carer such as a district nurse has to come in to give the insulin to someone who cannot inject their own, or for someone in whom the aim of treatment is not normoglycaemia but freedom from symptoms and avoidance of hypoglycaemia or marked hyperglycaemia. This regimen is not appropriate for the majority of patients. The insulins used are usually detimir or glargine. The insulin is usually added to the oral agents (but not rosiglitazone-📖 p.148).

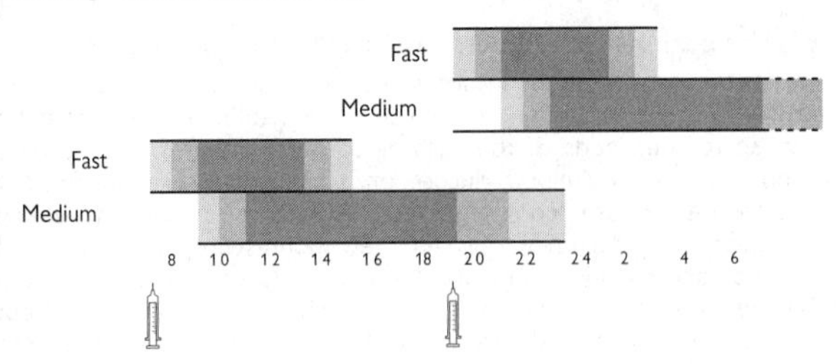

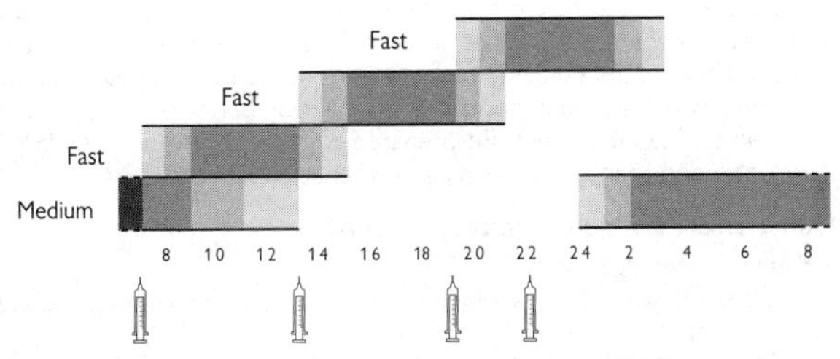

Fig. 9.5 Insulin injection regimens (dark shading, maximum glucose-lowering effect). The onset, intensity, and duration of insulin action varies from person to person and from day to day. Insulin action and duration is shorter with very-short-acting insulins. Long-acting insulins usually act throughout 24 hrs.

Monitoring people on insulin therapy

It is the patient who injects the insulin, not the doctor

The doctor prescribing the insulin is not the person who has to inject it and live with what happens thereafter. The insulin regimen must be tailored to the needs of the each person with diabetes. If the patient cannot control their blood glucose on a particular regimen, finds it hard to use, or loses confidence in it, it should be changed. Clearly, it is worth giving each new regimen a few months' proper trial with full education and continued support. If a patient moves to your clinic from elsewhere on a bizarre insulin regimen which seems totally illogical but appears to satisfy them, do not change it until you have had a chance to assess how it works for that person.

Honeymoon period

Warn patients about the possibility of a honeymoon period of diabetes in which the last remaining beta-cells, released from the effects of hyperglycaemia, produce some insulin before succumbing to the continuing autoimmune destructive process. Hypoglycaemia may occur and doses will have to be reduced rapidly. Patients may think that their diabetes has gone away. Warn them about the honeymoon period at the outset to avoid bitter disappointment. Be prepared to reduce insulin doses fast if this occurs, and to increase them again when it ends.

Clinic checks: insulin-treated patients

- Patient knowledge—theory
  - Does the patient know which insulins and how much of each he/she is taking?
  - What is the insulin for?
  - When is each insulin likely to act?
  - Does he/she know how to adjust the dose according to blood glucose levels, diet, and activity?
  - What should he/she do if he/she becomes ill?
  - What precautions should he/she take?
  - Is he/she aware of the risk and symptoms of hypoglycaemia?
- Patient knowledge—practical
  - Does the patient know how to check, store, and draw up his/her insulin? Does he/she know how to inject it?
  - Does he/she know what to do with unused and used sharps and syringes? Have you watched him/her draw up and inject insulin?
  - Does he/she know how to use his/her insulin pen, including changing cartridges? Have you watched him/her do this?
- Diabetes card? Ask the patient to show it to you.
- Carrying glucose? Ask to see it.
- Glucagon: Has the patient's partner or relative an up-to-date supply and does he/she know how to use it? (📖 p.209)
- Hypoglycaemia: Has the patient experienced this? Does he/she have warning symptoms? Does he/she have nocturnal hypoglycaemia?
- Blood glucose balance (Table 9.1): If the blood glucose is persistently outside your targets for that patient, his/her treatment needs adjusting.

- Type 1 patients: Ketone testing. Do they need blood ketone testing kit? Do they know how to use it? All patients who have had DKA should have a ketone testing kit at home.
- Clinical state: Apart from usual tissue damage monitoring, have any conditions arisen which would alter the insulin regimen? Is there any evidence of side effects of treatment? Have you examined the injection sites?
- Laboratory monitoring: Consider checking renal function as this will alter insulin clearance.
- Driving: Has the patient told the DVLA he/she is on insulin? Does he/she know how to drive safely on insulin? Has he/she told his/her vehicle insurance company?
- Take home message: What does should the patient be taking now? When should it be taken? Write it down.

Remember that the patients knows their diabetes far better than you do. Listen to their observations carefully and do not contradict them without due thought. They are usually correct in saying that a particular insulin does not suit them. Even if they do harbour misconceptions, correct them gently with an appropriate explanation.

The whole principle of insulin treatment is that the insulin is adjusted to the patient's lifestyle and not the other way around. People should not have to eat to keep up with their insulin—lower the dose to suit what they want to eat. People should not be prevented from doing particular things because they have to go home and inject their insulin—give them an insulin pen to carry with them. They should not be afraid that hypoglycaemia will ruin their work or a day out. Learn about your patient as a person and fit the diabetes treatment around his/her needs.

Box 9.2 Information for patients on insulin injections

Insulin name(s)

Dose injected before: breakfast / lunch / evening meal/ bed

Your insulin type is human/porcine/beef

Inject your insulin using.....................

Inject your insulin subcutaneously—this means into the fatty tissue under the skin of the thighs, abdomen, buttocks, or upper arms

Inject your pre-meal insulin…….minutes before food

Adjust your insulin dose for food, exercise, and current glucose as shown by your diabetes nurse or doctor

Eat three meals a day with mid-morning, mid-afternoon, and pre-bed snack unless otherwise advised.

Insulin lowers the blood glucose level and will help to control your blood glucose level.

Sometimes the blood glucose may fall too low (i.e. below 4 mmol/l). This is called hypoglycaemia and may happen if you are taking too big a dose, eat too little, or exercise more than you expect. If you feel muddled, slow-thinking, tingly, unduly emotional or cross, sweaty, or shaky, or notice your heart thumping fast, eat some glucose and then have a big snack. Contact your doctor or diabetes nurse. You may need to reduce your dose of insulin.

Insulin will work only if you inject it regularly as prescribed!

If you are unable to take your insulin for any reason, contact your doctor or diabetic nurse immediately.

Never stop your insulin. If you cannot eat, or are vomiting, contact your doctor immediately or follow the sick day rules he/she has given you.

Always carry a diabetic card and some glucose with you.

Inhaled insulin

Inhaled insulin (Exubera®) is licensed for the treatment of both type 1 and type 2 diabetes but was withdrawn by the manufacturers for financial reasons in 2007. At the time of writing other manufacturers have products in progress but none are licensed. This section has been left in the book for information as a few patients remain on the drug. Insulin is well absorbed via the lungs and has a more rapid glucose-reducing effect than injected insulin.

NICE (Technology Appraisal 113, 2006) has stated that inhaled insulin should be used as

'a treatment option for people with type 1 or type 2 diabetes mellitus who show evidence of poor glycaemic control despite other therapeutic interventions … and adequate educational support, **and** who are unable to initiate or intensify preprandial subcutaneous insulin therapy because of either:
a marked and persistent fear of injections that meet DSM-IV criteria for specific phobia "blood injection injury type" diagnosed by a diabetes specialist or mental health professional
or
severe and persistent problems with injection sites (for example, as a consequence of lipohypertrophy) despite with injection site rotation.'

NICE specify that inhaled insulin therapy should be carried out only at diabetes specialist centres, and require that the use of this product is audited (the national audit is via the Association of British Clinical Diabetologists)

Contraindications

- Age <18 yrs
- Age >75 yrs, limited experience
- Pregnancy
- Weight <30 kg
- Smokers (stop completely >6 months before starting inhaled insulin)—risk of hypoglycaemia with a cigarette.
- Passive smoking may impair absorption. Advise cohabitees to stop smoking in communal areas, or to stop altogether
- Asthma (poorly controlled, unstable, or severe)
- Chronic obstructive airways disease (severe)
- Congestive cardiac failure—avoid if significant impairment lung function
- Renal impairment—reduce dose
- Hepatic impairment—reduce dose
- Acute respiratory illness (e.g. respiratory tract infections, bronchitis)—monitor very carefully

Side effects

- Hypoglycaemia (as with all insulins).
- Risk of ketoacidosis in type 1 patients if not also taking longer-acting insulin.
- Respiratory: bronchospasm, fall in forced expiratory volume in 1 sec (FEV_1) cough, dry or irritated throat, pharyngitis, dysphonia, dry mouth. Concern has been expressed about deterioration of lung function with inhaled insulin, although studies so far suggest that this is not permanent or significant in most patients.
- Chest pain: data sheet indicates no increase in cardiac pain.
- As with other insulins: hypersensitivity, oedema, and effects of rapid glucose reduction.

Dose

- In type 2 diabetic patients, oral agents are usually continued.
- In type 1 diabetic patients, basal longer-acting SC insulin injection is nearly always required.

Oral insulin

Hitherto there has been no successful method of protecting swallowed insulin from digestive enzymes. Recent research has demonstrated that an enteric-coated capsule with an absorption enhancer and solubilizer (Capsulin™) can deliver insulin to the circulation in sufficient quantities to lower the blood glucose. This product has not yet reached production or licensing stage.

Summary

- If the patient needs insulin prescribe it—the sooner the better.
- Choose the insulin regimen that suits the patient's needs.
- An insulin regimen will succeed only if the person using it understands how their insulin(s) work and can adjust it according to insulin need.
- Remember the factors influencing insulin absorption from the injection site.
- Choose equipment appropriate to the patient's needs and keep up to date with advances in insulin delivery.

Further reading

Whitelaw, D *et al.* (2007) Absorption of orally ingested insulin in human type 1 diabetic subjects: proof of concept study. Presented at American Diabetes Association 2007. Available online at: http://www.diabetology.co.uk/ADA%20poster%20June%2005.pdf

NICE www.nice.org.uk

Chapter 10

Low blood glucose: hypoglycaemia

What is hypoglycaemia?

The price of normoglycaemia is often hypoglycaemia. Take care that your zealous quest for a normal glucose to reduce the likelihood of future tissue damage does not create problems now.

For the person who has diabetes, hypoglycaemia can be a terrifying experience to be avoided at all costs. The person may aim for persistent hyperglycaemia, preferring the absence of hypoglycaemia now to the vague and distant threat of long-term tissue damage. Many older patients still cling to old advice to 'keep a little sugar in your urine'. About one in three people with insulin-treated diabetes will experience hypoglycaemic coma; 2–3% of insulin-treated patients have frequent severe hypoglycaemia.

Hypoglycaemia occurs in sulphonylurea-treated patients—about one in three patients on glibenclamide experience hypoglycaemia. Patients taking metformin or incretin-effect drugs are rarely at risk of hypoglycaemia unless the drug is taken in overdose.

'When I feel my glucose is low'

For a person with diabetes, hypoglycaemia usually means 'when I feel that my glucose is low and I don't expect it to be'. Some patients discount symptoms before meals, or with exercise, when they expect to feel a little low, and report only episodes which have occurred at other times. Other patients discount episodes which they have successfully treated themselves—for them 'hypoglycaemia' means when someone else had to revive them. Many people with diabetes are unaware of some or all their hypoglycaemic episodes, and many have amnesia for severe hypoglycaemia. Some patients deny hypoglycaemia despite recording a value below 2 mmol/l because, to them, the only real hypoglycaemia is that which makes them feel unwell. Symptoms of hypoglycaemia are by definition subjective and vary from person to person and from episode to episode (Table 10.1). Symptomatic hypoglycaemia is not a good way to define hypoglycaemia.

Table 10.1 Common symptoms of hypoglycaemia

Sweating	Weakness
Trembling	Hunger
Inability to concentrate	Blurred vision
Any person with diabetes treated with glucose-lowering medication who behaves oddly in any way whatsoever is hypoglycaemic until proven otherwise	

Expanded from *Diabetic Medi* 1992; **9**:70–5

When counter-regulatory hormones are released

As the blood glucose falls, it stimulates release of adrenaline, noradrenaline, glucagon, cortisol, and growth hormone. Adrenaline causes tachycardia with palpitations and tremor. Glucagon stimulates glucose release from the liver. In people with diabetes the glucagon response may be blunted or absent, and excess insulin inhibits liver glucose release. The 'emergency' hormonal response to hypoglycaemia is called counter-regulation.

Hypoglycaemia could be defined as the blood glucose level at which the body initiates its emergency response. However, this point varies according to the prevailing blood glucose balance in that person. In people with persistently high blood glucose levels, counter-regulation may occur at a blood glucose of ≥5 mmol/l. This explains why some patients complain that they feel hypoglycaemic at blood glucose levels not normally regarded as hypoglycaemic. In those whose blood glucose is usually normal, significant counter-regulation may not occur until the glucose is <2 mmol/l. As patients tend to rely on autonomic symptoms to warn of hypoglycaemia, they may have little time to act before the falling glucose level incapacitates them.

Blood glucose concentration

Hypoglycaemia is usually defined as a venous plasma glucose <2.2 mmol/l. However, it is safest to tell patients on glucose-lowering drugs that if their blood glucose is <4 mmol/l it is too low. They should stop what they are doing and eat or drink glucose (see below). They should check their glucose again soon. In a potentially dangerous situation, or where rapid relief of symptoms of hypoglycaemia is required, they should stop and eat glucose, followed by a snack or meal, and check their blood glucose again soon (📖 p.208).

Signs and symptoms of hypoglycaemia

Any patient on glucose-lowering treatment who behaves oddly in any way is hypoglycaemic until proved otherwise.

The most frequently reported symptoms are sweating, trembling, inability to concentrate, weakness, hunger, and blurred vision (Table 10.1)

Changes in thinking and perceiving

- Subtle changes in mental function occur before the patient is aware that he/she is hypoglycaemic.
- Altered perception includes blurred vision, *déjà vu,* distancing from the world around, colour changes (e.g. everything turns pink), altered intensity of sound, or other sensation.
- Time slows. Time estimation is involved in assessment of speed and so hypoglycaemia may cause accidents to pedestrians and drivers/riders.
- Poor concentration, short attention span, easily distracted
- Slow decision-making is common.
- Conversation may be slow or hesitant.
- Once a task has been taken on, a hypoglycaemic person may not relinquish it—'I've started so I'll finish'. This can be dangerous, as in the hypoglycaemic driver who will not stop driving even though he realizes his blood glucose is low.
- As the blood glucose level continues to fall the person becomes increasingly confused, although they are often able to articulate this as it happens: 'I'm all anyhow, tee hee!'. The confusion may be patchy—e.g. the person may be unable to count his change but can steer a car (but not safely).

Emotions

- Any out-of-character behaviour may be due to hypoglycaemia: irritation and frustration worsened by attempts to help; fast-rising rage out of all proportion to the problem.
- Depression or tearfulness.
- Everything is wonderful, glorious, exciting, or hilariously funny.
- A change in personality may be an early and subtle sign.

Refusal of help

Patients commonly refuse help when hypoglycaemic. They may be convinced that they are coping well (but are not). Patients may also convince relatives that this is so.

Hunger with or without abhorrence of food

- Most symptomatic hypoglycaemic people complain of hunger, and will eat ravenously.
- Food may be rejected. Abhorrence of food is common and shows the split thinking of the hypoglycaemic person. Part of the brain may recognize the hypoglycaemia and the need to eat, while another part is revolted by the food, despite hunger.

Panic and hyperactivity

Cerebral irritation may combine with the stirring effects of catecholamines to produce panic, terror, and the desire to flee. Carers may be perceived as pursuers. The lack of glucose for muscle energy does not prevent considerable strength or stamina. Carers or staff may be injured.

Skin colour changes

Adrenaline causes skin pallor, but flushing or blotchy rashes may also occur in hypoglycaemia.

Sweating

- Some patients wait until they experience sweating before diagnosing hypoglycaemia.
- Sweating may be a late phenomenon.
- Sweating has been used in hypoglycaemia alarms which measure changes in skin resistance due to sweating and bleep to awaken a sleeping person (assuming that they are not already unconscious).

Palpitations and tachycardia

- Uncomfortable awareness of the heart's action
- Moderate increase in heart rate
- Systolic blood pressure may rise

Respiratory changes

- Apnoea
- Hyperventilation
- Uncomfortably awareness of breathing
- Cheyne–Stokes breathing, especially in comatose patients

Tingling

Unlike the prolonged paraesthesiae of severe recurrent spontaneous hypoglycaemia, the paraesthesiae of acute hypoglycaemia occur fleetingly, often around the mouth and lips. Paraesthesiae may also occur in the median nerve distribution in the hand, or elsewhere.

Tremor

A falling glucose level can induce a fine tremor of the hands which is not always noticeable unless sought.

Incoordination and unsteadiness

- A lack of coordination may combine with sweating and tremulous hands to cause spillages and breakages.
- Incoordination is observable in most hypoglycaemic people but they may not always realize it themselves.
- Patient feels unsteady and stumbles readily.
- Bumps into people.
- Occasionally patients exhibit considerable feats of balance, of which they are apparently incapable when not hypoglycaemic.

Weakness

- Generalized muscle weakness—'As if I've run out of petrol'
- Limb weakness
- Hemiplegia

Weariness, sleep, and coma

- Intense exhaustion and a compulsion to fall asleep can overwhelm the hypoglycaemic person.
- Increasing lassitude makes everything too much bother.
- A gradual descent through tiredness and sleep to coma.
- Sudden coma. People prone to the latter should not hold potentially hazardous jobs and should take especial care to avoid hypoglycaemia.

Tonic–clonic seizures or other epileptiform activity

- Fitting is relatively uncommon, usually with nocturnal hypoglycaemia.
- Sleep prevents recognition of early signs of a falling glucose.
- A person who has a fit only when hypoglycaemic is not epileptic and does not usually need anticonvulsants.
- People with epilepsy can fit when hypoglycaemic.

❶No symptoms—loss of warning

- Reduced warning occurs in ~25% of patients with 20 yr duration of diabetes.
- Symptomless hypoglycaemia is frightening for patients and carers.
- Near-normoglycaemia increases the risk of impaired warning.
- Warning may be restored by raising the average blood glucose for a few weeks and eradicating hypoglycaemia.
- Tell patients with poor warning of hypoglycaemia that they must not drive, operate machinery, or perform activities in which confusion or coma could put them or others at risk.

Diagnosis of hypoglycaemia

Diagnosis of hypoglycaemia

A person on glucose-lowering treatment (whether insulin or tablets) who seems unusual or behaves oddly in any way is hypoglycaemic until proved otherwise. Patients and carers should have a high index of suspicion. This can lead to friction: one of my patients pointed out that he can no longer express anger or impatience without being offered sugar.

Clinical suspicion—act in dangerous situations

In a potentially hazardous situation, e.g. swimming or rock-climbing, the person should eat glucose immediately they suspect hypoglycaemia. Delay caused by blood testing allows the glucose to fall further with worsening of symptoms and increased risk of inappropriate behaviour or coma. Rapid recovery proves the diagnosis.

Blood glucose <4 mmol/l

- Finger-prick blood glucose. Wash the finger well with water first. The patient may have been trying to eat glucose.
- If possible take a venous sample for laboratory blood glucose. There may be any diagnostic confusion or medico-legal implications. Do not delay treatment whilst awaiting the results.
- Remember that a finger-prick glucose may be misleading. If in doubt, or the patient is cold or vasoconstricted, take blood for laboratory venous glucose and give glucose.

Treatment of hypoglycaemia

In patients capable of swallowing

Glucose is absorbed most rapidly in liquid form. It is also best absorbed when swallowed alone—fat (e.g. in chocolate) slows absorption of glucose. As an approximate calculation, 10 g of glucose raises an adult's blood glucose by 2 mmol/l, and 20 g raises it by 4 mmol/l, but multiple factors influence this. Try not to overtreat hypoglycaemia. Patients on acarbose must use glucose to treat hypoglycaemia as they cannot break down sucrose.

Treat hypoglycaemia as soon as it is suspected. Check finger-prick glucose if possible. If not, give oral glucose immediately. Delay makes it harder to recover promptly.

The following contain about 10 g glucose:

- three glucose tablets (e.g. Dextrosol®)
- one tube 25 g Glucogel® (glucose gel)
- one-third of an 80 g bottle of Glucogel® (a whole bottle contains 32 g glucose)
- 50–60 ml or one-sixth of a 380 ml bottle of Original Lucozade® (a whole bottle contains 68 g glucose; other versions contain different quantities of glucose)
- 90 ml or one-third of a can of non-diet Coca Cola®
- Two spoonfuls of sugar
- Three sugar lumps
- Three or four sweets (e.g. fruit pastilles).

Patients who cannot, or will not, swallow safely

Conscious patients who refuse to swallow

Hypoglycaemic patients may irrationally reject food. Patients may spit out glucose or food and/or fight. Persistent firm encouragement usually works. This can usually be overcome by firm encouragement to eat. Glucogel® is best in this situation as it is difficult to spit out.

If the patient becomes violent, keep back to avoid personal injury and try to contain the patient in a safe area. Inject glucagon into whatever muscle bulk can be accessed safely. The alternative is to muster sufficient help to achieve robust venous access and give IV glucose (see below).

Unconscious patients, unsafe swallow, uncooperative

Profound hypoglycaemia is rare. It is most often seen in patients who have taken insulin overdoses, alcohol, or sulphonylureas, or in renal failure. 999 hospital admission is required.

- Risk of respiratory or cardiac arrest.
- Protect airway.
- Give oxygen if convulsing or hypoxic.
- Safeguard patient and staff from injury.
- Gain IV access via a large vein, tape in cannula securely (care—extravasated glucose can cause ulceration).
- Withdraw blood for laboratory glucose, urea and electrolytes, liver function, and perhaps thyroid function or cortisol.
- Give IV glucose (repeat once if not recovered within 15 min):
    - infuse 50 ml 20% glucose IV (adults)

  or
    - 25 ml 50% glucose IV (adults).
- Flush cannula with N Saline (IV glucose can cause thrombophlebitis).
- IV access impossible—inject glucagon IM (see below).
- If patient fails to recover consider steroid lack. Take blood for subsequent cortisol level and inject 100 mg hydrocortisone IV or IM.
- Monitor Glasgow coma scale, heart rate, BP, respirations, oxygen saturations.
- Feed patient if safe, or infuse 5% glucose slowly—rate depends on clinical situation.
- Monitor hourly until full consciousness regained and maintained. Keep under medical observation for at least 4 hrs and admit if any of the factors below ('after glucose given') apply.
- Do not remove IV cannula until patient ready for discharge

Glucagon (UK-GlucaGen®)

Use when IV access cannot be gained, e.g. in the home or if a vein cannot be found safely by a health professional. Glucagon releases glucose from the liver. However, the rise in blood glucose is temporary and there is considerable risk of recurrent hypoglycaemia. Feed the patient before they become hypoglycaemic again. This many be difficult as glucagon can cause nausea.

Contraindications to glucagon use

- Situations in which glucagon may be ineffective:
    - alcohol excess (chronic or acute)
    - fasting or very strict weight-reducing diet
    - anorexia nervosa
    - steroid lack
    - chronic or recurrent hypoglycaemia
    - chronic liver disease
- Sulphonylureas (caution—recurrent hypoglycaemia likely)
- Warfarin (increases plasma level of warfarin)
- Phaeochromocytoma (risk of hypertensive crisis)
- Indometacin (risk of worsening hypoglycaemia)
- Insulinoma or glucagonoma

Use of glucagon

- Teach families and carers how to use glucagon initially, and revise with each new prescription.
- Prescribe two kits in case of breakage.
- Storage—protect from light and store at 2–8°C. Can be stored at room temperature.
- Check expiry date regularly. Check fluid is clear and discard if not.
- Place patient in recovery position and protect airway (see above).
- Kit contains a 1mg glucagon powder vial and 1 ml water for injection in a pre-filled syringe.
- Inject water into glucagon vial and shake gently until dissolved. Clear air bubbles and inject.
- Adults and children >25 kg or >8 yrs inject 1 mg SC, IM, or IV
- Children <25 kg or <8 yrs inject 0.5 mg SC, IM, or IV
- Feed patient
- Beware recurrent hypoglycaemia

Insulin overdose

- Risk of death (especially if alcohol involved).
- Ice-packs on sites of injection of large insulin overdoses may slow insulin absorption to 'buy time' for treatment.
- Treat as above.
- Call diabetes registrar and consultant immediately.
- Admit to HDU/ITU.
- High risk of cardiac and/or respiratory collapse.
- Monitor potassium very carefully. Replace potassium according to potassium levels.
- Get all the old notes urgently.
- Treat concurrent disease with relevant specialist help.
- Obtain psychiatric help once patient able to talk and understand.
- Hypoglycaemic brain damage may take many months to recover and there is a risk of permanent damage.

After glucose or glucagon given

- Check the finger-prick blood glucose in 10-15 min (wash patient's fingers well). It should be ≥6 mmol/l.
- Feed patients with carbohydrate (biscuit, sandwich) after recovery from severe hypoglycaemia to sustain the recovery and prevent relapse.
- Wait a further 45 min to allow brain function to recover from hypoglycaemia before considering leaving the patient alone, or allowing him/her to drive or perform activities potentially hazardous to him/herself or others.
- Elderly people or those with cerebrovascular disease often take longer to 'come to' after hypoglycaemia than younger people.
- ❶Keep patients under observation for at least **1 hr** from glucose or glucagon treatment, and check glucose and mental function before allowing them to leave the clinic or hospital, or before leaving them alone.
- Check for injuries.

- Be particularly careful if the patient wishes immediately to drive or perform dangerous activities, activities which influence other people's safety, or activities which require concentration. If in doubt stop them.
- Hospitalize hypoglycaemic patients (after emergency treatment)
  - on sulphonylurea
  - elderly patients
  - those living alone and vulnerable
  - who have ingested alcohol or drugs of abuse
  - with renal disease, liver disease, or other significant disease
  - with psychiatric problems
  - with suspicion of overdose of insulin or glucose-lowering tablets
  - if you have concerns about their safety.
- Patients on long-acting insulin should be considered for admission unless they are fully conscious and capable of monitoring themselves and their finger-prick glucose, and adjusting their food and insulin safely.
- Patients on sulphonylurea treatment or long-acting insulin may have prolonged or recurrent hypoglycaemia until sulphonylurea-stimulated plasma insulin levels fall as the drug is excreted. Monitor finger-prick blood glucose 1–2 hourly for at least 24 hrs and until the glucose is stable. This may take several days with chlorpropamide or glibenclamide.
- Note that it is difficult to provide advice for all situations as the clinical effect and risk of hypoglycaemia varies considerably. If in doubt err on the side of caution. Remember that the patient's ability to judge their own cognitive function is likely to be impaired.
- Inform the diabetes team of the patient's admission.
- Diabetes team should check diabetes self-care, injection and blood-monitoring technique, and psychological issues. Change diabetes treatment as required (see below)
- Arrange psychological or psychiatric help if required
- **Follow-up appointment** with diabetes nurse or doctor in 1 month—or sooner if severe hypoglycaemia and vulnerable.

Prevention of further hypoglycaemia

- What glucose level is the patient aiming for? (📖 p.125, 161) Patients aiming for near-normoglycaemia are at risk of hypoglycaemia. Consider adding 2–4 mmol/l or more to the glucose targets, e.g. 4–7 mmol/l becomes 6–9 mmol/l or 8–11 mmol/l (the latter is safer).
- Immediate patient safety comes first.
- Be especially careful to prevent recurrence in patients with jobs or pursuits risking hazard to themselves or others.
- There is a high risk of recurrence in:
  - patients with previous hypoglycaemia
  - patients who are very frightened of diabetic tissue damage
  - elderly patients
  - those with erratic or small meals
  - renal disease
  - hepatic disease
  - those living alone
  - alcoholics
  - steroid-dependent patients
  - dementia
  - psychiatric or psychological disturbance
  - brittle diabetes.
- At what time of day did the hypoglycaemia originate?
  - Is there a pattern?
  - Beware nocturnal hypoglycaemia
  - Reduce daily dose by 25–50%
  - Reduce the tablet/insulin acting at the risky time of day
- Monitor finger-prick glucose before each meal, pre-bed, and during the night for a few weeks
- Monitor food intake and well-being

Children—emergency situations only

This book relates to adults only. However, health care professionals may encounter hypoglycaemia requiring immediate action in children. Note that using hypertonic IV glucose can be fatal in children. Read the BNF for Children (www.bnfc.org) which advises the following.

- By mouth: child 2–18 yrs ~10–20 g glucose (📖 p.208) repeated after 10–15 min if necessary.
- If still hypoglycaemic or oral route cannot be used: glucagon injection 1 mg/ml SC, IM, IV according to weight:
  - child body weight <25 kg 500 mcg (0.5 ml)
  - child body weight >25 kg 1 mg (1 ml).
- If prolonged hypoglycaemia or unresponsive to glucagon after 10 min:
  - glucose IV infusion 10%
  - by IV injection into large vein
  - child 1 month–18 yrs 2–5 ml/kg (glucose 200–500 mg/kg).

Recurrent hypoglycaemia in insulin-treated patients

Hypoglycaemia due to excess rapid-acting insulin usually responds rapidly to glucose treatment. However, if hypoglycaemia is due to longer-acting insulin it may recur after the initial dose of oral or IV glucose.

Recurrent hypoglycaemia may be seen in patients trying to normalize their blood glucose, in people whose lifestyle or eating patterns have changed, and in various other circumstances (Table 10.2). Recurrent severe hypoglycaemia may be due to manipulation by psychologically disturbed patients and can be hard to detect. General measures are as follows.

- First safeguard the patient.
- Stop them driving or doing dangerous jobs or pursuits.
- Refer to hospital diabetes team urgently.
- Remove all risk of hypoglycaemia by raising the blood glucose to a constant level of ~10 mmol/l.
- Reduce all insulin doses by 25–50%.
- Check insulin administration technique (from drawing up to injection, including timing—human insulin may need to be given closer to meals, even at the table).
- Ensure that food intake is evenly spaced throughout the day—three meals and three snacks (a pre-bed snack is vital).
- Test blood glucose before each meal and before bed (check technique), and during the night (about weekly or more often if severe nocturnal hypoglycaemia).
- Once the hypoglycaemia stops, the blood glucose will gradually be returned towards normal by gentle insulin adjustment.
- Sometimes such patients require hospital admission.

Causes of hypoglycaemia

Once the person is thinking clearly, review the sequence of events which led to the hypoglycaemic episode and derive lessons for future prevention. Often, the cause is obvious—late for work, no breakfast, running for the train, late business meeting, missed lunch, miscalculated insulin dose, unexpected activity (e.g. missed the bus, had to walk home), did not like lunch, so left it.

Patients may forget the incident entirely, and so it is important to inform diabetes carers what happened.

Too much insulin

- Deliberate overdose.
- Insulin dose excessive for patient's current needs
- Inappropriate increase in insulin dose by the patient or their carers.
- Check that the patient understands the time of maximum insulin action and its usual duration (Table 9.2 📖 p.168, Fig. 9.5 📖 p.191).

Unexpectedly rapid absorption of insulin

The insulin may arrive in the circulation earlier than expected—as from an IM injection, or if the circulation to a subcutaneous site is increased (e.g. by warmth or by exercising the muscle underneath). Absorption from an abdominal injection is faster than from the arm, which is faster than from the leg.

Too much sulphonylurea

Hypoglycaemia may arise early in treatment if a new patient is started on a weight-reducing diet and oral hypoglycaemics at the same time. It can also arise if the prescriber fails to appreciate that there is considerable variation in response to oral hypoglycaemics—2.5 mg glibenclamide may render one patient severely hypoglycaemic and have no obvious effect on blood glucose in another. Always start cautiously. The medication should be given with meals. Pay attention to the recommended dosage intervals and avoid large doses in the evening. Occasionally, sulphonylureas are taken in deliberate overdose by the patient, or by a depressed family member or friend. Newer glucose-lowering drugs may also cause hypoglycaemia.

Too little food

Probably the most common cause of hypoglycaemia. An accidentally missed meal, deliberate dieting (especially in young women), avoidance of disliked foods, missed snacks, and spoiled cooking can all contribute. The introduction of large amounts of fibre into the diet of someone usually on a low-fibre diet may also cause hypoglycaemia. This can occur in hospital, on a new diet, or on diabetic holidays.

Table 10.2 Causes of hypoglycaemia

Common	Uncommon
Too much insulin	Autonomic neuropathy
Too much sulphonylurea	Slow gastric emptying
Too little food	Liver impairment
Exercise	Steroid insufficiency
Alcohol	Hypothyroidism
Drugs (including street drugs)	Malignancy
Renal impairment	Severe infection

Exercise

Hypoglycaemia may be caused if the person has failed to eat enough to fuel the exertion or has too much insulin in their system, preventing glucose release by the liver. Planned exercise is best coped with by reducing insulin or hypoglycaemic tablets beforehand and, if the exercise is vigorous, by eating more. Unexpected exertion (e.g. the car running out of petrol so that it is necessary to walk to a distant garage) commonly causes hypoglycaemia. The hypoglycaemia can occur at the time of the exertion and for up to 48 hrs afterwards, e.g. at night. This can be explained to patients as 'the body reorganizing its glucose stores after exercise'. Eat carbohydrate to cover unplanned exertion. (📖 p.264)

Alcohol

People with insulin-treated diabetes who are also alcoholics run a high risk of severe, perhaps fatal, hypoglycaemia. What patients may not appreciate is that just one drink on an empty stomach may be enough to precipitate or aggravate hypoglycaemia. Every year patients find themselves guests of the constabulary who assume, at least initially, that a person who smells of alcohol, and is behaving oddly, is drunk. This is one reason why every person with diabetes who is on glucose-lowering treatment should carry a diabetic card and glucose.

Drugs

Beta-blockers, especially non-selective ones, may reduce the warning of hypoglycaemia. Beta-blockers and other hypotensive drugs, such as guanethidine and clonidine may reduce the response to hypoglycaemia. Some drugs potentiate the hypoglycaemic action of sulphonylureas and repaglinide (aspirin and NSAIDs, warfarin, sulphonamides, clofibrate, fenfluramine). ACE inhibitors may cause hypoglycaemia (Table 8.2 📖 p.142.)

Renal impairment

This can cause severe hypoglycaemia in both insulin-treated and sulphonylurea-treated patients. If a patient has falling insulin or tablet requirements check their renal function.

Autonomic neuropathy

This may lead to delayed gastric emptying. Pyloric obstruction can delay food digestion and absorption. Patients with severe autonomic neuropathy may not recognize hypoglycaemia.

Liver impairment

Can cause hypoglycaemia in a patient without diabetes. Its presence requires very careful insulin dose adjustment and frequent food intake (say, every 2 hrs). As most sulphonylureas and repaglinide are metabolized in the liver, they should be used with great caution in hepatic impairment or profound hypoglycaemia will ensue. Avoid rosiglitazone and pioglitazone.

Steroid insufficiency

Check for steroid lack (adrenal or pituitary) in patients with inexplicable recurrent hypoglycaemia whether or not they have diabetes.

Malignancy

This is another cause of spontaneous hypoglycaemia in non-diabetics, but it may precipitate puzzling recurrent hypoglycaemia in people with diabetes.

Severe infection

This is a rare cause of unexplained hypoglycaemia.

Hypoglycaemia and hypothermia

Hypoglycaemia and cold are a potentially lethal combination. Glucose is essential for normal thermoregulation—hypoglycaemic people cannot shiver (*Clin Sci* 1981; **61**:463–9). Check venous glucose in everyone with hypothermia. If this is difficult, give glucose anyway. This particularly applies to people suffering from exposure in the mountains, at sea, or in other cold/wet/windy situations.

Never do a finger-prick blood glucose on someone with cold vasoconstricted fingers, as the result, if obtained at all, will be hard to interpret. Use venous blood on a strip and send the sample to the laboratory as well (some glucose strips are not calibrated for venous blood).

Responsibility

Major efforts must be made to prevent hypoglycaemia. These include repeated patient and professional education. People with diabetes clearly have a choice about whether or not to accept medical advice. However, doctors and other health care professionals must ensure that patients understand that hypoglycaemia may not only cause them to injure themselves, but may also cause injury to others, e.g. while driving a car or operating machinery, or require the rescue services, perhaps risking the lives of rescuers.

Carry glucose and a diabetic card

People with diabetes on glucose-lowering treatment, whether insulin or pills, should carry glucose on their person. They must be taught when to take it and replenish it once eaten. A diabetic card may help others to help them.

Summary

- Hypoglycaemia frightens patients. It may cause harm to patients or others. Prevent it.
- Hypoglycaemia is common in people taking insulin or sulphonylureas.
- Hypoglycaemia is a laboratory venous blood glucose <2.2 mmol/l. Patients on insulin or glucose-lowering tablets with a blood glucose <4 mmol/l should stop and eat glucose or bring forward a snack or meal.
- Hypoglycaemia produces many symptoms, but patients can learn to recognize their early symptoms to allow prompt treatment.
- For practical purposes, anyone with diabetes on insulin or glucose-lowering tablets who behaves oddly in any way should be assumed to be hypoglycaemic. Staff and carers should have a high index of suspicion.
- The treatment of hypoglycaemia is glucose taken either by mouth or intravenously. Glucagon should be used only if glucose cannot be injected IV.
- After treatment the cause should be sought and preventive measures instituted. Re-educate the patient (and staff if appropriate).

Chapter 11

High blood glucose: hyperglycaemia

What is hyperglycaemia?

One aim of diabetes care is to restore the blood glucose towards normal. This is not the only aim—resolution of symptoms, prevention and treatment of tissue damage, control of other metabolic imbalance, and, above all, a good quality of life are also important.

Before defining hyperglycaemia, set the patient's blood glucose target zone. In most instances, the aim should be to maintain the blood glucose between 4 and 8 mmol/l most of the time without hypoglycaemia. The occasional random value up to 11.0 mmol/l is no worry. (Box 7.1 📖 p.112). Hyperglycaemia would usually be regarded as a glucose level >11.0 mmol/l.

These guidelines assume that the patient is capable of looking after themself and is not frail or vulnerable. In an elderly person with insulin-treated diabetes who lives alone aim for blood glucose levels of 6–11 mmol/l to avoid hypoglycaemia. Sometimes, e.g. if the patient is terminally ill, the aim is solely to avoid symptoms of uncontrolled diabetes with minimum discomfort to the patient. Tailor the target zone to the patient. Patients who keep their blood glucose <8 mmol/l all the time may suffer from frequent hypoglycaemia.

Hyperglycaemia is the blood glucose level above the target zone for an individual patient. However, most patients have 'one-off' levels above their target zone from time to time. Action is required only if hyperglycaemia persists. This may mean immediately in a patient in whom you are aiming for strict normoglycaemia (e.g. a pregnant woman with diabetes), or after observing the glucose levels for a few days in others. It is important not to cause hypoglycaemia by overzealous normalization of the blood glucose.

Causes of hyperglycaemia

Lack of insulin

- Insulin dose forgotten, omitted, too small, leaked out of the injection site, poorly absorbed from the injection site
- Insulin dose insufficient for everyday needs
- Insulin dose insufficient because of increasing insulin demands, as in any situation when the stress hormone response is triggered (e.g. in infection)
- Young girls may omit or reduce insulin to cause hyperglycaemia and hence weight loss
- Insulin omitted because of vomiting (usually wrongly, 📖 p.241)

Lack of non-insulin medication or failure to respond to it

- Failure to adjust oral hypoglycaemic drugs despite hyperglycaemia
- Dose of medication insufficient for everyday needs
- Forgotten tablets or exenatide
- Increasing insulin demands due to illness
- Medication may be vomited or pass through rapidly with diarrhoea
- Inadequate pancreatic insulin production—insulin treatment needed

Too much food

- One-off high due to large or unusual meal, e.g. Christmas (teach patients to increase glucose-lowering treatment relating to that meal)
- Slim or underweight patients may need both more food and more insulin
- Overweight patients should be encouraged to return to their diet

Too much IV glucose

Unmonitored glucose infusions in hospital are a frequent cause of hyperglycaemia in diabetic patients.

Too little exercise

Reduces energy expenditure, e.g. a previously active person changes to a sedentary job.

Infection

This is a common cause which should always be sought assiduously in a patient with unexplained hyperglycaemia. Insulin requirement rises rapidly with a developing infection, and then falls equally fast as it resolves.

Injury

May cause stress hormone release and increased insulin demands. Thus people with diabetes who have accidents or who undergo surgery require careful glucose monitoring.

Table 11.1 Causes of hyperglycaemia

Causes of hyperglycaemia
Lack of insulin
Lack of oral hypoglycaemic medication
Failure to respond to oral hypoglycaemics
Too much food
Too little exercise
Infection
Injury—accidental or surgical
Myocardial infarction
Menstruation
Pregnancy
Emotional stress
Drugs

Myocardial infarction

This may be the presenting feature of diabetes, especially in Asian patients. As the myocardial infarct can be silent or produce atypical symptoms, perform an ECG in any older patient with unexplained hyperglycaemia.

Menstruation

May be preceded by hyperglycaemia (📖 p.368) due to sex hormone fluctuations. Patients may not always volunteer this explanation of repeated hyperglycaemia.

Pregnancy

Can cause unexpected hyperglycaemia in young women, whether or not they are using contraception.

Emotional stress

This has unpredictable effects on the blood glucose. In theory, any stress which stimulates catecholamine release would be expected to raise the blood glucose. While hyperglycaemia is the usual response, some patients become hypoglycaemic under severe stress (e.g. fear) because of increased clearance of insulin from the injection site. Another effect of stress may be to influence the patient's management of their treatment. Anxieties about hypoglycaemia can lead to persistent hyperglycaemia. Severe psychological disturbance can be manifested by insulin omission or overdose.

Drugs

Hyperglycaemia may be caused by certain drugs, including steroids (e.g. in the management of asthma), thiazide diuretics, tricyclic antidepressants.

When to take action

The problem is that the blood glucose is only one factor to be considered. Review the duration of hyperglycaemia and its cause. A one-off high glucose following a birthday party is rarely a cause for concern, although the lesson learned is to increase the amount of insulin injected before another similar party. Persistent hyperglycaemia or hyperglycaemia in an ill person needs action immediately. Note that the level of the blood glucose may not match the patient's degree of illness. Patients can have life-threatening acidosis and a blood glucose of 12 mmol/l. Other patients walk into clinic, apparently well, with a blood glucose of 30 mmol/l.

Never consider the blood glucose without assessing the patient as a whole. This will also help you to identify patients whose general condition is such that they must be managed in hospital, those who need frequent assessments as their condition might deteriorate, and those in whom there is time to adjust the blood glucose balance gradually.

Is the patient ill?

First decide if the patient appears ill or not. Then consider the degree of hyperglycaemia. Your priority is to identify patients who should be managed in hospital. Then act to control the blood glucose concentration.

Check ketones (📖 p.126)

Check finger-prick blood ketones (best option) or urinary ketones:

- patient ill or vomiting, or emergency attender and glucose >11 mmol/l
- patient appears well and glucose >15 mmol/l.

If blood ketone ≥3 mmol/l or urinary ketones >++ treat for DKA (📖 p.237).

Box 11.1 Danger signs

❶Admit patients with these signs to hospital 999:

- Altered consciousness
- Confusion
- Vomiting
- Abdominal or chest pain
- Altered respiration
- Infection
- Dehydration
- Hypotension
- Blood ketones ≥3 mmol/l—DKA

❶Suspicion of diabetic ketoacidosis? HOSPITAL 999

DKA is still a major cause of death in people with insulin-treated diabetes <50 yrs old. The most prominent symptom is vomiting—a feature which always signals danger in diabetes Treat DKA promptly and effectively. It should always be managed in hospital (📖 p.237)

If blood glucose is >15mmol/l give 0.1 units/kg body weight of clear short-acting insulin (e.g. Actrapid®, Humulin S®, Apidra®, Humalog®, NovoRapid®) intramuscularly (📖 p. 241) while awaiting transfer. If available, infuse normal (150mmol/l, 0.9%) saline, 500 ml/hr IV during transfer (unless risk of fluid overload, e.g. heart disease).

Ill hyperglycaemic patients without ketones

These patients may also require hospital assessment. While arranging transfer to hospital start treatment for the high glucose—encourage oral water if safe to do so and inject one dose of clear short-acting insulin (e.g. Actrapid®, Humulin S®, Apidra®, Humalog®, NovoRapid®) intramuscularly.

- Adjust IM insulin dose to patient and situation.
- Do not inject insulin if blood glucose <15 mmol/l.
- Inject about 4 - 10 units insulin IM.
- Obesity—increase insulin dose.
- Known insulin-resistance—increase insulin dose.
- Infection—increase insulin dose.
- On steroids—increase insulin dose.
- Renal failure—reduce insulin dose.
- Do not give IM dose if patient has injected insulin within the past 2 hrs
- Make sure that your note for the admitting officer contains details of the blood glucose, the insulin dose, and the time it was given.

❶These suggestions must be adapted to each patient's clinical state

Infection

Evidence of infection anywhere is a danger sign. Infections in people with diabetes require prompt treatment which usually needs to be more intensive and longer lasting than in those without diabetes. As metabolic chaos can rapidly ensue during an infection, any patient with more than a minor infection should be assessed in hospital. Remember that blood glucose rises rapidly in the presence of infection. A patient's insulin dose may double, and people usually controlled on oral hypoglycaemic drugs often need insulin.

All patients with *any* evidence of foot infection should be assessed by the diabetes team (e.g. community diabetes team, podiatry or wound care, hospital diabetes foot team) on the same day. Check your local arrangements.

Pregnancy

Pregnant women should be managed by a specialist diabetes team. Any problems with diabetes management should be referred on the same day to the diabetes team. High glucose can damage the foetus acutely or chronically.

Elderly patients and children

It may be difficult to assess elderly patients clinically; they may have severe hyperglycaemia with little clinical evidence. Have a low threshold for seeking hospital assessment of a hyperglycaemic elderly person. The same applies to young children.

Non-diabetic illness

Diabetes can make the treatment of any other illness more difficult, and most other illnesses can cause hyperglycaemia. The presence of diabetes may determine the outcome of a coexisting illness. Such patients who become hyperglycaemic should be assessed in hospital. It is often better to refer the patient via the diabetes team who can then coordinate care with other disciplines. Alternatively, notify the diabetes team when referring a patient so that they can help to supervise the diabetes care.

Does the patient have symptoms of hyperglycaemia?

The symptoms of hyperglycaemia are mainly thirst, polyuria, and nocturia. The patient may also have general malaise and lethargy. These symptoms are unpleasant, so treat the hyperglycaemia quickly. The blood glucose level at which they occur varies from person to person and some people appear to adapt to persistently high blood glucose concentrations. If the patient's only problem is symptomatic hyperglycaemia and they are not ill in other ways, they can usually be managed at home by the GP and/or the diabetes team.

Start or adjust treatment on the day the patient is seen. Review the patient within a week. Provide a contact number for immediate help if their condition deteriorates. If there is no response despite further treatment adjustment, help seek help from the diabetes team.

Management of hyperglycaemia

It is assumed that other urgent treatment has been initiated and that other problems (see Table 11.1) have been addressed. This section is very difficult to write because management which seems appropriate in theory is not always practical. Assess each patient fully and adjust treatment to his/her particular situation. Remember that there are huge variations in the effect of blood glucose upon symptoms and clinical condition, and in the response of blood glucose to treatment.

Preventive vs reactive care

- ***React*** to a one-off high glucose with a one-off correction dose of insulin.
- ***Prevent*** persistent hyperglycaemia at a particular time of day by reviewing the HBGM diary and adjusting glucose-lowering treatment to reduce the glucose at that time.

(The same approach can be used to correct hypoglycaemia—react to a one-off low glucose with immediate treatment. Prevent repetition by reviewing the timing and circumstances of the hypoglycaemia and adjusting treatment.)

General measures

Check HBGM technique

Check that the patient is using their strips and meter correctly and that the results in the diary are at the times stated (patients often write in the wrong column in error). Review or download the glucose meter.

Check medication

Is the patient taking what you think they are—right amount, right time? Has other medication been started or stopped?

Check total calorie and CHO intake

Is the patient eating too much for his/her needs? If so, advise reduction. Refer to the dietitian.

Increase exercise

Regular exercise within the training zone (📖 p.263) which will help to reduce the blood glucose long term. Many people feel unable to make this commitment but it can be explored. Making an effort to walk regularly; using stairs will help. Patients unable to manage a full exercise programme can still increase their exercise level. (📖 p.74, 262).

Correct causes

Review the list of causes (Table 11.1) and treat any applying to your patient.

Insulin-treated patients

Check medication and technique

Check that you and the patient are both talking about the same insulin and the same doses. Observe insulin pen use or drawing up, injection sites, injection process (Is it too shallow? Does insulin leak out?).

If these are all satisfactory, consider whether it is appropriate to increase insulin, decrease food, or increase regular exercise—or all three.

Correction dose

Every person with diabetes has one-off highs. Patients using correction dosing can do so (📖 p.189). Others should consider missing the next snack, reducing the meal, or some exercise.

Adjust usual insulin

If the blood glucose is >11 mmol/l for ≥3 days and any underlying condition (e.g. premenstrual state) has not resolved, action should be taken.

Acute hyperglycaemia in ill people—increase insulin

Rapidly rising emergency hormones (e.g. bacterial or viral infection) can require rapid insulin increase. High-dose steroids for acute asthma require immediate insulin increase (or often insulin injections in those on other forms of hypoglycaemic treatment).This usually occurs in the context of illness, e.g. an infection. An example of sick day rules for a person with diabetes is shown in Table 11.2. Agree sick day rules for each patient on insulin before they need them.

Chronic hyperglycaemia in 'well' people - Increase insulin

Consider the time of peak action and length of action of the insulin acting at the time of hyperglycaemia. Increase one type of insulin at one injection time, wait 2 days for short-acting insulin, 3 days for intermediate-acting insulin, and 5 days for long-acting insulin, and then review. Make further changes as appropriate. It is usual to increase the insulin by 2 units at a time (1 unit in patients on <20 units/day or in patients especially sensitive to insulin) (see Table 11.3).

Reduce or redistribute carbohydrate food

Reduce CHO eaten at main meals or redistribute it to other times of day. Balance the calorie intake to the patient's dietary needs. It is unwise to stop snacks; and the pre-bed snack should never be stopped. People who have to get home from work (especially if driving or cycling) should always have a mid-afternoon snack. See Table 11.4.

Patients on non-insulin hypoglycaemic medication

Increase hypoglycaemic drugs

Unlike insulin, in which there is no upper limit, other hypoglycaemics have a maximum range. There is no benefit and possible harm in exceeding this. The dose should be increased gradually and with care not to induce hypoglycaemia. It is often better to look at the food pattern if there is isolated hyperglycaemia during the day. Most drugs should be given two or three times daily at meal times. Modified release drugs are usually given once daily. Add a second or third agent if on the maximum dose of existing treatment. (📖 p.132).

If the patient is persistently hyperglycaemic on maximum doses of non-insulin agents, they need insulin. This should be started without delay (📖 p.162).

Reduce carbohydrate food

Dietary changes are similar to those for insulin-treated patients, although people on oral hypoglycaemic drugs rarely need snacks. For people on oral hypoglycaemics who are overweight, reduction in food intake combined with increased exercise is the best way of improving glycaemic balance. See Table 11.4.

Table 11.2 Sick day rules for a person with insulin-treated diabetes

If you are ill your blood glucose will usually rise as your body releases emergency hormones. This means that you will probably need more insulin than usual, even if you are not eating.

1. Measure your blood glucose 6-hourly; that is, before each meal time and before bed. Test your blood or urine for ketones.

2. DO NOT STOP YOUR USUAL INSULIN

   Be prepared to inject extra insulin after each blood test.

Blood glucose	**Clear short-acting insulin (adapt dose to the patient)**
≤11 mmol/l	No extra units
11.1–15 mmol/l	4 extra units
>15 mmol/l	6 extra units

3. If you cannot eat, drink plenty of fluid. Try to keep your carbohydrate intake up by drinking milk with added sugar, Lucozade, Coca Cola, Pepsi Cola, or other sugary drinks, unless your blood glucose is >15 mmol/l.

4. CALL FOR HELP SOONER RATHER THAN LATER

   If your blood glucose is >25 mmol/l on two occasions

   If your blood glucose is >11 and your blood or urine shows ketones

   If you are vomiting and unable to keep fluids down

   If you feel too ill to measure your blood glucose

   If you do not know what to do

YOUR HELP TELEPHONE NUMBER IS ....

Table 11.3 Insulin increase to reduce blood glucose

Time of high blood glucose	Insulin dose to increase
Before breakfast	Pre-dinner or pre-bed intermediate/ long*-acting
Before lunch	Pre-breakfast short-acting
Before main evening meal (dinner)	Pre-breakfast intermediate/long*-acting Pre-lunch short-acting
Before bed	Pre-dinner short-acting Pre-breakfast long*-acting

*It is assumed that the patient is injecting a long-acting insulin (e.g. glargine) once daily.

Table 11.4 Carbohydrate reduction to reduce blood glucose

Time of high glucose level	Carbohydrate food to reduce
Mid-morning	Breakfast
Before lunch	Mid-morning snack/breakfast
Mid-afternoon	Lunch
Before main evening meal	Mid-afternoon snack/lunch
Before main evening meal	Mid-afternoon snack/lunch
Before bed	Main evening meal

Summary

- Hyperglycaemia means blood glucose concentrations above the target zone (normally 4-8 mmol/l) for each patient.
- In an acute situation, the level of blood glucose is less important than the patient's condition.
- Ill patients should be transferred to hospital regardless of their blood glucose. Hyperglycaemia in pregnant women, elderly patients, and children should be managed in hospital.
- Patients with severe symptoms need prompt treatment.
- DKA is a medical emergency requiring urgent treatment in hospital. It is preventable.
- Causes of hyperglycaemia are insufficient insulin or hypoglycaemic drugs, excess food, too little exercise, infection, injury (accidental or surgical), myocardial infarction, menstruation, pregnancy, emotional stress, and drugs.
- Treatment of hyperglycaemia includes treating the cause, if possible, and controlling the glucose by increasing hypoglycaemic therapy, reducing food, or increasing exercise.
- React to a one-off high glucose by adjusting hypoglycaemic treatment, food, or exercise that day. Prevent persistent high glucose levels by studying the pattern and adjusting hypoglycaemic treatment, food, and exercise.
- If the glucose cannot be controlled, seek the diabetes team's help early.

Chapter 12

Diabetic ketoacidosis (DKA) and hyperosmolar non-ketotic hyperglycaemic state (HONK)

DKA or HONK?

Diabetic high glucose emergencies are usually divided into acidotic and non-acidotic states, but some patients have components of both and the division is not rigid. It depends on the patient's body habitus (internal and external), the way in which fat and other body tissues respond to actual or relative insulin deficiency and dehydration, and the influence of coexisting conditions or medications. The division is useful to help plan fluid replacement, thrombosis risk, and prognosis. However, it is important to adjust treatment to each patient and to fine tune it according to clinical response. Rigid attempts to label the high-glucose problem are not always helpful. If in doubt, treat as HONK.

DKA is, by definition, a state in which high levels of ketones make the blood acid. Hyperosmolar non-ketotic hyperglycaemic state (HONK), also called hyperosmolar hyperglycaemic state and hyperosmolar hyperglycaemia non-ketotic state, is a situation in which the main problem is gross dehydration and high glucose levels producing hyperosmolar blood.

Table 12.1 DKA or HONK?

Test	DKA	HONK	Severely ill Contact ITU*
Blood glucose	>11 mmol/l	»11 mmol/l Usually>30 mmol/l	>40 mmol/l
Blood ketone	≥3 mmol/l	<3 mmol/l	>6 mmol/l
Arterial pH	<7.3	Normal	<7.0
Venous bicarbonate	<15 mmol/l	>15 mmol/l	<10 mmol/l
			Hyperventilating
			Confused or unconscious
			BP <90 systolic
			Pregnant
Calculated osmolality 2(sodium+potassium) + glucose		>350 mosmol	

*Consider contacting ITU for all patients with DKA or HONK.

DKA

- ❶Any suspicion of DKA requires immediate transfer to hospital.
- Caused by absolute or relative insulin lack.
- A major diabetic emergency—preventable, predictable, treatable.
- Mortality 7%—the most common cause of death in diabetic patients <50 years of age.

This chapter relates to adults >16 years (for guidance on DKA in children see 📖 p.256). Doses of fluid and insulin are given for guidance but treatment must be tailored to the individual patient. Seek senior advice if unsure.

Symptoms

- Vomiting (most common symptom)
- Tiredness, malaise, weakness
- Thirst, polyuria
- Weight loss
- Air hunger
- Anorexia, abdominal pain, diarrhoea, or constipation
- Symptoms of diabetic complications
- Symptoms of precipitating condition
- May be few symptoms

Signs

- Ketotic breath, hyperventilation.
- Tired, unwell
- Dehydration, weight loss.
- Tachycardia, hypotension.
- Hypothermia
- Vomiting ± coffee grounds (due to haemorrhagic gastritis)
- Abdominal tenderness
- Gastric retention
- Full bladder or polyuria (if not, very dry)
- Evidence of diabetic complications
- Evidence of precipitating condition
- Coma (rare—either very ill or other cause)

Causes

- Infection (most common cause)
- Too little insulin
- Psychological factors
- Too much food, especially sugars
- Lack of education (patient or staff)—inexperienced nurses or junior doctors often omit insulin in vomiting patients!
- New diabetes mellitus
- Alcohol abuse
- Exercise with insulin lack
- Myocardial infarction
- Stroke
- Gangrene
- Surgery
- Trauma
- Any illness
- Gynaecological problems
- Pregnancy
- Manipulation
- Stress (exclude other causes)

Diagnosis

- History—exclude DKA in any **vomiting** insulin-treated diabetic patient.
- Examination—may find little, may be dehydrated and hypotensive.
- Capillary glucose >11 mmol/l (if shut down use venous blood on strip).
- Urine ketones positive. Blood ketones ≥3 mmol/l.
- Arterial pH <7.3.
- Bicarbonate <15 mmol/l.

❶DO NOT DELAY TREATMENT AWAITING LABORATORY RESULTS

Management

Initial management

- Resuscitation : airway, breathing, circulation.
- Aim door to needle time <15 min.
- Good IV access.
- Take venous bloods
- 1000 ml 0.9% NaCl IV over 1 hr
- One IV or IM bolus of 0.1 units/kg soluble insulin, maximum 10 units (e.g. Actrapid®, Humulin S®) unless infusion pump ready immediately.
- Insulin infusion 0.1 units/kg/hr soluble insulin (e.g. Actrapid®, Humulin S®) up to a maximum of 6 units/hr.
- Inform diabetes registrar or consultant diabetologist.

Tests

- Finger-prick capillary blood glucose + ketone (beware cold fingers)
- Arterial blood pH and gases
- Urgent laboratory venous glucose, U&E, creatinine, FBC
- Later LFT, TFT, lipids, blood cultures
- Dipstick urine
- MSU, throat swab, microbiology swab any lesion
- Pregnancy test
- ECG
- Chest X-ray
- Consider abdominal X-ray

Aims of treatment

Start initial resuscitation within 15 min. Then:

- Gradual return to normal
- Rehydrate over 24 hr; use IV fluid and insulin to correct DKA
- Aim for a glucose fall of 4–6 mmol/hr
- Aim for the arterial pH to rise gradually over 24 hr

Actions

- Consider ITU/HDU for each patient
- Good IV access
- Consider CVP monitoring if very ill, cardiac disease, elderly
- Oxygen 35% (unless respiratory disease risking CO_2 retention)
- Nasogastric tube if severe vomiting, gastric retention, coma
- Urinary catheter if not passed urine within 2 hr, elderly, immobile, coma
- IV fluids and electrolytes
- Insulin
- Treat precipitating condition (e.g. antibiotics for infection)
- Prophylactic low molecular weight heparin
- Contact seniors and diabetes team

Treatment

Insulin

- Use soluble insulin (e.g. Actrapid® or Humulin S®).
- One IV or IM bolus of 0.1 units/kg soluble insulin (e.g. Actrapid®, Humulin S®) (maximum 10 units) unless insulin infusion pump ready within 15 min of arrival. Avoid SC insulin in shocked patients—absorption may be delayed.
- Insulin infusion 0.1 units/kg/hr soluble insulin (e.g. Actrapid®, Humulin S®) to a maximum of 6 units/hr.
- Continue fixed continuous infusion until pH >7.3 (use IV glucose to fuel ketone clearance by insulin, and to slow rate of fall of glucose).
- IV sliding scale (📖 p.181) if glucose <15 mmol/l *and* pH >7.3 or finger-prick blood ketones <0.5 mmol/l.
- If glucose <12 mmol/l and ketones >0.5 mmol/l change to 10% glucose IV (5–50% depending on volume requirements) to allow higher insulin dose to clear ketones.
- Continue IV sliding scale until patient eating properly.
- Restart usual insulin at next appropriate meal.
- Continue sliding scale (reduced if necessary) until meal after that.

Fluids (depends on patient—beware fluid imbalance)

- Fluid deficit averages 6 litres, but may be as much as 10 litres. Rate of infusion must be tailored to each patient's clinical condition, age, and comorbidities.
- Reduce rate in elderly, cardiac disease, if bicarbonate >10 mmol/l (mild acidosis).
- Use 0.9% NaCl to correct fluid deficit.
- If BP <90 systolic consider a plasma expander.
- Infuse:
  - 0.9% NaCl 1000 ml in 1 hr (once or twice according to clinical need)
  - 0.9% NaCl 1000 ml in 2 hr (once or twice according to clinical need)
  - 0.9% NaCl 1000 ml in 4 hr
  - 0.9% NaCl 1000 ml in 6–8 hr, continued as needed.
- Use IV glucose to keep the blood glucose 8–12 mmol/l:
  - if glucose <12 mmol/l and pH <7.3 add 5–50% glucose infusion in parallel with other fluids (adjust glucose concentration to fluid needs and metabolic state); no more than 2 litres of 5% glucose solution per 24 hr.
  - infuse glucose to keep blood glucose 8–12 mmol/l until blood ketones <0.5 mmol/l.

Potassium

- Patients are potassium depleted
- Give potassium in second NaCl bag onwards (40 mmol/l)
- Stop potassium if K > 6.0 mmol/l or anuric
- Beware known renal failure—care with potassium replacement

Bicarbonate

- There is no benefit from using bicarbonate if pH >6.9
- There is no evidence that bicarbonate helps with pH <6.9
- Bicarbonate causes hypokalaemia.
- Do not use bicarbonate unless in cardiac arrest situation or peri-arrest.

HONK

- Phone consultant diabetologist.
- Often hard to manage. May be confused and aggressive.
- May be misdiagnosed as stroke.
- Manage as for DKA at first, but be aware that HONK patients may be, or may become, more insulin sensitive than expected and so the 6 units/hr insulin infusion may need halving to 3 units/hr.
- If no fall in glucose in 2 hr and all lines are working, double insulin infusion rate (but beware changes in insulin sensitivity as blood glucose levels fall).
- High risk of thromboembolism. Fully anticoagulate with low molecular weight heparin provided that there are no contraindications.
- Most patients with HONK need ITU/HDU.
- Mortality up to 15%.
- Most patients elderly.
- Many have infections (e.g. urinary tract).
- Many are on diuretics.
- Many have cardiac disease.
- Usually have type 2 diabetes.
- Blood sodium level often rises. If sodium >155 mmol/l consider 0.45% NaCl infusion (discuss this with consultant diabetologist).

Monitoring DKA and HONK

Bedside monitoring

- **LOOK AT THE PATIENT** (hourly at first) Can they talk normally?
- Pulse, BP, respirations (hourly).
- Fluid input/output – hourly
- Neurological observations if impaired conscious level (Glasgow coma scale chart)
- CVP hourly if used
- Urine/blood ketones
- ECG monitor—look at T waves (peaked if high potassium) and rhythm

Laboratory monitoring

- Arterial pH every 2–4 hr until pH >7.3
- U & E every 2–4 hr
- Laboratory glucose every 2 hr until <30
- Finger-prick glucose hourly unless BP low/cold; if so use laboratory venous reading
- Finger-prick ketone every 2–4 hr until <0.5

Lessons learnt the hard way

Take it seriously

- Take DKA/HONK seriously. Don't delay!
- Put all patients with suspected DKA/HONK into the resuscitation area
- One-to-one nursing until stable, or longer if very ill
- Call medical registrar and/or diabetes registrar
- Make diagnosis and start treatment within 15 min

Get the old notes

Previous clinical records must be available within an hour of patient's arrival in hospital. Many patients admitted with DKA/HONK will be under your local diabetes service. Many will have had previous admissions with DKA. Old clinical records may indicate risk (e.g. known cardiac or renal disease), and speed diagnosis and management.

Admit the patient to the diabetes ward or ICU/HDU

Patients should be cared for by staff expert and experienced in their management. They are more likely to spot problems, or unusual clinical responses. Patients usually go home sooner.

Review the patient yourself

Patients with DKA/HONK should improve gradually from your first intervention. A doctor should talk to the patient once an hour for at least the first 6 hr, and 4 hourly thereafter. If the patient cannot talk there is a serious problem. The most common reason for failure to improve is treatment not happening e.g. cannula fallen out. Medical wards are busy places and nurses are stretched to the limit.

Patients who do not look ill—but are!

Patients who usually run high glucose levels tolerate them well. They may have problems with self-care or manipulate their management. Although you often see them in clinic with glucose >20 mmol/l, always check their ketone levels—you may be able to pre-empt an admission in DKA. Some patients tolerate DKA remarkably well. They may be vomiting and a little dry but with no other signs. However, they may still be significantly acidotic and dehydrated. Always take a vomiting or sugary diabetic patient seriously.

Use blood ketone strips to assess ketosis

- Use blood ketone strips to diagnose DKA and monitor progress.
- The predominant ketone in DKA is β-hydroxybutyrate. This is what the blood ketone strips measure.
- Blood ketones 1.5–2.9 mmol/l and not acidotic may progress to DKA. Give insulin *immediately* to prevent DKA. Consider admission, fluids and insulin infusion (see 📖 p.181).
- Urine ketone strips measure acetone, which is a less helpful indicator of ketosis. Also, the urine will have been in the bladder for varying lengths of time and indicates past, but not necessarily present, ketosis.

Missed infection

- Infection is the most common cause of DKA/HONK and patients may not have a fever.
- Most patients with DKA will have a slightly raised WBCC—this cannot be used as a marker for infection. Marked elevations usually indicate infection.
- Viral infections can trigger DKA/HONK.
- Bacterial infections may be due to multiple organisms.
- If in doubt give broad-spectrum antibiotics—the patient is too ill to await microbiological results
- Fungal infections may be hard to diagnose, and may be systemic and not just superficial. Candida is the most common.

Hypothermia

- The temperature in DKA/HONK may be normal or low.
- Hypothermia is common in DKA/HONK and has a high mortality.
- Measure temperature with a low-reading thermometer.
- Lack of fever does not rule out infection.

Glucose 'not high enough'

Patients who have eaten little for some time, or who have liver disease, can have severe DKA with a glucose of as low as 12 mmol/l. Look at the whole picture, not just the glucose level.

Normal or low potassium on admission

The potassium should be raised in insulin lack. Normal or low potassium usually means severe, often chronic, potassium lack (do not forget laxative abuse). Give potassium in the first bag of saline. Such patients may need large doses of potassium IV and therefore may need HDU nurses to administer this. Watch the T waves on the ECG to monitor the effect of the potassium on the heart.

Normal or high sodium concentration on admission

- The sodium should be low if the glucose is high due to insulin lack.
- If the sodium level appears normal or high the patient may be severely dehydrated.
- The calculation to correct the sodium for glucose concentration is about 0.4 mmol/l sodium per mmol of glucose (Am J Med 1999; 106: 399–403). But the relationship between sodium and glucose is non-linear as the glucose rises so the correction should be regarded as approximate only. Example: plasma glucose 30 mmol/l and sodium 135 mmol/l corrects to sodium ~147 mmol/l (0.4 x 30=12, 135 + 12 = 147).
- Infuse IV 0.9% saline initially in all patients but if hypernatraemia develops consider 0.45% NaCl after discussion with a consultant (see 📖 p.244).

Raised urea and creatinine

Dehydration can cause marked rises, e.g. creatinine >500 micromol/l. Some of these patients will have acute-on-chronic renal disease. Proteinuria suggests the latter (in the absence of a UTI). Also, low urine output despite plentiful fluid replacement may indicate poor renal function. Check the past notes or previous laboratory results.

Bizarre or dramatic changes in glucose levels

- Check cannula and lines. Has there been a delay in refilling an empty insulin pump?
- Check that insulin has been given—and at the right dose.
- Suspect manipulation, especially if the patient is psychologically disturbed. Rarely, patients substitute water for insulin in the pump.

Abnormal oxygen or carbon dioxide concentrations

- The arterial oxygen level should be normal. If the patient is hypoxic, they have cardiac or respiratory disease or fluid overload, or are developing very severe complications of DKA such as adult respiratory distress syndrome (ARDS). Urgently seek and treat the cause of hypoxia.
- The arterial CO_2 should be low because of hyperventilation. If is it not, the patient may have respiratory disease causing CO_2 retention, or they may be so ill that they have respiratory depression.

Complications of DKA and HONK

❶Cardiac arrest

- Institute all usual cardiac arrest procedures
- Call diabetes registrar or consultant diabetologist
- Patients may arrest because the severity of their condition has not been appreciated
- Check for hypoglycaemia immediately
- Ensure insulin and fluids (e.g. plasma expanders) have been given
- Give bicarbonate unless pH normal or alkalotic
- DKA causes major potassium shifts—check it
- Ensure infection and other precipitants have been treated
- Even young patients with DKA may have had a myocardial infarct
- Consider aspiration of gastric contents
- Even if the situation appears hopeless carry on full resuscitation for at least twice the usual time to allow some correction of the metabolic issues—remarkable recoveries can occur
- Transfer to ICU if resuscitation successful

Patient not recovering

- Each time you see the patient he/she should have improved clinically.

If not:

- Check treatment: Is IV cannula still in and working? Are infusion lines patent? Have all drugs/fluids all been given according to prescription?
- Check diagnoses: Consider other causes of acidosis. Other cause(s) of DKA/HONK. Missed infection? Silent myocardial infarct?
- Further events (e.g. silent myocardial infarct or stroke).
- Additional new or existing diagnoses.

Hypoglycaemia

- Common and dangerous
- Caused by over-enthusiastic insulin infusion
- Aim for glucose fall of no more than 4–6 mmol/l
- In DKA infuse glucose when glucose <12 mmol/l until blood ketones <0.5 mmol/l

Cerebral oedema

- Needs ICU/HDU
- Can be fatal
- Has been linked to use of concentrated bicarbonate solutions, over-rapid fall of glucose, excessive use of hypotonic electrolyte infusions
- Signs/symptoms:
  - headache
  - drowsiness
  - irritability
  - bradycardia
  - hypertension
  - slowing of respiratory rate
  - reduced Glasgow coma scale
  - neurological signs (e.g. cranial nerve abnormalities, papilloedema, seizures)
  - hypoxia
  - respiratory arrest
- Management:
  - slow insulin infusion rate.
  - give mannitol
  - get consultant diabetologist help
  - transfer to ICU

Persistent hypotension

- Consider ICU/HDU
- Too little fluid—or not enough to overcome glycosuric effect.
- May be due to cardiac dysfunction, including silent myocardial infarct
- Is it solely DKA? Consider lactic or renal acidosis
- Consider septic shock
- Consider excessive/persistent hypotensive medication or overdose of any drug

Pulmonary aspiration

- Needs ICU/HDU
- Why did you not insert nasogastric tube before!
- Has patient's risk of aspiration changed since your initial assessment because of vomiting with impaired gag reflex (stroke, reduced conscious level), or gastric retention and massive vomiting
- Management:
  - oxygen
  - empty stomach via nasogastric tube
  - vigorous chest physiotherapy and suction as appropriate
  - antibiotics (e.g. cephalosporin and metronidazole)

Pulmonary oedema

- Needs ICU/HDU
- Too much fluid, too fast
- Cardiac disease—new or existing
- Early ARDS (see below)
- Low albumin (patient very ill or prolonged illness)
- Management:
  - slow or stop IV infusion
  - consider diuretics or cardiac support medication
  - may need non-invasive or invasive ventilation

Adult respiratory distress syndrome (ARDS)

- Needs ICU/HDU
- Hypoxia and crackles in very sick patient
- Usually patient obviously very ill on admission and already on ICU
- Requires ventilation
- High mortality

Thromboembolism

- Dehydrated sugary patients have hypercoaguable blood and don't move much
- Are you giving enough fluid?
- Patient should have been on prophylactic low molecular weight heparin
- Increase this to treatment dose if safe in HONK and for proven thromboembolism

Rhabdomyolysis

Can occur after HONK and cause renal failure.

Fetal distress/death

In pregnant women with DKA obtain obstetric opinion as soon as initial resuscitation is done. There is a risk of fetal death in maternal DKA.

A fetus of viable age should be monitored as it may need to be delivered if the fetal heart slows unduly. However, the risk of *any* surgery in an acidotic patient is huge, and the mother must be resuscitated and her pH improved before any surgery can be contemplated.

The next stage

- Review usual diabetes treatment. Is it the right treatment for this patient? Did the treatment contribute to the DKA/HONK?
- Change glucose-lowering treatment if it has been inappropriate.
- In patients on very-long-acting insulin (e.g. glargine) some diabetologists continue a reduced dose throughout with mild DKA. This speeds return to normal treatment but may cause later hypoglycaemia as it must be given subcutaneously and therefore could be absorbed later than expected. Care needed.
- Start SC insulin. An episode of DKA demands long-term insulin treatment in most patients. Some patients with HONK may return to oral hypoglycaemics.
- Elucidate cause (gather evidence from patient, relatives, health professionals inside and outside hospital, social services).
- Once the patient is recovering, the problem (DKA) and its cause must be fully explained and steps taken to prevent recurrence.
- Note that the DKA may have been precipitated by inappropriate insulin reduction by a health care professional who should be identified and constructively educated.

Follow-up

- Every patient admitted with DKA must be followed by the specialist diabetes service.
- All such patients should be seen by a DSN.
- Follow-up appointment intervals vary according to the patient and local arrangements, but a month is reasonable.
- African Caribbean patients may have ketosis-prone type 2 diabetes (📖 p.16) and about half will subsequently be able to manage on diet and oral hypoglycaemic agents for some years.

Prevention of DKA

- Education of patients and staff.
- Monitor glucose and adjust treatment.
- If ill—never stop insulin, monitor glucose, monitor ketones, ask for help.
- Address psychological problems.
- Plan surgery.
- Plan pregnancy.
- Treat infection promptly and fully.
- Identify high-risk patients—previous DKA, brittle diabetes, youthful non-attenders. The DSN should keep in touch with them.
- Always admit vomiting type 1 diabetics unless you or the patient are very experienced

DKA/HONK in children <16 yrs of age

- Diagnostic features are similar in adults and children.
- HONK is rare but may occur in African Caribbean teenagers.
- Treatment of DKA in children demands specialist paediatric expertise.
- Contact on-call paediatric registrar or consultant paediatrician immediately.
- Guidelines for the management of DKA in children can be found at: http://www.bsped.org.uk/professional/guidelines/docs/BSPEDDKAApr04.pdf

Summary

- DKA and HONK are potentially fatal.
- DKA and HONK are usually preventable.
- The most common cause is infection.
- DKA and HONK are medical emergencies requiring immediate treatment—door to needle time <15 min.
- DKA and HONK are the product of insulin deficiency and tissue (especially fat) response to this.
- Vomiting in insulin-treated patients is a key symptom of DKA.
- Blood ketones ≥3 mmol/l = DKA.
- DKA and HONK. Infuse IV insulin, 0.9% saline, then potassium, and ultimately glucose.
- HONK—start treatment as for DKA but beware greater insulin sensitivity and greater dehydration. Sodium usually rises.
- Treat precipitating cause
- Monitor the patient very closely, both clinically and with bedside or laboratory tests
- The most common cause of failure to respond to treatment is failure of treatment to be given.
- Complications of DKA/HONK include cardiac arrest, hypoglycaemia, cerebral oedema, hypotension, aspiration, pulmonary oedema, ARDS, thromboembolism, rhabdomyolysis, fetal distress/death. Many of these complications are preventable.
- Start or restart insulin therapy carefully to avoid a return of DKA/HONK
- Educate patient and staff to prevent recurrence
- Ensure diabetologist follow-up

Further reading

ABCD guidelines for the management of hyperglycaemic emergencies in adults. Available online at: http://www.diabetologists.org.uk/Position%20Paper%20on%20Hyperglycaemic%20Emergencies.pdf

Chapter 13

Exercise

Prevention of type 2 diabetes

Regularly supervised exercise programmes ± dietary advice has been shown in international studies to reduce the risk of developing type 2 diabetes in people with impaired glucose tolerance (*BMJ* 2007; **334**:299–302). This effect was as good as, or better than, giving metformin. Successful participants required frequent (e.g. every 1–2 months) individualized advice and encouragement from physical trainers ± dietitians and other health care professionals.

Exercise is good for people with diabetes

Regular exercise:
- improves blood glucose balance in both type 1 and type 2 diabetes although the benefit appears greater in the latter
- increases insulin sensitivity
- improves glucose tolerance
- aids weight reduction.
- reduces the risk of coronary heart disease
- makes many people feel good.

Exercise, insulin, and glucose

In a non-diabetic, exercising muscles first use their stored glycogen. Glucose is then taken up from the bloodstream as required for continued exercise. As the blood glucose concentration falls, pancreatic insulin release is reduced, glucagon rises, and glucose is released from the liver glycogen stores to 'top up' the blood glucose concentration. If CHO has been eaten, this will be absorbed into the bloodstream and insulin will be released, if necessary, to store it in the liver and/or facilitate its use by the exercising muscles. Liver glycogenolysis will cease while the glucose derived from the meal is distributed. However, if exercise continues and the blood glucose level falls, insulin release will fall and liver glycogenolysis will again release glucose into the circulation.

This process can still occur in a person with diabetes treated by diet alone, and to a large extent in patients being treated with metformin. However, as soon as sulphonylureas or, particularly, insulin injections are introduced, the fine tuning of glucose balance in exercise is disturbed.

The effects on blood glucose and other biochemistry, such as lipids, in a person with insulin-treated diabetes who exercises depend on the amount of circulating insulin and how much food has been eaten. The crucial difference between the diabetic and non-diabetic athlete is that there is no fine on–off control of insulin release.

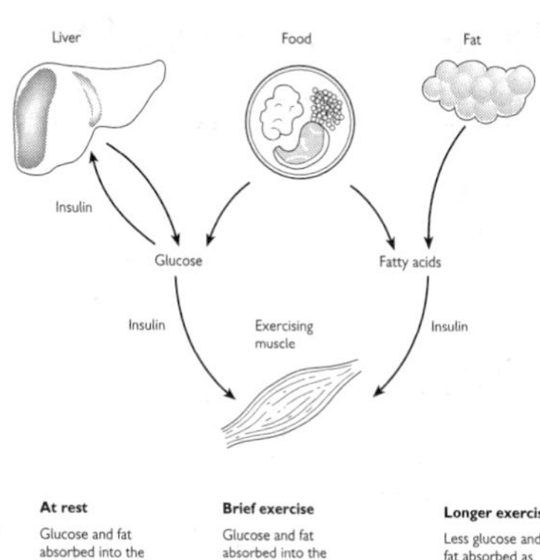

	At rest	Brief exercise	Longer exercise
Food	Glucose and fat absorbed into the blood	Glucose and fat absorbed into the blood	Less glucose and fat absorbed as some blood diverted to muscle
Insulin normal	Released from the pancreas according to blood glucose	Less insulin released from pancreas as glucose falls	
diabetic	Released from the injection site	More released from injection site as circulation to muscles and skin increases	
Liver	Stores glucose as glycogen*	Starts to release glucose ^	Releases a lot of glucose ^
Fat	Stores fatty acids*	Starts to release fatty acids ^	Releases a lot of fatty acids ^
Muscle	Stores glucose as glycogen*	Converts glycogen to glucose for energy ^	Takes up glucose and fatty acids and uses them for energy*

* Needs insulin
^ Blocked by insulin

Fig. 13.1 Exercise, food, and insulin.

Someone who is insulin-deficient is likely to have a high blood glucose. Exercise will further increase the blood glucose as the stress hormone response releases glucose from the liver. As exercise continues, the muscles take up glucose from the bloodstream. However, this effect is unlikely to outweigh that of hepatic glucose release. Lipolysis, which occurs in prolonged exercise to provide free fatty acids as an additional fuel, may be followed by ketone formation in insulin deficiency. Any food eaten will merely serve to exacerbate the hyperglycaemia. Thus exercise may worsen hyperglycaemia and promote ketosis in an insulin-deficient person.

Hypoglycaemia may ensue in someone who has a large subcutaneous reservoir of injected insulin. As before, the exercising muscles will use their stored glycogen. The presence of insulin ensures good glucose uptake by the exercising muscles. However, high plasma insulin concentrations inhibit glucose release from the liver, further reducing the blood glucose concentration. Hypoglycaemia rapidly ensues. This situation can be prevented by eating CHO which will be absorbed and top up the blood glucose level as exercise proceeds.

In patients taking sulphonylureas, the drugs enhance pancreatic insulin release, as well as improving tissue glucose uptake. Thus they may produce hyperinsulinaemia and can cause exercise-induced hypoglycaemia.

Which form of exercise and how much?

To derive full benefit from exercise it should be regular—at least 20–30 min on at least 5 days each week. The aim should be to keep the heart rate within the training zone, i.e. between 60% and 85% of the maximum heart rate (Table 13.1). The heart rate should not exceed the maximum, which is calculated by subtracting the age from 220. Two or three 10 min episodes are nearly as good as one longer one. Obese patients who are not reducing calorie intake may have to do double this exercise requirement to lose weight.

Exercise does not have to be weight-lifting or marathon running. A brisk walk will maintain the pulse rate within the training zone. Furthermore, exercise which does not reach the training zone, such as gardening or gentle swimming, can be helpful in improving well-being and maintaining a full range of joint movement.

Exercise may be aerobic (e.g. running, swimming, dancing) or resistance (e.g. weight-training) or a combination of these. Either form of exercise has been shown to improve glucose levels, but aerobic physical exercise is likely to reduce the HbA_{1c} more.

Table 13.1 The training zone

Age (years)	Heart rate (beats/min)		
	Training zone		Maximum
	60%	85%	
15	123	174	205
20	120	170	200
25	117	166	195
30	114	162	190
35	111	157	185
40	108	153	180
45	105	149	175
50	102	145	170
55	99	140	165
60	96	136	160
65	93	132	155
70	84	119	140
75	87	123	145
80	84	119	140

To derive greatest benefit from exercise the heart rate should be within the training zone for at least 20 min on most days. First aim for the lower end of the training zone (60%), or lower in someone who has not exercised recently. Do not use for people with autonomic neuropathy.

Helping people with diabetes to exercise safely

Use common sense. Start gradually. The exercise activity(ies) chosen must be practical and fit in with everyday life in all seasons. Patients should seek expert advice (e.g. a trainer or join a club/gym) for activities that are out of the ordinary for them. If it hurts, stop.

Controlling the blood glucose

Diet-treated diabetes

No special measures need to be taken regarding blood glucose balance if the glucose is well controlled on diet alone.

Non-insulin-treated diabetes

Metformin alone usually presents no problem, although if insulin sensitivity increases and weight is lost, the metformin dose may be reduced. Exenatide and sitagliptin should not require adjustment for exercise as the insulin release they promote is stimulated by glucose. These drugs are new agents and experience of vigorous exercise when on them is limited.

Unexpected or vigorous exercise in patients taking sulphonylureas occasionally causes hypoglycaemia, which may be prolonged. In this case, the person should check his/her blood glucose during or after exertion and eat some CHO if necessary. If hypoglycaemia ensues, the person should eat a series of small snacks until he/she is sure that the blood glucose has stabilized. The blood glucose must be checked regularly for at least 24 hr.

If the exercise is planned, it is better to reduce the dose of sulphonylurea before the exertion so that hypoglycaemia is prevented. If too much CHO is eaten to cover the exertion, excess insulin will be released and this may compound any late exercise-induced hypoglycaemia. If the exercise is regular, a long-term reduction in sulphonylurea dosage may be possible.

Insulin-treated diabetes

Exercise is a common cause of hypoglycaemia. It is preferable to reduce the insulin acting during the exertion (and afterwards if exercise is vigorous or prolonged exercise). Eating extra can result in an increase in weight, especially in type 2 diabetes.

In general, advise 15–30 g glucose before exercise. If the exercise is very vigorous, unusual, or hazardous take about 15–45 g every 30–60 mins and afterwards. Tailor advice to the individual patient and situation. Encourage blood glucose testing as the symptoms of hypoglycaemia can be hidden by the sweating, tachycardia, and breathlessness of exercise. For prolonged exertion it is theoretically helpful to eat some high-fibre CHO as well.

For planned exercise, the insulin acting during the time of exertion should be reduced beforehand. If the extent of the exertion is unknown (as in learning a new sport) it is better to reduce the insulin by about 20–40% for the first few occasions. Inject the insulin away from any exercising muscle. Take care to avoid the risk of hypoglycaemia while swimming or driving home. The next meal should contain extra high-fibre CHO to prevent subsequent hypoglycaemia. The next dose of insulin may also need to be reduced after vigorous or endurance exercise. Hypoglycaemia may occur up to 24 hr after exercise.

There is no simple calculation for the amount of insulin dose reduction and the amount of extra CHO. Each person has to work it out for themselves. The key is finger-prick blood glucose estimation. This should be done four times a day (before each meal and before bed) and also immediately before and after the exercise until it has become familiar. As people train regularly, they will need less extra food for exercise and less insulin reduction.

Glucose control in dangerous activities

This applies mainly to people on insulin injections. In some sports (e.g. subaqua diving, hang-gliding) a person could die if he/she becomes confused or comatose. Other sports involve taking responsibility for others, as either coach or leader, or in sharing safety (e.g. belaying a climber). There is little or no margin for error and the individual must ensure that hypoglycaemia will not occur.

Reduce the insulin dose which acts during the activity by 20% (50% if hypoglycaemia prone or no warning of hypoglycaemia). The last meal before the activity should contain more CHO than usual. If there has been a long preparation time for the activity, and especially if this in itself has involved exercise (e.g. rowing out to a diving point, walking to the base of a climbing route), an appropriate double snack should be eaten. Before starting the hazardous activity the blood glucose must be checked. If it is <6 mmol/l an additional snack must be eaten and the blood glucose should be rechecked after 15–30 min. Immediately before starting the activity (e.g. just before putting foot to rock) 15 g glucose should be eaten. The aim is for the activity to take place on a rising glucose from gut absorption which is independent of insulin concentration.

The same principles can be applied for situations in which hypoglycaemia could let the person down (e.g. in a competition) or let others down (e.g. team games). The difficulty lies in balancing freedom from hypoglycaemia, safety, and impairment of performance because of hyperglycaemia. Each sportsperson has to spend some time experimenting for themselves. Start sugary and then fine tune with experience.

There are few activities which are unsuitable for people with diabetes. Only patients who are competent and confident in glucose self-management and who have informed support from a diabetologist should undertake high-risk activities such as scuba diving or ice climbing. Unplanned 'one-off' holiday activities are particularly dangerous as equipment and supervision are very variable, food may be unfamiliar, and communication with supervisors may be difficult (📖 Chapter 444).

Fit to exercise?

Doctors and nurses are frequently asked to confirm fitness to exercise. In general, if the patient can walk briskly without problems they are usually fit to start an exercise programme. Areas to consider are:

- hypoglycaemia awareness or not (see advice above about glucose safety)
- heart
- feet
- eyes
- autonomic neuropathy.

Heart

- No symptoms. As diabetes may modify cardiac symptoms these cannot necessarily be used as a guide to the degree of exercise that can be undertaken. The American Diabetes Association (ADA) state (2007): 'A graded exercise test with electrocardiogram (ECG) monitoring should be seriously considered before undertaking aerobic physical activity with intensity exceeding the demands of everyday living (more intense than brisk walking) in previously sedentary diabetic individuals whose 10-year risk of a coronary event is likely to be ≥10%'. In practice, this includes many patients. A simpler and more practical view may be to do exercise ECGs on all those aged >40 yrs who wish to perform exercise more strenuous than brisk walking or more strenuous than that individual's usual maximum exercise level. Discuss this with your local diabetologist and cardiologist.
- Known cardiac disease. Ask a cardiologist's advice. Appropriate exercise is good for people with coronary heart disease, but only with the advice of a cardiologist after any treatment required has been instituted.

Foot

- All patients should have appropriate footwear for their chosen activity. Ask the podiatrist if advice is needed.
- Neuropaths must be careful to avoid rubs and blisters, and increased callus formation on pressure areas.
- Charcot feet—avoid weight-bearing exercise. Risk of multiple fractures.
- Foot ulcers—avoid weight-bearing exercise.
- Patients with peripheral vascular disease should keep their feet warm in cold weather.
- Seek and treat athletes' foot.

Eyes

Unstable proliferative retinopathy is a contraindication to exercise. Exertion could cause blindness from vitreous haemorrhage. Arrange treatment and follow the ophthalmologist's advice. Especial care with resistance exercise.

What to tell a trainer or exercise supervisor

Patients should tell anyone supervising their exercise that they have diabetes. If they are on non-insulin treatments there are unlikely to be any significant issues. Insulin-treated patients should explain that they have adjusted their diet and treatment for the exercise and that problems are unlikely. However, they should ensure that the supervisor knows the symptoms of hypoglycaemia and where the patient's glucose is kept.

Most national sporting bodies are aware of diabetes and will have guidance. Diabetes UK can also help.

Summary

- Regular exercise can prevent diabetes in people with impaired glucose tolerance.
- Regular exercise is good for people with diabetes.
- Patients on insulin (and sometimes sulphonylureas) should reduce their medication for planned exercise. They need to eat extra CHO to fuel exercise.
- Take care to avoid hypoglycaemia, especially in high-risk sports and in those with poor warning.
- Check cardiac fitness for exercise more vigorous than brisk walking.
- Give appropriate advice to patients with diabetic tissue damage.
- Consult Diabetes UK for further advice about individual sports.

Chapter 14

Diabetic tissue damage

Diabetic tissue damage

In most people's minds diabetes is sugar trouble. Yet most of the problems of diabetes arise not from the ups and downs of the glucose concentration, but from its many tissue complications. Diabetes is a chronic multi-system disorder of which one manifestation is hyperglycaemia.

The tissue complications of diabetes are preventable and although we still have much to learn about the causes of diabetic tissue damage, we can at least work on reducing the damage due to factors we have identified. Diabetes is for life. The quality of that life and its extent will be largely determined by the development of tissue damage and its extent.

Diabetic tissue damage is usually divided into that which occurs only (or predominantly) in diabetes and that which is more common in people with diabetes but does occur in others.

Microvascular disease—thickening of the basement membrane of capillaries causing leakage or blockage to the transfer of nutrients and waste substances—is virtually specific to diabetes. This is associated with retinopathy, nephropathy, and neuropathy. These and other changes, such as cheiroarthropathy and dermopathy, may be linked to glycosylation of proteins (📖 p.124).

Macrovascular disease—atherosclerosis—is common in the non-diabetic population, but is much more frequent in people with diabetes.

Life expectancy

WHO has estimated that in the year 2000 there were 2.9 million excess deaths among people with diabetes, equivalent to 5.2% of all deaths. Having diabetes shortens patients' lives by about 8 yrs, depending on age at onset and other risk factors. However, the mortality and morbidity of diabetes is improving with modern care.

Type 1 diabetes

- In 23 752 diabetic patients '62% of male deaths and 75% of female deaths would not have occurred if the general population mortality rates had applied' (*Diabetic Med* 1999; **16**:459–65).
- Standardized mortality ratio (SMR) 4. 0 men, 2.7 women (compared with non-diabetic population SMR 1.0).
- Cardiovascular death can occur at any age but is more common if longer duration of diabetes.
- Renal death is a more common cause in shorter duration.

Type 2 diabetes

- About double the mortality of the non-diabetic population.
- In an 8 yr study follow-up after diagnosis of diabetes (mean age 56 yrs) one in five of all UKPDS patients had died (*BMJ* 1998; **317**:703–12).
- Older patients (diagnosed at any age) have an excess mortality of 9% compared with non-diabetic patients (*Arch Intern Med 2007;* **167:921–7)**
- Patients diagnosed >age 60 yrs have only a slightly worse mortality rate than the non-diabetic population (*Age Ageing* 2006; **35**:463–8).
- Mortality is inversely related to educational attainment (*Diabetes Care* 2003; **26**: 1650).

As most medical and nursing training relates to body systems, the following discussion of tissue damage is considered by system rather than by aetiology. In most instances symptoms are a late feature of diabetic complications. By the time the patient is aware of a problem it may be too late to treat it. Therefore a major part of diabetes care is screening patients for evidence of tissue damage and for risk factors of tissue damage (Box 14.1).

Table 14.1 Tissue complications of diabetes

Eyes	Retinopathy, maculopathy, cataract, squint
Ears	Deafness
Smell and taste	Reduced
Kidneys	Nephropathy, renal failure, chronic pyelonephritis
Nervous system	Peripheral neuropathy, autonomic neuropathy, mononeuropathy, proximal motor neuropathy
Heart	Ischaemic heart disease, cardiac failure
Lungs	Impaired function
GI tract	Oral and dental problems, dysmotility.
Liver	Non-alcoholic fatty liver
Peripheral vascular disease	Especially legs
Feet	Ulcer, infection, gangrene, amputation
Brain	Stroke, transient ischaemic attack
Skin and soft tissue	Dermopathy, necrobiosis lipoidica, mastopathy
Ligaments	Dupuytren's contracture, cheiroarthropathy
Skeletal system	Charcot joint, osteopenia, osteosclerosis
Cancer	Increased risk of some cancers

Box 14.1 Prevention of diabetic tissue damage

- Treatment must be safe and practical for each patient
- Help people with diabetes to learn how to work with the diabetes team:
  - to reduce the risk of developing diabetic tissue damage
  - to recognize tissue damage early, if present
  - to slow deterioration of existing tissue damage
- Reduce risk factors
- Stop smoking
- Exercise regularly
- Keep BP <130/80 without hypotension
- Keep $HbA1_c$ between 6.0% and 6.5% without hypoglycaemia 📖 p.125
- Keep BMI between 18.5 and 25 kg/m^2
- Keep cholesterol <4 mmol/l, LDL cholesterol <2 mmol/l
- Keep triglyceride <1.7 mmol/l
- Treat microalbuminuria
- Avoid added salt

See Chapter 3 for detailed discussion of rise factors and targets

Cardiovascular disease

- Heart
- Hypertension
- Peripheral vascular disease
- Cerebrovascular disease

Cardiovascular disease is two to three times as common in people with diabetes as in the general population. Premenopausal diabetic women are about as likely to have a myocardial infarct as diabetic men. Diabetic men are more than twice as likely and diabetic women more than three times as likely to die from cardiovascular causes as the general population. About 70% of people with diabetes die from cardiovascular disease (mostly coronary artery disease).

Advanced glycosylation end-products (AGE) are implicated in atherogenesis in diabetes. Raised insulin levels are associated with increased cardiovascular risk. Diabetes is a procoagulant state. Additionally, diabetic patients have dyslipidaemia and hypertension, and may be obese.

Prevention and reduction of cardiovascular risk

People with diabetes should pay attention to the same risk factors as those without diabetes. It seems likely that all these risk factors have a more detrimental effect on people with diabetes. The main risk factors are smoking, hypertension, obesity, and hyperlipidaemia.

Glucose

It used to be thought that glucose concentrations were not directly linked with large vessel disease. However, the DCCT (📖 p.39) showed a reduction in plasma cholesterol concentrations in the intensively treated patients and a trend towards less cardiovascular disease in those with near-normoglycaemia. In UKPDS (📖 p.39) patients with intensive glucose control on metformin had a lower risk of fatal myocardial infarct than these on conventional glucose control. However, the sulphonylurea and insulin groups did not show a significant reduction in cardiovascular events with intensive glucose lowering. More detailed studies in patients with cardiovascular disease have shown that outcome is worse with hyperglycaemia, e.g. sugary patients have larger myocardial infarcts.

Smoking

Smoking shortens the life of a person with diabetes by about 6 yrs. Diabetic smokers have a similarly increased risk of cardiovascular disease to non-diabetics. Overweight hypertensive diabetic women who are taking oral contraceptives are at especially high risk of cardiovascular complications. Studies have also shown that smokers were more likely to have nephropathy and retinopathy than non-smokers.

Obesity

Obesity is common in people with type 2 diabetes and can occur in insulin-treated patients, especially if they are eating to keep up their insulin. To help patients lose weight safely, reduce their glucose-lowering treatment as they start their reduced calorie diabetes diet. Patients must be aware of the risk of hypoglycaemia. Some patients on insulin or oral hypoglycaemic drugs may be able to stop them if they lose weight. Patients treated by diet alone may need medication if they gain weight. Beware of the weight loss of uncontrolled diabetes. Remember to measure the patient's height—it is often forgotten (📖 p.41).

Hypertension

📖 p.36

Hyperlipidaemia

Glucose is not the only biochemical problem in diabetes. Both cholesterol and triglyceride may be raised. In addition, lipoproteins are glycosylated and this process may be involved in atherogenesis. Hyperlipidaemia can be defined as follows:

- Cholesterol > 4.0 mmol/l
- HDL cholesterol < 0.9 mmol/l
- LDL cholesterol > 2.0 mmol/l
- Triglyceride > 1.7 mmol/l

These values relate to a sample after an 8 hr fast (Joint British Societies' Guidelines on the Prevention of Cardiovascular Disease in Clinical Practice: Risk Assessment (JBS2), British Heart Foundation 2006). (Joint British Societies: British Cardiovascular Society, British Hypertension Society, Diabetes UK, Heart UK, Primary Care Cardiovascular Society, The Stroke Association)

Triglyceride

The main lipid abnormality in diabetes is hypertriglyceridaemia. Plasma triglyceride is elevated in about one in three patients with type 2 diabetes. Patients with type 1 diabetes who are insulin deficient also have high triglycerides. A few patients have extremely high plasma triglyceride levels and their serum is milky with chylomicrons. These patients may have eruptive xanthomata, abdominal pain, and pancreatitis, with malaise, tingling, and impaired cerebral function.

Cholesterol

Total cholesterol is more likely to be raised in type 2 than in type 1 patients. HDL cholesterol has the same inverse relationship to coronary heart disease and other conditions due to atheroma as in non-diabetic people. HDL cholesterol is more often reduced in women with type 2 diabetes than in men. The abnormalities related to HDL cholesterol are more closely linked with triglyceride than with total cholesterol

Seek and treat secondary causes of hyperlipidaemia

- Factors affecting triglyceride levels:
  - glucose control
  - alcohol
  - obesity
  - liver disease
  - chronic kidney disease
  - nephrotic syndrome
  - thiazides
  - beta-blockers
  - myeloma
- Factors affecting cholesterol levels:
  - hypothyroidism
  - cholestasis
  - nephrotic syndrome
  - eating disorders
  - diuretics

Raised triglyceride and reduced HDL cholesterol (<1 mmol/l) increase the risk of CVD. For triglyceride levels >1.7 mmol/l, institute rigorous blood glucose control and reduction of alcohol intake. If the triglyceride is between 2.3 and 5 mmol/l use atorvastatin or 80 mg doses of simvastatin. Triglyceride levels >5 mmol/l are unlikely to respond to a statin so use a fibrate e.g. fenofibrate. Monitor liver function with both statins and fibrates.

Cardiovascular screening

There is less consensus about the timing and frequency of some screening for cardiovascular disease and its risk factors in diabetes than there is for microvascular disease. What is suggested is a compromise. (See *National Service Frameworks for Coronary Heart Disease* 2000.)

Box 14.2 Cholesterol lowering

Give simvastatin or atorvastatin (or follow local statin protocol) to:

- All diabetic patients aged > 40 yrs*
- Diabetic patients 18-40 yrs with any of:
  - retinopathy
  - nephropathy
  - HbA_{1c} >9%
  - BP >130/80
  - Total cholesterol ≥6 mmol/l
  - Waist circumference
    >102 cm in men (>92 cm in Asian men)
    >88 cm in women (>78 cm in Asian women
  - Triglyceride >1.7 mmol/l (fasting), >2.0 mmol/l (random)
  - HDL cholesterol <1.0 mmol/l (men), <1.2 mmol/l (women)
  - Family history of premature CVD in first-degree relative

Add ezetimibe if cholesterol still above target despite full-dose statin or unable to tolerate statin or increased dosage.

Joint British Societies *Heart* 2005; **91**(suppl V):v1–52

* NICE (2008) advocates statin if CV risk >20% 10 yrs

(See www.dtu.ox.ac.uk/index.php?maindoc=/riskengine)

**Consider fibrate 📖 p.275 see Chapter 3

Heart

People with diabetes are more likely to have coronary atheroma than the general population. A third of newly diagnosed type 2 diabetic patients will have an abnormal ECG at diagnosis. They also have cardiac small vessel disease with basement membrane thickening as in the retina. This probably contributes to the higher frequency of cardiomyopathy in people with diabetes, with or without coronary artery disease.

Checklist on diagnosis of diabetes check:

- Symptoms of cardiovascular disease (e.g. angina, intermittent claudication)
- Smoking history
- Family history of heart disease
- Height and weight
- BP
- Pulse
- Heart size, sounds, and evidence of failure
- Peripheral pulses
- ECG if hypertensive or evidence of cardiac disease (some doctors would screen all those with type 2 diabetes)
- Chest X-ray if smoker, hypertensive, evidence of respiratory or cardiac disease, tuberculosis prone
- Fasting cholesterol and triglyceride

Screen patients annually (or as stated) thereafter

- Cardiovascular symptoms
- Smoking
- Family history—new events?
- Weight (assess in relation to height)
- BP
- Peripheral pulses
- Cardiac examination if symptoms, otherwise every 5 yrs
- ECG if symptoms and every 5 yrs routinely
- Cholesterol and triglyceride (2 monthly if elevated, every year if normal)

Angina

- Some patients will present with classic symptoms of angina pectoris
- Silent ischaemia is common
- In autonomic neuropathy the symptoms may be different or less pronounced, and there is a greater likelihood of silent ischaemia
- Have a low threshold for requesting exercise ECGs or thallium scans
- As these patients may be difficult to diagnose and treat, seek a cardiologist's advice early
- If the exercise ECG is positive it should be followed by coronary angiography
- Diabetic patients usually have diffuse and extensive coronary atheroma

Acute coronary syndrome (ACS)

This includes acute myocardial infarction (AMI), both ST elevation (STEMI) and non-ST elevation (NSTEMI).

General

- Have a very low threshold for urgent hospital referral with any symptom which might indicate AMI or acute coronary syndrome.
- Presenting symptoms may be atypical, including painless breathlessness or acute malaise or tiredness, pain anywhere in the chest, right arm pain, and chest tenderness as well as traditional presentations.
- About one in four patients with ACS have diabetes (*Arch Intern Med 2004*; **164**:1457–63). As many as half of South Asian ACS patients may have diabetes.
- One in three deaths of diabetic patients are due to AMI.
- The risk is twice to four times greater than that of the general population.
- Patients under 30 yrs old may have AMI.
- Women with diabetes of any age are at risk of AMI, which is less likely to be diagnosed and treated adequately.
- Diabetic patients have a higher mortality from ACS than other patients. In one study, those with NSTEMI had about an 80% increased risk of death within 30 days, and those with STEMI a 40% increased risk (*JAMA* 2007; **298**:765–75).
- It has been suggested that having diabetes is equivalent to having had a myocardial infarct in terms of risk of further cardiac event, but this is disputed.
- Acute hyperglycaemia or DKA may be due to AMI.
- Perform a troponin test in all diabetic inpatients whose condition deteriorates without good cause

Care in hospital

- Give diabetic patients standard treatment for ACS. They may gain even greater benefit than those without diabetes.
- Do not give thrombolytic therapy to patients with unresolved proliferative retinopathy or current vitreous haemorrhage (rare).
- Every patient with ACS should have a fasting blood glucose test.
- Patients with any glucose reading >11 mmol/l should have intensive glucose control using IV insulin infusion with an appropriate concentration of IV glucose depending on fluid needs and eating ability. Monitor and replace potassium as necessary.
- The DIGAMI study (*BMJ* 1997;**314**:1512–15) initially suggested that a year of intensive insulin therapy reduced mortality after AMI. Later studies were not convincing, and patients often suffered hypoglycaemia when this was attempted under non-study conditions
- Control blood glucose with usual medication appropriate to the patient once the acute phase of ACS is over.
- Avoid hypoglycaemia which can cause dysrhythmias or cardiac arrest. This means meticulous blood glucose monitoring, including at 2 a.m. and especially at weekends.

Cardiac failure

- Two to five times more common in people with diabetes than in those without, with or without symptoms of myocardial ischaemia
- Diabetic cardiomyopathy is due to both microvascular disease and ischaemia. There may be interstitial and perivascular fibrosis.
- Hypertension causes left ventricular hypertrophy.
- Silent AMI can cause both impairment of ventricular function and increased risk of dysrhythmia.
- May be preceded by a reduction in left ventricular function which can be found in asymptomatic young people and children with diabetes.
- May have both diastolic and systolic impairment.
- Failure diastolic relaxation of the left ventricle. Reduced ejection fraction on exercise causes exertional dyspnoea.
- Autonomic neuropathy may be associated with inability to raise a tachycardia when appropriate, and dysrhythmia. Postural hypotension may be severe with low cardiac output and diuretic treatment.
- Cardiac failure can cause hyperglycaemia and rising insulin requirements.
- Diuretic treatment of cardiac failure may worsen renal function, especially if there is pre-existing diabetic nephropathy.
- Hepatic congestion may worsen the effects of non-alcoholic steatohepatitis (NASH)—hopefully temporarily.

Treatment of cardiac disease

- Drugs as for non-diabetic patients (see warnings 📖 p.284 on). As cardiac disease is more severe and more likely to prove fatal in people with diabetes it should be managed with greater therapeutic 'aggression' than in non-diabetic people, with earlier intervention including coronary artery bypass grafting if indicated.
- Stop smoking.
- Healthy eating with low salt intake.
- Alcohol <21 units/week men, <14 units/week women.
- Resume appropriate weight for height.
- Exercise safely (📖 p.266).
- Vigorous statin therapy for all unless contraindication to reduce total cholesterol to <4 mmol/l and LDL cholesterol to <2 mmol/l.
- Control hypertension.
- Control hyperglycaemia as this may improve cardiac function.

Hypertension

There is debate about why people with diabetes are about twice as likely to have hypertension as non-diabetic people. Hypertension is found in one in three people with diabetes—or more. As with other tissue damage, hypertension is uncommon in people with newly diagnosed type 1 diabetes but is frequent in those with type 2 diabetes at diagnosis. Hypertension is three times more common in type 2 diabetes than in the non-diabetic population. Rare causes of hypertension (e.g. Cushing's syndrome, phaeochromocytoma, acromegaly) will be found more often in people with diabetes than in the general population. Non-diabetic renal causes should be considered.

Table 14.2 Tests in people with hypertension

Electrolytes
Urate
Creatinine + eGFR
Cholesterol and triglyceride
Full blood count
Urine—microalbumin, microscopy, culture if indicated
ECG (seeking left ventricular hypertrophy; echocardiogram is better but more expensive)
Chest X-ray if clinically indicated
Consider renal ultrasound
(Urinary catecholamines and free cortisol etc. if indicated)

The British Hypertension Society (BHS) (🕮 p.283) advises two or three readings per visit in a seated relaxed patient, taken at monthly intervals over a 4–6 month period before diagnosing hypertension. Always use phase V (disappearance of sound) to determine diastolic pressure. The aim in the general population is BP <140/90. NICE (2008), and hence primary care, targets are <140/80 in uncomplicated diabetic patients and <130/80, in those with kidney, eye or cerebrovascular damage. However, the Joint British Societies (2005) (🕮 p.48) advise <130/80 in diabetic patients, which is more likely to protect the patient from cardiovascular and renal disease. This more rigorous level is harder to achieve and carries greater risk of postural hypotension and side effects of medication. Set a realistic and safe target for each patient (🕮 p.32).

Patients can self-measure BP, although this intervention has not been proven to improve outcome in diabetic patients. They should check the BHS website (http://www.bhsoc.org/blood_pressure_list.stm) for their list of approved devices and follow the instructions with the device meticulously. Self-measurement is not suitable for patients in atrial fibrillation.

Treatment of hypertension

Follow NICE guidelines for management of hypertension but aim for a BP <130/80 if safe (www.nice.org.uk/nicemedia/pdf/CG66diabetesfull-guidelinepdf).

- Drugs
  - Use ACE inhibitor. Use ARB if patient intolerant of ACE inhibitor.
  - African Caribbean: use ACE inhibitor and calcium-channel blocker.
  - Any age or ethnicity:

    BP not controlled—add calcium-channel blocker or thiazide diuretic

    BP not controlled—use ACE inhibitor/ARB with calcium-channel blocker and thiazide diuretic

    BP not controlled—more diuretic or alpha- or beta-blocker.

    Woman of child-bearing potential—advise contraception before treating hypertension. If the patient is planning conception refer to specialist diabetic preconception service. NICE (2008) CG 66 (📖 p.48) advocates using calcium-channel blockers in women who may conceive but CG63 is more cautious as is the BNF. (📖 p. 382. Labetalol is used in pregnancy but does cross the placenta. Methyldopa is not known to be harmful but has multiple long-term side effects.
- Statin for all unless contraindication. Aim for total cholesterol <4 mmol/l, LDL cholesterol <2 mmol/l
- Stop smoking.
- Healthy eating.
- ↓Salt intake.
- Alcohol <21 units/week men, <14 units/week women.
- Regular exercise.
- Resume appropriate weight for height.
- Stress reduction and relaxation.
- Check lying and standing BP and seek symptoms of postural hypotension, especially in neuropathic patients.
- Warn patients on beta-blockers that they may have reduced warning of hypoglycaemia.
- Check concordance. The most common cause of failure to reach the desired target is failure to take the tablets.

Drugs in management and prevention of diabetic cardiovascular disease and hypertension

For all these drugs please read the current BNF and SPCs for full information. They all have extensive lists of interactions and side effects. This section specifically notes issues important in diabetic patients but is not exhaustive.

Angiotensin-converting enzyme (ACE) inhibitors (ARBs if ACE-inhibitor intolerant) are the first-line treatment, followed by calcium-channel antagonists, thiazides, and beta-blockers.

- Avoid all these drugs in pregnancy, and in women of child-bearing potential not using contraception except possibly calcium channel blockers 📖 p.283.
- Avoid all in breastfeeding women.
- Once-daily preparations are more likely to be remembered than multiple-dosage regimens.
- Beware hypotension, particularly postural hypotension, which may be worse in patients with autonomic neuropathy. Ask about postural dizziness or light-headedness, and measure lying and standing BPs.
- ACE inhibitors, beta-blockers, and diuretics can all cause fluid or electrolyte imbalance
- Drug interactions are common. Check them before prescribing.
- ACE inhibitors, beta-blockers, calcium-channel antagonists, and diuretics can cause erectile dysfunction

ACE inhibitors

Captopril, enalapril, fosinopril, lisinopril, perindopril, and ramipril have all been shown to be effective in reducing adverse measures in people with diabetes. The benefits shown with different drugs in different trials in diabetic patients in reducing BP, improving the outcome of AMI, preventing cardiovascular events, and reducing microalbuminuria are likely to be a class effect. However, their licensed indications vary, and at the time of writing the only ACE inhibitors which specifically mention diabetes in their SPCs are ramipril and captopril. This does not mean that other ACE inhibitors cannot be used for hypertension, and treatment of cardiac disease in diabetic patients. However, it seems sensible to use those which have been studied in diabetic patients. Captopril is less commonly used nowadays than other ACE inhibitors.

Ramipril has been studied extensively and the SPC advises that it should be used for reducing the risk of myocardial infarction, stroke, cardiovascular death, or need for revascularization procedures in diabetic patients:

- ≥55 yrs of age

or

- who have one or more of the following clinical findings:
  - hypertension (systolic BP> 160 mmHg or diastolic BP> 90 mmHg)
  - total cholesterol >5.2 mmol/l
  - HDL <0.9 mmol/l
  - current smoker
  - known microalbuminuria
  - clinical evidence of previous vascular disease.

Cautions

- Check U&E pre-treatment and regularly on treatment
- Renal impairment: seek specialist advice before prescribing. Dosage reductions shown on SPCs.
- Beware renal artery stenosis: most likely in hypertensive patients with severe peripheral vascular disease. If BP uncontrolled on three agents consider renal artery stenosis. Danger of renal failure.
- Avoid in aortic stenosis, mitral stenosis and hypertrophic cardiomyopathy.
- First-dose hypotension varies with different agents but is more likely in fluid-depleted patients (e.g. those on diuretics) or in autonomic neuropathy.
- ACE inhibitors can occasionally induce hypoglycaemia in patients on glucose-lowering treatment. Warn patients.

Angiotensin II receptor antagonists

Have also been shown to be of benefit in diabetes (losartan and irbesartan are licensed for nephropathy). They appear to have a better side-effect profile with less likelihood of cough than ACE inhibitors but require the same cautions.

Calcium-channel antagonists

Amlodipine, felodipine, nifedipine (long-acting), and others. Calcium-channel antagonists do not cause fluid, electrolyte, or glucose changes. They do cause vasodilatation, and this may result in headache, flushing, or ankle swelling. Class II agents (such as those above) are less likely to depress cardiac contraction than Class I agents such as verapamil. Avoid these drugs in pregnancy.

Diuretics

Bendroflumethiazide and hydrochlorothiazide have both been shown to be safe and effective in diabetes. Thiazides were used in UKPDS (📖 p.36). Although they may increase blood glucose, this was not a problem and neither was electrolyte disturbance. Measure U&E pre-treatment and regularly thereafter. Diuretics combined with beta-blockers seem particularly likely to cause hypokalaemia in clinical practice. Bendroflumethiazide 2.5 mg is usually sufficient to achieve a hypotensive effect. Thiazides should be used with care in pregnancy (and only in a specialist centre).

Beta-blockers

Not first line. Atenolol was shown to be safe and effective in UKPDS, but has since been shown to be inferior to loasartan in reducing cardiovascular mortality and morbidity in diabetic hypertensive patients (LIFE, RENAAL 📖 p.48)

Cautions

- Warn patients (especially if on insulin) that beta-blockers reduce warning of hypoglycaemia.
- Avoid in patients with asthma or chronic obstructive pulmonary disease,
- Avoid if bradycardia or heart block.
- Avoid in uncompensated heart failure.
- Avoid in severe peripheral vascular disease.
- May cause exertional tiredness, cold extremities, sleep disturbance, and bradycardia.

Aspirin

- Control BP to <145/90.
- Exclude contraindications.
- Prescribe aspirin 75 mg daily post-prandially for the following diabetic patients:
  - all patients >50 yrs old
  - Patients <50 yrs old with significant cardiovascular risk factors

Clopidogrel

Clopidogrel has been shown to reduce CVD rates in diabetic patients. Adjunctive therapy in very-high-risk patients or as alternative therapy in aspirin-intolerant patients should be considered (*Am J Cardiol* 2002; **90**:625–8).

Glycoprotein IIb/IIIa inhibitors

Glycoprotein IIb/IIIa inhibitors have been shown in a meta-analysis to reduce 30-day mortality after non-ST segment ACS (*Circulation* 2001; **104**:2767–71).

Lipid-lowering drugs

The Heart Protection Study (HPS) (*Lancet* 2003; **361**:2005–16) demonstrated convincingly that simvastatin reduced major coronary and vascular events, strokes, and revascularization requirement in people with diabetes regardless of initial lipid values. Similar results were obtained for atorvastatin and pravastatin. Advice at the time of writing is to use the most cost-effective statin initially, moving to atorvastatin if maximum doses are ineffective or not tolerated.

Statins

Atorvastatin, fluvastatin, pravastatin, rosuvastatin, and simvastatin. Simvastatin, pravastatin, and atorvastatin have been used in large lengthy studies which included people with diabetes (📖 p.38). Statins can lower LDL cholesterol by up to 40% with a slight increase in HDL and reduction in triglyceride. Atorvastatin is the most potent triglyceride-reducing statin. Simvastatin at a dose of 80 mg daily can also lower triglyceride. Pravastatin is less likely to interact with warfarin than other statins. These drugs work best if taken before bed.

NICE 2006 recommend the statin with the lowest acquisition cost, taking into account required daily dose and product price per dose.

Diabetic patients who should have statins (see Box 14.2 📖 p.277):

- age over 40 yrs
- age under 40 yrs and
  - microvascular or macrovascular complications
  - HbA_{1c} >9%
  - hypertension
  - metabolic syndrome
  - total cholesterol >4 mmol/l
  - HDL cholesterol <0.9 mmol/l
  - LDL cholesterol >2 mmol/l
  - triglyceride >1.7 mmol/l
  - family history of premature cardiovascular disease.

Precautions for statins and fibrates

- Stop/do not give statins if creatine kinase (CK) >5 times ULN.
- Check liver function before starting statins and at 1 month, 6 months, and 1 yr. Stop/do not give statins if any liver function test >3 times ULN.
- Do not give statins to women of child-bearing potential unless they are using reliable contraception, although cholestyramine has been used in severe hypercholesterolaemia in pregnancy.
- Hyperlipidaemia in transplant patients should be managed by specialist centres, as should familial hypercholesterolaemia

Side effects of statins

Statins are for life. Long-term studies show that there are few side effects. A review (*Am J Cardiol 2006;* **97**(suppl):52–60C) estimated the following incidence per 100 000 person-yrs:

- statin alone—rhabdomyolysis 3.4 (x10 with fibrate)
- myopathy—11
- peripheral neuropathy—12
- liver failure—0.5 (as for general population).

Fibrates

Now second-line agents. Bezafibrate, ciprofibrate, fenofibrate, and gemfibrozil. These drugs reduce both cholesterol and triglyceride. Control glucose first. Use as first-line agents in patients whose genuinely fasting triglyceride is >4.5 mmol/l with or without elevated cholesterol. Also use in those with isolated hypercholesterolaemia who cannot tolerate statins.

They may also be added to statin in patients with raised cholesterol and a triglyceride >2.3 mmol/l,. This increases the risk of rhabdomyolysis and should be done under specialist supervision.

Bile-acid sequestrants

Colestyramine or colestipol. Rarely used nowadays. Use if patients cannot tolerate other agents, or in combination for severe hypercholesterolaemia. Bile-acid sequestrants often cause gastrointestinal side effects and are poorly tolerated. Use in patients with high cholesterol but avoid if triglycerides are raised. Start very cautiously with half a sachet before a meal and increase gradually. Other medication should be taken 1 hr before or 4 hrs after the bile-acid sequestrant. This medication may cause reduction in absorption of fat-soluble vitamins.

Soluble fibre

Ispaghula husk increases soluble fibre in the gut and can reduce cholesterol. It may cause gastrointestinal side effects but can be used as a 'natural' lipid-lowering agent for patients who prefer this or who cannot tolerate other drugs. Ispaghula should be introduced gradually. It may slow glucose absorption and cause hypoglycaemia.

Young diabetic women with hypertension

- Most hypotensive agents are contraindicated in pregnancy.
- Not planning pregnancy—advise reliable contraception while taking hypotensive drugs.
- Planning pregnancy (📖 p.372)—refer immediately to specialist peri-pregnancy diabetes clinic. Methyldopa is usually advised but should be discontinued post-partum as it has long-term adverse effects (e.g. depression).

Peripheral vascular disease

After 20 yrs of diabetes, half of men and two-thirds of women over 60 yrs old have no foot pulses. People with diabetes are 2–4 times as likely to experience intermittent claudication as non-diabetics, and 4–6 times as likely to have an amputation. Up to 50% of people requiring amputation have diabetes.

Screening

- Screen all patients on diagnosis and annually thereafter.
- Check smoking history. Ask about intermittent claudication.
- Look at the feet for evidence of ischaemia and feel the anterior and posterior tibial pulses.
- Measure cholesterol and triglyceride (📖 p.39).

Assessment

Patients may have calf or buttock pain. If the patient has symptoms or absent pulses, check with a Doppler probe if you have one. Palpate the popliteal and femoral pulses and listen for femoral bruits.

Warning signs

- Gradually worsening symptoms. Refer the patient to a vascular surgeon.
- Rest pain. Telephone the diabetologist or vascular surgeon to arrange for admission under their joint care.
- Critical ischaemia—red, painful. Poor capillary refilling. Same day review—diabetologist or vascular surgeon.
- Acute ischaemia—white/blue, cold, pulseless, painful foot/limb. Transfer to hospital immediately 999 to be seen by the vascular and diabetes teams.
- Gangrene—transfer to hospital same day to be seen by the vascular and diabetes team.
- Any foot problem in addition to peripheral vascular disease (📖 p.325).

Treatment

Insist that the patient stops smoking and vigorously support his/her efforts to do so. Encourage exercise (take care that this does not exacerbate other foot problems such as pressure areas). Encourage a low-fat diet and control hyperlipidaemia if present. Stop beta-blockers. Naftidrofuryl oxalate may relieve symptoms but resolution can occur spontaneously as collaterals open up.

The consequences of peripheral vascular disease are disastrous and all patients should be assessed jointly by a vascular surgeon and diabetologist. Angiography is performed in patients with worsening symptoms or whose limb is at risk and who would be suitable for surgery. It usually reveals multiple stenoses with diffuse distal disease. Angioplasty is sometimes possible and both proximal and distal arterial bypass are being used increasingly. Amputation is discussed on 📖 p.337.

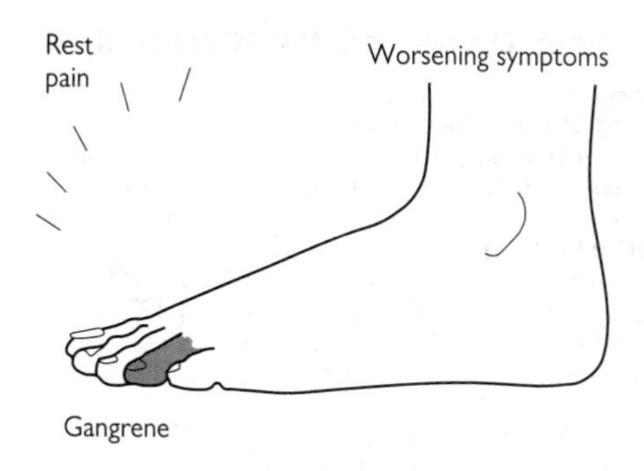

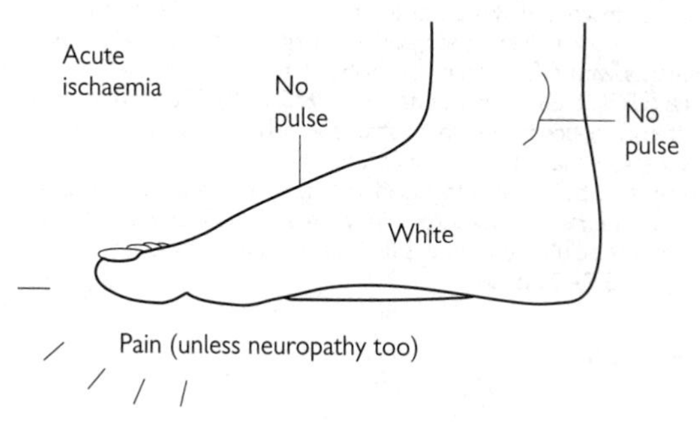

Fig. 14.1 Warning signs of peripheral vascular disease.

Stroke and transient ischaemic attacks

Both transient ischaemic attack (TIA) and stroke are common in people with diabetes. Stroke is four times more likely in women with type 1 diabetes and twice as likely in type 2 diabetes than in non-diabetic women (*Diabetes Care* 2007; **30**:1730–6). The relative risk of stroke in diabetics compared with non-diabetics was 3.70 for men and 4.35 for women (*Stroke* 1997; **28**:1142–6).

Diabetic patients are more likely to die or be disabled after a stroke than those without diabetes (*Diabetes Res Clin Pract 2005;* **69**:293–8). In a European study 'Diabetic patients, compared with those without diabetes, were more likely to have limb weakness ($P < 0.02$), dysarthria ($P < 0.001$), ischemic stroke ($P < 0.001$), and lacunar cerebral infarction ($P = 0.03$)'. They were also more likely to be disabled (*Stroke* 2003; **34**:688–94).

Several studies of people with or without known diabetes have shown that a high admission glucose predicts poor clinical outcome.

'Admitting hyperglycemia was common among patients with acute ischemic stroke and was associated with increased short- and long-term mortality and with increased inpatient charges' (*Neurology 2002;* **59**:67–71).

Patients with fatal stroke had higher HbA_{1c} than those with non-fatal stroke (UKPDS 66 *Diabetes Care 2004;* **27**:201–7). There are current trials on intensive glucose control in stroke—early results show increased risk of hypoglycaemia with insulin infusion.

'Type 2 diabetic patients found to have incidental carotid bruits have >6 times the risk of first stroke in the first 2 yrs than patients without a bruit and should receive intensified management of vascular risk factors'. (*Stroke* 2003; **34**:2145–51.

Management of TIA and stroke in diabetic patients

- Check finger-prick and laboratory glucose to exclude hypoglycaemia which can mimic stroke.
- If glucose <3 mmol/l give 100 ml 10% glucose IV (📖 p.209) and reassess patient.
- Manage as for non-diabetic patients with prompt referral to the specialist stroke team and transfer to the stroke unit. See guidelines:

NICE CG 68 (2008)
www.nice.org.uk/nicemedia/pdf/CG68FullGuideline.pdf.

- Assess for other cardiovascular disease—patients may have had an ACS as well.
- Assess for other diabetic tissue damage—visual problems and neuropathy make rehabilitation more complex.
- Contact diabetes team promptly.
- Control blood glucose with usual medication if oral agents, patient can swallow, glucose <11 mmol/l, and tablet dose can be adjusted to control glucose.
- If unable to swallow or glucose ≥11 mmol/l set up very careful IV insulin infusion sliding scale (📖 p.181) with slow 5% or 10% glucose infusion IV. Monitor finger-prick glucose hourly. Do not allow patient to become hypoglycaemic.
- Glucose control is difficult with nasogastric (NG) feeding. Start with IV sliding scale as above. The patient will need a rate while feed is running and being absorbed, and a rate for no feed.
- Once the patient has stabilized it may be possible to use SC insulin for NG feeding. This should be prescribed and monitored by the diabetes team. Glucose control can be difficult in such patients.
- Pressure sores are more likely in diabetic patients, especially if they have PVD or neuropathy. Be very careful to protect pressure areas.

Eyes

Diabetic eye disease is the most common cause of blindness among people of working age in the Western world.

The Diabetes NSF requires all patients in the UK to be offered digital retinal photographic screening via programmes sufficiently large for quality assurance. Make certain that all your patients are enrolled in the local screening programme and vigorously encourage them to attend. If there is no local scheme, make arrangements for your patients to be seen in the local eye clinic or by local optometrists. Only if you are fully trained in diabetic ophthalmoscopy should you screen the patient's eyes yourself.

Diabetic eye disease is common. After 20 yrs of diabetes virtually every type 1 patient, and most with type 2 diabetes, will have retinopathy. Before this, the incidence depends largely on the age of onset of diabetes and the type of diabetes. Type 1 patients diagnosed under the age of 30 yrs are unlikely to have retinopathy on diagnosis but develop it steadily after ~3 yrs. About one in five patients with maturity-onset type 2 diabetes will have retinopathy at diagnosis.

Table 14.3 Eye problems in diabetes

Orbits	Fungal infections via sinus (rare)
Lids	Ptosis, inflammation
Eye muscles*	Mononeuropathy causing squint
Cornea	Reduced sensitivity, scratches, ulcers
Iris	Rubeosis iridis, neovascular glaucoma
Lens	Cataract, refraction problems
Vitreous	Posterior detachment
Retina	Diabetic retinopathy, lipaemia retinalis, central retinal vein occlusion
Optic nerve*	Swelling (papilloedema), optic atrophy

*Exclude other causes before attributing to diabetes

Adapted from *J Am Optom Assoc* 1990; **61**:533–43, and Ariffin A, Hill RD, Leigh O, 2002. *Diabetes and primary eye care*. Blackwell Scientific, Oxford

Preventing diabetic eye disease

Factors which have been implicated are high blood glucose, hypertension, smoking, the contraceptive pill, and alcohol. High blood glucose and hypertension have definite links; the others are less clear. Diabetic retinopathy may progress rapidly during pregnancy.

Hyperglycaemia

Patients with persistent hyperglycaemia are much more likely to develop diabetic retinopathy than those with near-normal blood glucose levels. Normalization of the blood glucose slows the rate of development of retinopathy. However, it seems sensible to reduce the blood glucose gradually, over ~4–8 weeks, as a sudden return to normal may worsen retinopathy in the short term.

Hypertension

This can cause a retinopathy in its own right, but uncontrolled hypertension may be associated with severe diabetic retinopathy. It has been suggested that lisinopril may reduce retinopathy.

Other factors

Pregnant women must have their eyes screened as soon as pregnancy is diagnosed and again later in pregnancy. It is probably sensible to avoid oral contraceptives in women with a marked background of proliferative retinopathy. Smoking should be stopped anyway, and excess alcohol intake is inadvisable.

Screening

Every patient with diabetes should attend their free annual digital retinal photographic eye check. If they have not been offered one, register them with the local scheme. If there is no local digital photographic scheme, patients' eyes should be examined for diabetic eye disease by a doctor, optometrist, or nurse specifically trained in diabetic eye examination.

- Try to alternate appointments so that someone checks the patient's eyes every 6 months.
- Screen all patients on diagnosis of diabetes and annually thereafter.

Warning symptoms (Table 14.4)

- Deterioration in vision. Check the patient's visual acuity with a Snellen chart. Use pin-hole correction if acuity is worse than 6/6 in either eye.
- If the visual acuity is worse than 6/9 despite pin-hole correction, refer the patient to an ophthalmologist. (NB If the patient is hyperglycaemic, it is advisable to retest the eyes after the blood glucose has returned to normal—hyperglycaemia may cause temporarily blurred vision.) If the pin-hole resolves the impairment of visual acuity, advise the patient to visit an ophthalmic optician or optometrist. Patients should not buy new spectacles until their blood glucose level is stable, preferably near normal.
- 'Floaters', blobs, or wisps across the vision. The patient may have had a vitreous haemorrhage (Fig. 14.2). Examine the eye and refer to an ophthalmologist for urgent assessment.

Table 14.4 Eyes —urgent action (the retinal screening service will make most of the referrals directly)

Problem	Ophthalmologist review
Sudden loss of vision	Same day
Retinal detachment	Same day
Central retinal vein occlusion	Same day
New vessels	Within 1 week
Haemorrhage inside eye (vitreous/ pre-retinal)	Within 1 week
Rubeosis iridis (new vessels on iris)	Within 1 week
Cataract in patients under 30 yrs old	Within 1 week
Macular oedema	Within 1 month
Unexplained fall in visual acuity	Within 1 month
Hard exudates near fovea	Within 1 month
Severe retinopathy	Within 1 month
Dilated/tortuous veins	Within 1 month
Soft exudates	Within 1 month
Unexplained findings	Within 1 month
New squint or eye movement problems	Refer to medical on-call team or neurologist same day

Sources of information include Ariffin A, Hill RD, Leigh O, 2002. *Diabetes and primary eye care*. Blackwell Scientific, Oxford, Kritzinger EE, Taylor KG, 1984. *Diabetic eye disease*. Kluwer Academic, Lancaster, NICE Clinical Guideline E (2002), and Royal College of General Practitioners (2002).

Squint

This may occur acutely, often with associated pain, as a sign of diabetic mononeuropathy. The 3rd, 4th, or 6th nerve may be affected. In 3rd nerve palsy due to diabetes, pupillary function is often intact. The squint may gradually resolve. Beware the coincidental brain tumour. Refer patients with a new squint to the medical on-call team or a neurologist on the same day.

Lens

If the patient has a cataract in either eye and they have impaired visual acuity or you cannot see the retina, refer them to an ophthalmologist. Patients under 30 yrs old with cataracts should be seen by an ophthalmologist that week; acutely developing juvenile cataract can cause blindness within days.

The macula

This is the area of best vision so problems here require urgent treatment.

Macular oedema

If the little pink dot which marks the fovea is blurred or if the whole macula appears swollen, the patient should be seen by an ophthalmologist within a month. Because the patient's problem is at the fovea, using a pin-hole to correct visual acuity may make it worse.

Macular exudates

If there is a ring of hard yellow exudates around or near the macula this may impair the best vision. The patient should be seen by an ophthalmologist within a month.

The optic nerve

Rarely, diabetes can cause optic neuritis visible as papilloedema. Refer to an ophthalmologist but also consider other causes of papilloedema.

The retina

Microaneurysms and blot haemorrhages

These red dots and blots indicate background retinopathy (Fig. 14.2). This will not impede vision but may progress. If visual acuity is impaired despite pin-hole correction, refer to an ophthalmologist. Otherwise, keep it under review every 3–6 months.

Hard exudates

These are shiny, clearly defined, yellowish fatty exudates. It may be difficult to assess the degree of severity. Refer the patient to an ophthalmologist. An urgent referral is needed if these exudates are at the macula (see above).

Dilated veins

A sign of diabetic ophthalmopathy. If the veins also have bulges and extra loops on them this means pre-proliferative retinopathy. Such patients should see an ophthalmologist within a month.

Soft exudates

These are like blobs of cotton wool—pale and poorly defined. Like veins with blobs and extra loops with which they are often seen, soft exudates are usually a sign of pre-proliferative retinopathy and such patients should see an ophthalmologist within a month.

New vessels

These fine tangles of tiny vessels are most often seen near the optic disc but can occur anywhere, including at the periphery of an otherwise normal-looking fundus. Disc vessels are particularly likely to bleed. Neovascularization indicates proliferative retinopathy. Contact the ophthalmologist—the patient should be seen within a week.

(a) CATARACT

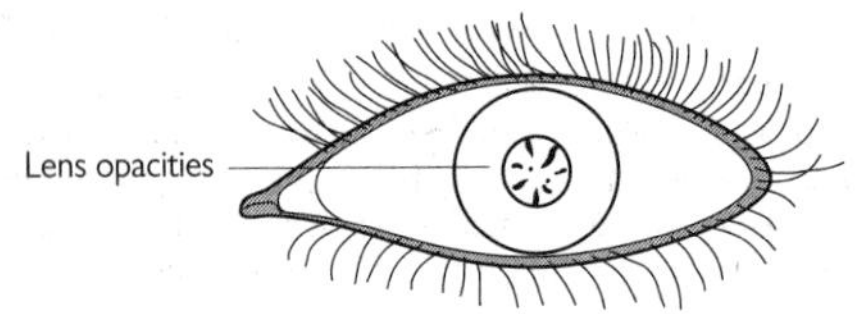

(b) RETINOPATHY

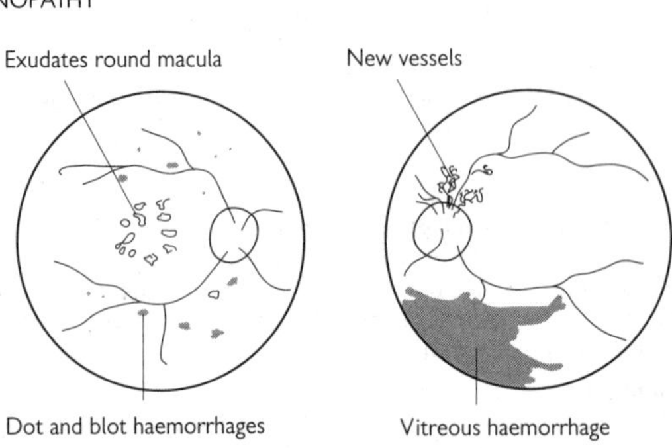

Fig. 14.2 Diabetic eye problems: (a) cataract; (b) retinopathy.

Vitreous haemorrhage

Vitreous haemorrhage (Fig. 14.2) should not happen—it is largely preventable. Bleeding occurs when the fragile new vessels are damaged. Red or black blobs ('tadpoles', 'floaters') or wisps float across the patient's vision. A big bleed may be like a curtain. The haemorrhage may clear, but some people may develop severe permanent visual impairment. Telephone the ophthalmologist for a same-day appointment. The more bleeding, the harder it may be to visualize the bleeding vessels and attempt to photocoagulate them.

Advanced eye disease

Even if the interior of the eye appears completely disorganized with fibrous bands pulling on the retina and detaching it, vitreous surgery and other specialist techniques may be helpful. Rubeosis (i.e. new vessels on the iris causing glaucoma) may occur, but it may be treatable. Such patients should be seen by an ophthalmologist within a week.

Other retinal problems

Thrombosis of retinal arteries and veins, and glaucoma are more common in people with diabetes than in the general population. They all require prompt ophthalmological advice.

Laser photocoagulation

The aim is to induce regression of new vessels and sometimes to seal leaking new vessels. It is also used to treat maculopathy. Laser treatment prevents severe visual impairment in the majority of patients, although the results for maculopathy are less predictable because treatment is close to the macula. Patients should understand that laser treatment may not improve vision but it should stop major deterioration. The treatment is usually given in one or more 30–60 min sessions as an outpatient. Modern equipment is quicker than this. Local anaesthetic and dilating eye drops are used, and the patient has to remain still and concentrate while the treatment is given. Afterwards there is blurring of vision, photophobia, and sometimes eye discomfort or headache. Patients who complain of severe pain should be referred to the eye emergency service.

Hearing, smell, and taste

Hearing

Studies have shown inconsistent results in hearing loss in diabetes. A study using audiometry found no overall association between diabetes and hearing loss, although there was a weak link in a subset (*Diabetes Care* 1998; **21**:1540–4). A Dutch study (*Diabetes Care* 1999; **22**:180) found hearing aids in 24% of diabetic and 7% of non-diabetic patients >55 yrs old. Patients with auditory neuropathy may also have balance and coordination problems.

Two rare forms of diabetes are associated with deafness:

- Wolfram's syndrome (diabetes insipidus, diabetes mellitus, deafness and optic atrophy)—very rare.
- Maternally inherited mitochondrial DNA abnormality causing deafness and diabetes. Affects about 0.1% of the diabetic population. Associated with mitochondrial encephalomyopathy, lactic acidosis, and stroke-like episodes

Patients with hearing loss should always have a formal auditory assessment. It seems sensible to ensure that blood glucose balance is good as this is implicated in other microvascular disease.

Some patients will require a sign language interpreter in clinic. Record this need in their notes.

Smell

The sense of smell may be diminished in diabetes. This appears to be associated with vasculopathy. (*Physiol Behav* 1993; **53**:17–21.)

Taste

A few studies have reported reduction in taste in people with diabetes. 73% of a diabetic group had impaired taste vs 16% of the non-diabetic controls in a French study This appeared to be linked with neuropathy. (*Ann Otolaryngol Chir Cerivicofac* 1989; **106**:455–61)

Kidneys

After 15 yrs of diabetes approx. one in three people with type 1 diabetes will have evidence of diabetic nephropathy. Fewer people with type 2 diabetes are affected (estimates vary). Renal failure is the cause of death in 10–20% of people with type 1 diabetes, but only 1–2 % of those with type 2 diabetes.

Preventing or slowing renal impairment

Hyperglycaemia (📖 p.39)

Persistent hyperglycaemia is linked with increased likelihood of developing nephropathy. Normalization of the blood glucose slows the rate of deterioration of renal function. This may be difficult to achieve without hypoglycaemia in patients with impaired renal function, who should perform frequent HBGM. Most of these patients will end up on insulin although 50% of people with diabetes who develop endstage renal failure have type 2 diabetes.

Hypertension (📖 p.36)

Tight control of hypertension slows deterioration of renal function in nephropaths. This means treating people whose BP would not normally fall into the treatment range for non-diabetic people. In patients with known diabetic kidney disease the aim is to keep BP <125/75, (NICE CG66 2008 says <130/80). but be careful to avoid dizziness and falls in patients with severe postural hypotension due to autonomic neuropathy. ACE inhibitors (e.g. captopril, ramipril) or ARBs (e.g. losartan, irbesartan) are licensed for use in diabetic nephropathy. Check U&E + creatinine before starting, after 2 weeks, and after changing dose. Other hypotensive drugs can be used (e.g. amlodipine, which does not need reduction in renal impairment).

Treating microalbuminuria (📖 p.37)

ACE inhibitors (captopril, ramipril) and ARBs (losartan) slow the progression of diabetic nephropathy if initiated when persistent microalbuminuria is detected. Test for ACR or PCR annually. If the ratio is raised in two of three samples collected consecutively within 1 month, prescribe an ACE inhibitor (e.g. ramipril) and increase to maximal tolerated dose.

Low-salt diet

Reduced sodium chloride intake may help control hypertension and reduce fluid retention. Once the patient has significant renal impairment a low protein and/or low phosphate diet may help. Seek a renal physician's advice before prescribing such diets via a dietitian.

Stop smoking (📖 p.36)

Screening—kidneys

- Screen every patient at diagnosis of diabetes and annually thereafter
- Screen by measuring urinary microalbumin concentrations (📖 p.104)
- Screen by measuring plasma creatinine concentrations

Warning symptoms or signs

- None: by the time symptoms and signs develop, severe renal impairment is present
- Hypoglycaemia or falling insulin or non-insulin hypoglycaemic dose
- Rising BP
- Oedema

Diabetic nephropathy

It may take several years for microalbuminuria to progress to overt albuminuria and for other signs of renal impairment to develop. The rate of deterioration of renal function can be slowed down.

Evidence of nephropathy

- Raised ACR or PCR (>3.5 mg/mmol in men, >2.5 mg/mmol in women)
- Dipstick proteinuria
- Haematuria: microscopic rare in purely diabetic nephropathy, seek other cause; macroscopic (exclude menstruation), refer to urology
- Low eGFR (see Table 14.5)

If nephropathy check:

- Personal history of renal or urinary disease (e.g. recurrent UTIs)
- Family history of renal disease
- BP (lying and standing)
- Heart (high cardiovascular risk)
- PVD (severe PVD increases likelihood of renal artery stenosis)
- Fundi (no retinopathy seek other causes nephropathy)
- Urine microscopy and culture
- Urine 24 hr protein (unless your laboratory uses ACR/PCR instead)
- Blood U&E, creatinine, eGFR, lipids, calcium, albumin, phosphate, FBC, HbA_{1c}

Tell patient to drink plenty of water but avoid food for fasting sample

- Renal ultrasound if CKD 3+
- Appropriate tests if non-diabetic cause suspected

Action

- See Table 14.5.
- Refer all patients with raised ACR/PCR to the diabetes team.
- Vigorous renal and cardiovascular risk reduction:
    - ACE or ARB first line (captopril, ramipril, losartan, irbesartan)—watch for ↑potassium, renal function
    - diuretic—thiazide CKD 1 + 2; loop diuretic CKD 3–5 (beware dehydration); watch for ↓potassium, check renal function
    - amlodipine: beware oedema.
- Vigorous and careful glucose control: risk of hypoglycaemia with worsening eGFR—HBGM four times daily.
- Check Renal Association website: http://www.renal.org/eGFR/index.html
- Keep monitoring ACR/PCR long term

Table 14.5 Stages and management of chronic kidney disease

CKD stage	eGFR ml/min/ 1.73m^2	Kidney function	Management
1	>90	Normal but urine abnormality including ACR/PCR >3.5 mg/mmol men, >2.5 mg/mmol women or structural abnormality or genetic trait renal disease	Monitor Refer diabetes team? BP<125/75 if safe HbA_{1c} 6.0–6.5% if safe. Avoid hypo. Cholesterol <4 mmol/l ACE I or ARB titrate to full dose Statin Aspirin 75 mg once daily Stop smoking *Renal referral if:* ACR>100 mg/mmol or >45 mg/mmol + microscopic haematuria
2	60–89	Mildly reduced kidney function + above (but eGFR calculation less accurate in this zone, so repeat with patient well hydrated)	As CKD 1 Refer diabetes team
3	30–59	Moderately reduced kidney function	As CKD 1, but HbA_{1c} 6.5–7.3% Check for sepsis, CCF, big bladder Renal ultrasound *Renal referral if:* Progressive fall in eGFR or rise in serum creatinine Microscopic haematuria ACR/PCR >100mg/mmol Unexplained anaemia Abnormal potassium, calcium, or phosphate Suspected systemic illness Uncontrolled BP (>150/90 on three agents)
4	15–29	Severely reduced renal function	As CKD 3 + urgent renal referral
5	<15	Endstage/established kidney failure	As above + same-day renal referral

Adapted from Renal Association guidelines: www.renal.org/eGFR/eguide.html

Patients with evidence of nephropathy should be seen by a diabetologist and also referred to a renal physician (see Table 14.5). Several centres now have joint renal diabetes clinics. Patients may need continuous ambulatory peritoneal dialysis (CAPD) or haemodialysis. CAPD has a 60% 3 yr survival rate in diabetes. A quarter of patients entering some renal transplant programmes have diabetes. Transplants have >60% 5 yr survival.

Patients with diabetic nephropathy always have retinopathy and often have foot problems, neuropathy, vascular disease, and ischaemic heart disease. Many die from the latter rather than from their renal impairment.

Diabetic neuropathy

Diabetes can produce virtually any peripheral (sensory or motor) or autonomic neurological deficit. Because it is difficult to measure minor degrees of neuropathy, its frequency is difficult to establish. After 20 yrs of diabetes most people have evidence of impaired nerve function on detailed testing. About one in 12 people with newly diagnosed type 2 diabetes have clinically detectable neuropathy.

Preventing or improving neuropathy

Hyperglycaemia

People with persistently high blood glucose levels are more likely to have peripheral neuropathy than those with normal glucose levels. Normalization of the glucose concentration (some authorities believe insulin should always be used) may relieve severe pain or abnormal feelings in neuropathy. Returning the glucose to normal slows worsening peripheral neuropathy, and may also improve it, but may have little effect on autonomic neuropathy.

Screening—nerves

- Screen every patient at diagnosis of diabetes and annually thereafter
- Symptoms: numbness, tingling, weakness; there are often no symptoms
- Examination: muscle wasting
- Muscle weakness (if symptoms/wasting)
- Feet: light touch—cotton wool
- Pressure—monofilaments (≤10 g is normal)
- Pin-prick—Neurotips (Owen Mumford)
- Vibration—tuning fork (C_0 pitch)
- Position sense
- Tendon reflexes—ankle, knee
- BP: lying and standing

Peripheral neuropathy

There are several nomenclatures which can be confusing. In practice they are not always clearly definable. From the patient's point of view it is important to know if any sensory modality is missing so as to be careful to avoid injury, if it hurts or feels peculiar, or if a muscle is weak or does not work.

Sensory peripheral neuropathy ('glove and stocking')

The most common form of neuropathy is loss or blunting of sensation in a 'sock' or sometimes 'glove' distribution. Different modalities may be differently affected. Problems that arise are:

- numbness so that rubbing or injury is not noticed
- loss of temperature discrimination with a risk of burning
- loss of position sense which, if severe, can make walking and balance difficult.
- loss of vibration sense (an early sign of neuropathy with little clinical impact)
- tingling or actual pain.

Mononeuropathy(ies)

Single-nerve lesions, with or without entrapment, are quite common. They include median and ulnar nerves and those serving eye movement (📖 p.296). Several single nerves in different parts of the body may be affected in one patient.

Neuropathic muscle weakness

Muscle weakness may be secondary to an individual nerve lesion (as above) or more diffuse. It can affect the thighs with marked wasting, weakness, and pain, or rarely be more extensive.

Symptoms of neuropathy (or not)

Many patients are unaware of the extent of their neuropathy until they are affected by one of its consequences, such as a foot ulcer at the site of an unnoticed injury. A few are severely disabled by pain. Refer such patients to a diabetologist. The pain is sometimes relieved by minor analgesics but if not tricyclic antidepressants, duloxetine, gabapentine or pregabalin may help.

Check for non-diabetic causes of neuropathy

Obviously the most likely reason for neuropathy in someone with diabetes is diabetic tissue damage. However, it is important not to miss other treatable causes which may coexist including:

- vitamin B_{12} deficiency
- vitamin B_6 deficiency
- alcohol excess
- drugs
- uraemia
- collagen-vascular disease

Warning for neuropathic patients

- Never walk barefoot
- Check shoes and socks for foreign bodies every time you put them on
- Never use a hot water bottle
- Check the bathwater temperature with a bath thermometer
- Always use an oven glove
- Inspect your feet every day

Autonomic neuropathy

Two in five patients with diabetes have some evidence of autonomic neuropathy when tested in detail, but symptoms are uncommon. If the patient does have symptoms, they may be unpleasant and the prognosis is poor. One in two patients with symptomatic autonomic neuropathy will be dead within 5 yrs. Symptoms include:

- postural hypotension
- altered sweating
- gastropathy (📖 p.311)
- diarrhoea or constipation (📖 p.312)
- urinary retention
- erectile dysfunction (📖 p.386)
- ankle swelling
- loss of hypoglycaemia warning (📖 p.204)
- sudden death.

Refer all patients with evidence of autonomic neuropathy to a consultant diabetologist. Investigation and treatment are complex, and these patients have multiple complications.

Postural hypotension

- May be severe, even on sitting up in bed
- May be immediate on rising or delayed for some minutes
- Symptoms:
  - none
  - dizziness or faintness
  - confusion
  - sudden collapse
  - falls in elderly
- Worsened by:
  - fluid depletion
  - excessive treatment of hypertension
  - diuretics
  - nitrates and other vasodilators
  - psychotropic drugs (such as tricyclics)
- Management
  - seek non-diabetic + diabetic causes
  - ensure adequate hydration
  - remove or reduce drugs worsening hypotension
  - consider compression stockings (check arterial circulation)
  - consider fludrocortisone (beware oedema)
  - warn patient to get up slowly and exercise calf muscles before walking.

Altered sweating

Patients may sweat less on the feet but more in the upper half of the body. This may cause dry skin—advise emollient cream but not between the toes.

Gustatory sweating—facial sweating precipitated by spicy or highly flavoured foods. Avoiding these foods may help

Urinary retention

This occurs imperceptibly. The bladder slowly enlarges with an increasing post-micurition volume. This forms a reservoir for infection. Regular urination with pressure in the suprapubic region may help. If the person suffers recurrent UTIs, prophylactic antibiotics such as trimethoprim may be required. Other causes of urinary retention, such as prostatism, must be excluded. They may coincide.

Sudden death

May occur at any time. People with autonomic neuropathy are at especial risk of sudden death if they become hypoxic or during anaesthesia. Always tell the anaesthetist that the patient has autonomic neuropathy. Anaesthesia should be performed only in a hospital with full resuscitation and medical support.

Screening—autonomic neuropathy: symptomatic patients

Apart from BP, tests for autonomic neuropathy are usually reserved for symptomatic patients. Some are complex. The following can be done with a sphygmomanometer and an ECG machine.

- Lying and standing systolic BP. Wait 2 min for delayed fall. Normal fall ≤ 10 mmHg; abnormal fall ≥ 30 mmHg.
- Heart rate during and after Valsalva manoeuvre. Find pulse, ask patient to breathe in and then to try to push the breath out hard against a closed glottis for as long as they can. Count the pulse once they have started. Then count the rate as they relax afterwards. It is much easier with an ECG machine. Rate during/rate after: normal ≥ 1.21; abnormal ≤ 1.20. Do not do this in people with proliferative retinopathy.
- Heart rate after standing ('30:15 test'). Attach the ECG and make sure the patient will be able to get up easily. Once the ECG is recording continuously ask the patient to stand and mark the ECG as they start to do so. Calculate the ratio of the longest R–R interval (about the 30th beat after they start standing) to the shortest R–R interval (~15th beat after they start standing): normal ≥1.04; abnormal ≤1.0.

These tests are fraught with practical difficulties (patients who find it hard to stand up, ECG leads fall off, etc.).

Gastrointestinal problems

Mouth

Diabetes is associated with an increased likelihood of both oral and dental problems. Most of these conditions are more likely with smoking ± hyperglycaemia (*Clin Diabetes* 2005; **23**:171–8

Oral problems

- Dry mouth—lack of saliva. More likely with hyperglycaemia, and with neuropathy. Worsens other oral/dental problems. Advise saliva substitute or stimulant.
- Parotid enlargement found in 25% of diabetic patients.
- Bad breath—periodontal disease, oral hygiene problems.
- Oral candida—risk 2–5 times, particularly with dentures. Treat with improved oral hygiene and nystatin or .fluconazole (beware interactions)
- Tongue—glossitis, atrophic patches, fissures.
- Angular cheilosis.
- Denture stomatitis.
- Lichen planus—risk of cancer and candida. May need steroid treatment.
- Poor wound healing in mouth.
- Burning mouth syndrome
- Fibromas.

Dental problems

- Periodontal disease. This infection is especially linked with hyperglycaemia. Treatment of periodontal disease with antibiotics (e.g. amoxicillin) may improve glucose balance. Mouthwashes such as Listerine® or chlorhexidine may prevent periodontal disease. Some authors suggest that periodontal disease increases the risk of atherosclerosis.
- Gingivitis—plaque irritates the gums. Good tooth brushing to remove plaque reduces the risk. Symptoms are red, swollen, painful, and bleeding gums.
- Dental caries—painful damaged teeth impair healthy eating.
- Loss of teeth.

Practical and financial issues

Every diabetic patient should have regular dental checks. Unfortunately, there is a shortage of NHS dentists in the UK. Diabetic patients may already find that their condition makes life more expensive (costlier insurance, travel to hospital, etc.). They may be reluctant to pay for dental care. Some patients with diabetes have severe oral and dental disease which worsens their glucose balance and can seriously risk their general health.

Box 14.3 Recommendations for oral health

- Ask people with diabetes about their oral health, specifically if they have noticed any signs of infection, bad breath, or a bad taste in their mouth, or if they have any other symptoms.
- Ask about the last dental check-up.
- Remind all diabetic patients to register with a dentist.
- Remind diabetic patients to have dental and periodontal check-ups every 6 months or more frequently if needed.
- Tell patients to see their dentist straightaway if they notice signs of infection such as sore, swollen, or bleeding gums, loose teeth, mouth ulcers, or pain.
- Look in their mouth—soft tissues and teeth.
- Advise regular tooth brushing and flossing An electric oscillating toothbrush may clean teeth better—ask the dentist.
- Regular mouthwash (e.g. chlorhexidine) may help—ask the dentist.
- Stop smoking.
- Keep HbA_{1c} 6.0–6.5% if safe.

Adapted from American Diabetes Association guidelines. *Clin Diabetes* 2005; **23**:171–8.

Stomach and oesophagus

The main problem is gastric or oesophageal dysmotility.

Oesophageal dysmotility

- About 60% of diabetic patients with gastrointestinal symptoms have oesophageal motility problems
- Abnormal oesophageal motility may impair swallowing
- Due to autonomic neuropathy
- Must exclude other causes
- Refer patients with swallowing problems to gastroenterology

Diabetic gastropathy

- Gastroenteritis is a more common cause of vomiting than gastropathy. Exclude DKA in a vomiting, insulin-treated patient (📖 p.240)
- Caused by autonomic neuropathy but made much worse by hyperglycaemia
- Stomach emptying may be delayed for ≥12 hrs (e.g. breakfast vomited in evening)
- Symptoms include:
  - feeling full early
  - abdominal discomfort (gastric distension)
  - vomiting—may be debilitating and require hospital admission
  - bloating, belching
  - hypoglycaemia—insulin arrives in bloodstream before food)
  - failure to recover from hypoglycaemia (oral glucose remains in stomach and so is not absorbed)

- Investigation
  - seek non-diabetic + diabetic causes (e.g. opiates, calcium blockers, alcohol, smoking, hypothyroidism, renal impairment, electrolyte impairment, high glucose).
  - upper GI endoscopy in all—strict 8 hr fast; if food found, diagnosis confirmed—may need other tests via specialist (gastric cancer is more common in type 1 diabetes than in non-diabetics)
  - check for *Helicobacter pylorii*
  - refer to gastroenterology
- Treatment
  - difficult—share care with gastroenterology
  - frequent small meals—solid food may pass more readily than liquids (counter-intuitive)
  - avoid exenatide or sitagliptin, and acarbose
  - metoclopramide or domperidone; ?erythromycin (*Am J Gastroenterol* 2003; **98**:259–63)
  - optimize glucose balance
  - very careful insulin therapy—do *not* use rapid-acting insulin analogues (arrive in bloodstream long before food does); insulin pump therapy may be required
  - tricyclic antidepressants may help
  - pancreatic enzyme supplements (worth a trial even if no proof of malabsorption)
  - electrical stimulation has been used (gastric pacing)
  - in severe cases percutaneous jejeunal feeding may be required

Atrophic gastritis

Atrophic gastritis may occur in patients with autoimmune diabetes and is associated with iron and vitamin B_{12} deficiency. 15–25% type 1 diabetic patients have parietal cell antibodies (*Diabetes Care*, 2000; **23**;1384–8).

Helicobacter pylorii

This infection appears to be more common in diabetic patients than in non-diabetics.

Diarrhoea

The most common causes of diarrhoea in diabetic patients are gastroenteritis or metformin. Diarrhoea and constipation due to bowel dysmotility may alternate in the same patient. The problem is caused by autonomic neuropathy but other factors such as hyperglycaemia may worsen it.

- Symptoms of diabetic diarrhoea:
  - may be sudden with urgency
  - may cause faecal incontinence
  - often nocturnal or early morning
  - may come in bouts of days or weeks
  - may seriously limit going out

- Causes and investigation
  - Is the patient on metformin? If so, stop it and start another oral hypoglycaemic. Exenatide and sitagliptin can also cause GI side effects.
  - Consider coeliac disease, pancreatic insufficiency, thyrotoxicosis.
  - Investigate as for non-diabetic patients. If you think the diarrhoea is due to metformin, request a GP review for the patient 2 weeks after stopping the metformin to check if the symptoms have settled.
  - Refer to gastroenterology.
  - Colonoscopy—colon cancer is more common in diabetic patients than in non-diabetics.
- Treatment
  - Refer to diabetologist who should share care with gastroenterology.
  - Avoid metformin, acarbose, sitagliptin, and exenatide.
  - Soluble fibre.
  - Anticholinergics.
  - Colestyramine.
  - Erythromycin (to eradicate bacterial overgrowth and improve motility).
  - Pancreatic enzymes.
  - Octreotide (but beware hypertensive crisis).
  - Clonidine (but beware worsening postural hypotension).

Constipation

- Common—up to 60% of patients.
- Often due to dehydration from hyperglycaemia.
- Autonomic neuropathic constipation less common than dehydration.
- May be presenting feature of diabetes due to dehydration.
- Management
  - Investigate as for non-diabetic patients.
  - Consider hypothyroidism. Analgesics, tricyclic antidepressants used for painful peripheral neuropathy.
  - Consider colon and pancreatic cancer.
  - Refer to gastroenterology.
  - Colonoscopy:- NB will need extra bowel preparation for good view—discuss with gastroenterology team first. This also applies to radiological investigations (e.g. CT pneumocolon).
  - High-fibre diet and bulking compounds, e.g. ispaghula (not if gastroparesis).
  - Metformin for glucose control.
  - Laxatives, e.g. lactulose (a non-absorbed osmotic laxative).
  - Care with stimulant laxatives.

Liver

See *Diabetes Care* 2007; **30**:734–43

Liver problems associated with diabetes or more prevalent in diabetic patients include the following.

- Elevated liver enzymes (LFTs) (mostly due to NAFLD)
- Non-alcoholic fatty liver disease (NAFLD)
  - non-alcoholic steatohepatitis (NASH)
  - cirrhosis
  - hepatocellular carcinoma
  - liver failure
- Hepatitis C
- Adverse reactions to hypoglycaemic drugs (rare)

Also, patients with liver disease often have diabetes (12–57%). Cirrhosis is associated with insulin resistance.

Raised liver enzymes

Should not be ignored. 2–24% of type 2 diabetic patients have raised LFTs (ALT, AST) depending on the inclusion or exclusion of patients with known liver disease (about 5%). 98% of type 2 diabetic patients with raised liver enzymes have liver disease, usually NAFLD or chronic hepatitis.

NAFLD and NASH

Diabetes is now the most common cause of liver disease in the USA. Diabetes and metabolic syndrome are associated with the development of NAFLD. Prevalence estimates vary (34–74%) but 100% of obese type 2 diabetic patients have some evidence of NAFLD. Insulin resistance increases lipolysis and fat is deposited in the liver. In some, but not all, patients this leads to liver cell damage and fibrosis (NASH). This process may then continue to cirrhosis and liver failure. It may progress to cancer. Hepatocellular carcinoma is four times more common in diabetics than in non-diabetics.

In one study of NAFLD, 40% of NASH patients had progressive fibrosis. Progression was more likely with weight gain. 5% had endstage liver disease, and half of these had hepatocellular carcinoma. The presence of NASH reduced survival. The absence of periportal fibrosis on liver biopsy indicated low risk of liver complications. Most patients with NAFLD who are not diabetic initially will become so with time. *Hepatology* 2006; **44**:865–73

Hepatitis C

Hepatitis C infection is three to four times more common in the diabetic population than in non-diabetic people.

Management of liver abnormalities in diabetes

Refer patients with abnormal LFTs to the diabetologist. The diabetologist should agree guidelines with their local hepatologist/gastroenterologist and radiologist. Suggestions for the management of raised LFTs in diabetic patients are as follows.

Tests

- Check for non-diabetic causes (e.g. alcohol, drugs, gall bladder disease).
- Blood (fasting):
  - ALT, alkaline phosphatase, bilirubin, albumin, INR
  - lipids—for triglyceride
  - ferritin (haemochromatosis)
  - hepatitis A, B, C screen
  - HbA_{1c} if not done in last 2 months
  - tests for non-diabetes-related causes.
- Liver ultrasound (suggestion: do ultrasound if any LFT >3 × ULN ± age >50 yrs ± abdominal or gastrointestinal symptoms ± triglyceride >1.7 mmol/l ± any non-diabetes-related cause likely).
- Liver biopsy (risk of morbidity small, but risk of death present) after review by hepatologist/gastroenterologist unless otherwise agreed.

Treatment

Treat non-NAFLD causes as usual. The management of NAFLD is controversial.

- All patients:
  - Monitor LFTs regularly
  - If BMI >25 kg/m^2, diet and exercise to lose weight gradually—over-rapid weight loss may worsen NASH
  - If HbA_{1c} >6.5%, control glucose carefully avoiding hypoglycaemia which is a risk in patients with severe liver disease (NB glucagon may not elevate glucose if there is severe liver disease). Use metformin unless there is a risk of liver decompensation and hence lactic acidosis. Some authors have used glitazones to reduce insulin resistance. There was an improvement in LFTs. However, glitazones are under review by safety authorities so it may be prudent to avoid them in this situation. Nateglinide has been shown to improve LFTs
  - If triglyceride >1.7 mmol/l and all LFTs <3 × ULN, consider atorvastatin or gemfibrozil which have been used in NAFLD
  - Avoid alcohol completely.

Lungs

Diabetic microangiopathy can affect the lungs, causing thickening of basal lamina in all parts of the lung—diabetic pulmopathy. Also infection risk is greater and infections may be prolonged and severe,. This can lead to residual damage. Type 2 diabetes is more common in people with chronic obstructive pulmonary disease (COPD) than those without, but not in asthma.

Direct or indirect pulmonary complications

- Reduction in forced expiratory volume in 1 sec (FEV_1), forced vital capacity (FVC), vital capacity (VC), and peak expiratory flow (PEF) by about 10% compared with non-diabetic population. All measures gradually worsen. 'Absolute measures continued to decline at an annual rate of 68, 71, and 84 ml/year and 17 l/min for FVC, FEV_1, VC, and PEF, respectively' (*Diabetes Res Clin Pract* 2000; **50**:153–9, *Diabetes Care* 2004; **27**:752–7)
- Decline in pulmonary function could be predicted by poor glycaemic control
- Decreased FEV_1 has been associated with increased mortality
- Reduced diffusing capacity in type 1 diabetes with less adverse effects on volume functions
- Bacterial lung infections are common
- Tuberculosis
- Fungal lung infections
- Pulmonary oedema (secondary to cardiac disease)
- Respiratory arrest
- Pneumothorax, pneumomediastinum, pneumopericardium (rare)
- Adult respiratory distress syndrome (ARDS)
- Aspiration of gastric contents (with gastroparesis)

Cystic fibrosis

- Autosomal recessive, 1:2500 Caucasian incidence, less in other ethnic groups
- Defect in gene regulating salt and water balance in secretory tissues which causes thickened secretions
- Chronic suppurative lung disease
- Failure of pancreatic enzyme production (exocrine function)
- Severe pancreatic damage causing diabetes
- Liver disease
- Gatrointestinal bleeding
- Osteoporosis
- Infertility
- 70–90% adults with cystic fibrosis have diabetes (usually diagnosed around age 18–21 yrs)
- Glucose intolerance is influenced by lung infections and other complications
- Diagnosis of diabetes should be made by OGTT, not one-off glucose levels
- Most need insulin
- Continue high-fat diet
- Cystic-fibrosis-related diabetes is difficult to manage and every such patient should be referred to a specialist unit. Guidelines available at: http://www.cftrust.org.uk/aboutcf/publications/consensusdoc/diabetes.pdf

Diabetic skin and soft tissue problems

Infection

- Minor skin infection may be the first clue to diabetes and can remain a problem
- Boils to carbuncles
- Pustules (especially on the legs) may be staphylococcal
- Cellulitis, often streptococcal or staphylococcal, can spread very fast
- Paronychia, especially related to ingrowing toenails, is common
- Fungal infections, usually candida, affect the perineum and produce intertrigo in the groin and elsewhere in obese patients
- Overweight patients may develop chronic sweat gland infections, cavities, and scarring in axillae and groin (hidradenitis suppurativa)

Diabetic dermopathy

Shin spots are flat reddish-brown marks in the pretibial region. They may follow trauma but can emerge spontaneously. They do not require treatment. Protect legs.

Necrobiosis lipoidica diabeticorum

Is not common. Refer to a dermatologist. It occurs in about three patients with diabetes per 1000 per year. The lesions are red plaques with a purple edge and a yellowish centre which gradually becomes atrophic. They usually occur on the pretibial area and may remit spontaneously. The main concern is cosmetic effect. Lesions may become infected. Treatment is not always satisfactory. Steroids can be used on non-atrophic lesions and some authorities advocate nicotinic acid orally. Skin grafting may be successful.

Itching

Localized itching may be associated with perineal candidiasis. Generalized itching may be due to uraemia or jaundice.

Diabetic mastopathy

Occurs in women with long-standing type 1 diabetes (less often with type 2) with long-term high glucose levels. A painless irregular hard breast lump can be felt which may be hard to differentiate from cancer. These lumps consist of lympocytic infiltration and fibrous tissue on biopsy. Mastopathy is often bilateral and frequently recurs after surgery. It has been suggested that it should be followed by ultrasound with ultrasound-guided biopsies if required. Refer to breast clinic. A painful breast lump is probably infected.

Diabetic musculoskeletal problems

Ligaments

Skin thickening can occur in diabetes but connective tissue thickening is more obvious in ligaments. Diabetes is associated with the following.

- Dupuytren's contracture and similar problems in the feet
- Carpal tunnel syndrome
- Cheiroarthropathy—a tightening of the tendons in the hand so that fingers can no longer be pressed flat against those of the other hand when opposed
- Limited joint mobility
- Frozen shoulder
- Trigger finger

Bones

Osteopenia

People with diabetes can develop marked osteopenia. Loss of bone density may be most evident in the first few years after diagnosis of type 1 diabetes. It seems to be linked to poor blood glucose balance—improve this. Treat as for non-diabetic patients.

Increased bone density

Patients with type 2 diabetes may show diffuse interstitial skeletal hyperostosis with osteophytes and new bone, e.g. in the vertebrae. Although they may have increased bone density in some areas, they also at risk of osteoporosis (*Clin Diabetes* 2002; **20**:153–7).

Fractures

Fractures of the femur and proximal humerus are more common in women with diabetes than in non-diabetic people. Patients on insulin have more than double the risk of foot fractures compared with the non-diabetic population (*J Clin Endocrinol Metab* 2001; **86**:32–8). Fractures are also more common in patients on glitazones.

Charcot joints

Severe neuropathy and trauma may cause bone destruction in feet and Charcot joints. Refer to orthopaedics and specialist podiatry.

Osteoarthrosis

Osteoarthrosis also appears to be more common.

Rheumatoid arthritis

13% of people with rheumatoid arthritis also have diabetes. Check glucose with steroid treatment. Screen for hypothyroidism and B_{12} deficiency. Refer to podiatry for preventive foot care advice.

Cancer

Several studies have reviewed cancer incidence and prevalence in diabetes. A large prospective US study of about a million people with 16 yrs mortality follow-up showed an increased frequency of cancer in patients with any form of diabetes of colon, pancreas, female breast; and liver + bladder in men (*Am J Epidemiol* 2004; **159**:1160–7).

Patients with newly diagnosed diabetes have twice the risk of pancreatic cancer compared with non-diabetics, especially if young with gastrointestinal symptoms (*Clin Gastroenterol Hepatol* 2006; **4**:1366–72).

A Swedish study showed a 20% increase in frequency of cancer in type 1 diabetes, with cancer of stomach, cervix, and endometrium being more common.

An increased risk of liver (hepatocellular), pancreas, kidney, and endometrial cancer has been described in type 2 diabetes. Obesity may confound the issues (*J Nat Cancer Inst* 2003; **95**:1797–1800).

Summary

- Diabetes is a multisystem disorder of which one manifestation is hyperglycaemia.
- Diabetic tissue damage is largely preventable.
- If present, tissue damage can be treated, and its progress slowed.
- Tissue damage can affect every part of the body:

• Eye	Retinopathy, maculopathy, cataract, squint
• Ear	Deafness
• Smell/taste	Reduced
• Kidneys	Nephropathy, renal failure, chronic pyelonephritis
• Nerve	Peripheral neuropathy, autonomic neuropathy, mononeuropathy, proximal motor neuropathy
• Heart	Ischaemic heart disease, cardiac failure
• Lungs	Impaired function
• GI tract	Oral + dental problems, dysmotility.
• Liver	Non-alcoholic fatty liver
• Peripheral vascular disease, especially legs	
• Feet	Ulcer, infection, gangrene, amputation
• Brain	Stroke, transient ischaemic attacks
• Skin + soft tissue	Dermopathy, necrobiosis lipoidica, mastopathy
• Ligament	Dupuytren's contracture, cheiroarthropathy
• Skeletal system	Charcot joint, osteopenia, osteosclerosis
• Cancer	Increased risk of some cancers

Chapter 15

Diabetic foot problems

Why are the feet so vulnerable?

We bear our entire weight on our feet, subjecting their components to enormous stresses every day. Early warning of problems helps us to protect our feet.

Diabetic foot problems are largely preventable. Assal *et al.* (1982) dramatically reduced the amputation rate in a Swiss diabetes service by introducing an intensive patient education and foot care programme (📖 p.340, Useful reading).

Neuropathy

Diabetic neuropathy reduces sensation of pain, touch, temperature, and position. Rubs, scrapes, and knocks are ignored because they cannot be felt. Patients may walk around with a pebble in their shoe all day without realizing it. Skin may be burned by near-boiling water with no sensation of heat or pain. If you do not know where your foot is in space, you cannot keep it in the best position for safe weight-bearing. Patients buy overtight shoes because they feel loose on neuropathic feet. Callus can build up under the metatarsal heads and elsewhere. Neuropathy may alter the circulation, causing arteriovenous shunting and increasing bone blood flow.

Microvascular disease

Small vessel disease may damage the healing response, so that minor injuries are not repaired and infections may eventually spread to threaten the viability of deeper tissues.

Vascular disease

Atheroma is common in diabetes, affecting not only large vessels but also smaller ones, e.g. those supplying the legs and feet, in which calcification may be seen on X-ray. Poor circulation causes symptoms of its own: intermittent claudication, rest pain, and finally gangrene. In addition it worsens other problems by depriving injured or infected areas of oxygen, slowing healing, and allowing anaerobic bacteria to flourish. Antibiotics may not reach the areas of infection in sufficient concentrations to be effective.

Deformity

Diabetes can cause ligamentous changes. In the feet this may lead to clawed or hammer toes. This causes further abnormalities of weight-bearing, and the curled toes may develop corns on top as they rub against shoes. Neuropathy, vasculopathy, and infection may cause damage leading to deformity, as can surgery. The foot then develops multiple pressure points and callus builds up.

Bones

Bone density is reduced in people with diabetes, more so in those with type 1 than in type 2. Diabetic autonomic neuropathy intensifies this process in the feet with increased vascularity and shunting. When this is combined with peripheral neuropathy, small injuries can initiate bony destruction and distortion, which extends rapidly with continued weight-bearing or repeated injury. The bones and joints are gradually destroyed, causing Charcot joints.

Infection

Hyperglycaemia reduces white cell mobility, and a poor blood supply slows delivery of white cells and nutrients, thereby impeding the body's defensive response to infection. Via areas of callus, pockets of infection can extend deep into the foot and thence into the tissue planes and bones. Infections there and elsewhere do not hurt and progress rapidly.

Other problems

If they cannot feel pain, even those who can see or smell a problem may not treat it with the seriousness it deserves: 'If it doesn't hurt it can't be too bad'; 'It can't be happening to me'. Those who are aware of the seriousness may be so frightened of losing their foot or leg that they conceal the problems. Partially sighted patients may not be able to see trouble developing on their feet.

> Marion was a 60-year-old woman with long-standing type 1 diabetes. She attended diabetic clinic between annual reviews. 'Are your feet all right?' asked the doctor. 'Yes, thank you', she replied. Three weeks later she was admitted with infected gangrene of her toe. At that point she confessed that she had gangrene at the time of her clinic visit but had been so terrified of being admitted to hospital that she had lied to her doctor.

Prevention of diabetic foot problems

Patient and staff education are crucial. Many people know that diabetes can lead to leg amputation, but patients may still fail to take the practical steps to prevent themselves ending up in a wheelchair too. Health care professionals, whether in hospital or in general practice, fail to take the time to check patients' feet themselves, and often fail to act sufficiently vigorously when patients present with what look like minor foot problems. A small blister on a little toe can lead to amputation.

Examine the feet

Examine every diabetic patient's feet on diagnosis and annually. On examination check the following.

- Skin: colour, ulcers, rubs, blisters, corns, calluses, etc.
- Shape of feet and toes: hammer or claw toes, bunions, missing toes, surgery, deformities
- Swelling
- Pulses: anterior and posterior tibial
- Sensation: light touch, monofilament, vibration, position
- Hygiene
- Shoes and hosiery

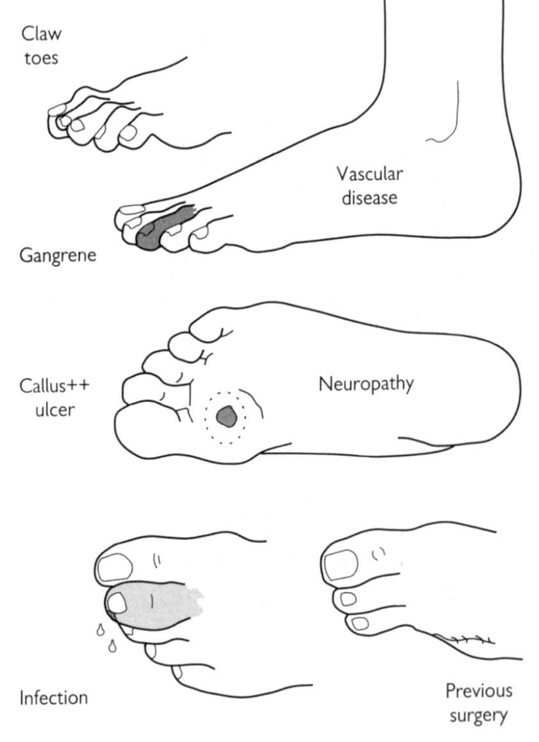

Fig. 15.1 The diabetic foot: warning signs during examination.

Table 15.1 Look after your feet: guidelines for patients

1.	Look at your feet every day. Use a mirror or ask someone else to help if you have difficulty seeing.
2.	If you have any of the following see your doctor (or chiropodist or diabetic clinic) within 24 hrs:
	any colour change
	any new pain or unusual feeling
	any sore places (corns, blisters, cracks, calluses, ulcers, bunions)
	swelling anywhere
	any break in the skin (ulcers, cracks, blisters)
	a strange smell from your feet
3.	Treat any skin break by washing with dilute antiseptic (follow the instructions on the container), drying gently with sterile gauze, and covering with a dry non-adherent dressing. Use non-allergic tape (e.g. Micropore) and never wind it round a toe. Then contact help
4.	Wash your feet daily in lukewarm water. Dry carefully, especially between the toes
5.	If you have dry skin use a moisturizing cream or emollient lotion, but not between the toes
6.	Cut toenails in a gentle curve and file smooth without leaving sharp edges to dig in to that or other toes
7.	Wear clean socks, stockings, or tights every day
8.	Buy shoes which do not squeeze your foot, and which do not hurt or rub anywhere the first time you try them on. Low-heeled lace-ups with plenty of toe room are best
9.	Do not walk bare foot.
10.	Do not use corn cures, or cut corns or callus
11.	Do not use a hot water bottle
12.	Do not use vibrating foot massagers or baths
13.	Do not smoke
14.	See a state registered chiropodist (SRCh) or podiatrist regularly

Patient foot care advice leaflets in 30 languages can be printed off from www.diabeticfoot.org.uk

Who should treat foot problems?

Any patient with a foot problem is at risk of further trouble and it is sensible to examine their feet whenever you see them (a) to reinforce the message of foot care to patients and (b) to spot early trouble. All diabetic patients should have priority access to chiropody and those with any foot problem should have regular chiropody.

The best place to treat such patients is at a diabetes foot clinic where all the relevant specialists see the patient together. If this is not available, the diabetes team have the most experience of dealing with such problems and it is usually best to refer foot emergencies directly to the diabetes service. Check your local arrangements before you need them. The diabetologist will then coordinate all care with vascular surgery, orthopaedics, chiropody, wound care, special shoes, rehabilitation, etc. It is vital that good communication is maintained with GP and that he/she is fully informed about the care plan.

High-risk patients should remain under the care of the diabetic foot team. One person should act as keyworker to make sure that all facets of care are actually happening—gaps are common because of lapses in communication or transport failures. One missed treatment may be disastrous.

All diabetic inpatients with foot or leg problems should be referred to the inpatient specialist diabetes team. This particularly includes those in care of elderly or rehabilitation/long-stay wards, and patients on vascular or orthopaedic wards.

Assessment of diabetic patients with foot problems

Always remove dressings, having first warned the nursing staff that they will need to be redone. Inspect the whole of both feet and legs.

The foot/leg

- Look
- Smell
- Touch
- Test
- Assess skin colour
- Seek skin damage: rubs, blisters, scratches or ulcers, calluses
- Fungal infections? Verrucas?
- Assess shape: deformities, scars, surgery, amputations
- Oedema
- Fluid? Clear ooze, pus, blood?
- Check for pressure discoloration or sores (if present on heels, check the sacral area)
- Look for gross distortion of foot anatomy with warmth, swelling, and neuropathy—Charcot foot, but these feet can also be infected.
- Note malodour—usually very bad = anaerobes ± other organisms
- Note dryness (neuropathy)
- Note heat or cold to touch
- Measure monofilament sensation, light touch, vibration (and temperature with cold tuning fork), position sense, ankle and knee reflexes
- Palpate peripheral pulses: dorsalis pedis and posterior tibial
- Digital photograph of foot lesion with ruler (and patient consent)
- Wash hands before and after (use gloves if broken skin) and using medical cleaning wipes or sterilise for all equipment after each patient

The rest

- Review glucose control
- Most patients with diabetic foot problems have diabetic tissue damage elsewhere—seek it (use gloves)
- Employ single-use equipment
- When admitting patients with foot problems for admission, fully clerk patient including neurology (📖 p.25)

❶Danger signs

Patients with any of the following features should be referred promptly to the specialist diabetes team or diabetic foot team for a full assessment. They may need admission.

Colour change

Refer to hospital same day.

- Red foot (infection or 'sunset' ischaemic foot)
- White (no circulation)
- Blue/black (gangrene)

Blisters/crepitus

Due to subcutaneous infection, oedema, or diabetic dermopathy. Crepitus indicates gas gangrene which is usually due to multiple organisms, but exclude *Clostridium welchii*.

Infection

Treat any foot infection in patients with neuropathy or vascular disease vigorously. If you suspect any infection is major or extends below the immediate subcutaneous tissues, refer the patient to hospital immediately. Superficial infected areas should be cleaned and dressed (📖 Table 15.1, p.329) and seen daily by a nurse or doctor until healed. Any infection which is not healing in 3 days should be referred to hospital. Refer patients with worsening foot or leg infection to hospital immediately. NB Infected diabetic patients are often apyrexial.

Ulceration

- Clean punched-out ulcers are usually neuropathic but some will also have peripheral vascular disease
- Irregular-edged ulcers are usually neuro-ischaemic (it is rare to find any purely vascular ulcers in diabetic patients)
- Exudate or frank pus, odour, surrounding erythema, oedema, pain indicate infection
- If you can feel bone at the bottom, there is osteomyelitis
- There may be a sinus

Swelling

This may mean infection, autonomic neuropathy, Charcot joints, cardiac failure, or nephrotic syndrome. Swelling is often a danger sign in people with diabetes. Consider referral to a diabetologist.

Pain

Pain requires urgent investigation. It may represent an easily treatable problem, e.g. tight shoes, or it may represent major trouble such as infection. Neuropathy may blunt pain but can also cause pain. Charcot joints develop in neuropathic limbs, but may be painful while evolving. Repeat X-rays in diabetic neuropathic patients with persistent pain, swelling, or heat after an injury.

Heat

A hot area may indicate infection or an active Charcot joint. Such 'hot spots' should always be investigated.

Cold

A cold foot or leg strongly suggests vascular insufficiency. Rapidly developing coldness indicates acute vascular block and the need for immediate inpatient vascular care (📖 p.467).

Absent foot pulses *(📖 p.467)*

Neuropathy ***(📖 p.306).***

Investigations

Blood tests

- Full blood count—white count may be normal despite infection
- C-reactive protein (CRP) —may be normal despite infection
- U&E
- LFT
- Calcium
- Thyroid function tests

Infection screen

- Ulcer/pus swabs, bone debris, slough—always send sample to microbiology in appropriate medium/container
- NB Remind surgical teams to send samples from debridement or amputation specimens to microbiology
- Blood culture
- MRSA screen

Cardiac

- ECG in all. Very high risk of coronary artery disease
- Echocardiogram if possible cardiac failure and not done recently

Radiology

- Tell the radiologist exactly where the ulcer or colour change is or draw a picture on the request form
- Always X-ray the foot even though there may be little superficial evidence of problems. Patients with neuropathy can have multiple fractures with little or no pain. Osteomyelitis can lurk beneath subtle superficial change.
- Consider MRI to differentiate between osteomyelitis and Charcot change
- CT can be used but MRI is often more helpful
- Consider labelled white cell scan to seek concealed infection
- Technetium bone scans are rarely helpful as they 'light up' with both infection and Charcot change.

Vascular

- Ankle–brachial pressure index: measure this in all patients but remember that it can appear falsely normal as highly calcified blood vessels do not compress.
- Venous and/or arterial duplex scans: have a low threshold for requesting detailed vascular imaging. Patients with diabetes may have venous ulcers. Peripheral vascular disease is very common.
- Angiography—after review by vascular team.

Treatment of diabetic foot problems

- ❶Treat promptly and vigorously. Review frequently (daily if inpatient)
- Pain relief may be needed even in neuropathic patients. The pain of critical ischaemia is agonizing and relentless, and prevents sleep. Such patients hang their foot out of bed for some relief and opiates are usually needed.
- Suspect infection in all patients. Treat if any evidence or strong clinical suspicion. Use your district or hospital antibiotic protocol. Several organisms and anaerobes may often be present. Screen all diabetic foot patients for MRSA when first seen. Consider MRSA screening once or twice annually thereafter if recurrent infections. In general, antibiotics such as co-amoxiclav, penicillin with flucloxacillin, or clindamycin are used, in combination with metronidazole in many cases. Many patients referred to hospital will already have failed to respond to one or more courses of oral antibiotic so consider IM or IV antibiotics, especially if osteomyelitis is present. As these patients may have significant neuropathy and slow gastric emptying, as well as poor circulation, the highest safe concentration of antibiotics should be sought. Many of these patients will have renal impairment and may need dose reduction. Patients with osteomyelitis may need several months of antibiotics (usually oral). Take great care to prevent MRSA or *Clostridium difficile* infection.
- Debridement/excision is essential if there is dead tissue or such grossly infected tissue that antibiotics will not penetrate. Podiatrists or nurses experienced in wound care will remove slough. Debridement must be thorough. More extensive surgical excision may also be needed. In patients with vascular disease perform angioplasty or vascular surgery promptly first.
- Larva therapy can be used to clean up sloughy ulcers.
- Avoid occlusive dressings—these can worsen diabetic ulcers
- Avoid further pressure on the affected area(s). This may mean complete non-weight-bearing. A total contact cast or boot can remove the pressure but allow walking. Such treatment needs to be applied by experts or further damage can ensue.
- Elevation—unless there is severe arterial insufficiency, swollen feet or legs should be elevated to reduce fluid and aid healing. Be very careful to avoid heel pressure ulcers.
- Most hospitalized diabetic foot patients need thromboembolism protection with low molecular weight heparin. Thromboembolism prevention stockings are not a good idea unless one is certain that arterial function is reasonable, as ischaemia can ensue. Also, neuropathic patients may develop sores in the creases under such stockings.
- Good nutrition is essential. Many of these patients have not eaten properly for months and have lost weight. They may have vitamin deficiencies. Refer to the dietitian.
- Psychological support is also essential. Depression and anxiety are common.
- Optimize glucose control
- See other complications and comorbidities and treat vigorously.

- Vascular treatment. Review arterial and venous circulation in all patients. Ideally, all patients with any vasculopathy should be seen by the vascular team on the day of admission and urgent vascular investigations arranged. Check renal function, and stop metformin, ensuring that patients are well hydrated before angiograms. Monitor renal function in all patients after any contrast is used. If stenoses (above or below the knee) are amenable to angioplasty or surgery, this should be performed promptly, with referral to centres of expertise if necessary. Ensure that a senior anaesthetist assesses the patient. Warn of autonomic neuropathy (risk of cardiac arrest) if present. Regional blocks are often used. Remember that these can be frightening and often painful for patients.
- Amputation—nowadays we try and try to preserve limbs. However, this may mean months in hospital with deteriorating physical and emotional health. Patients with severe infection or gangrene often do better with early rather than late amputation (after vascular intervention if appropriate). Address psychological problems before and after this mutilating surgery. Refer all amputees to the rehabilitation team before surgery if possible.

Preventing further foot problems

- The greatest risk factor for diabetic foot problems is a previous foot problem.
- Such patients must remain under specialist diabetes care.
- These patients should be monitored for life by a podiatrist experienced in complex diabetic foot care as signs of early trouble may be subtle. If possible, the same podiatrist should monitor the patient so that they know their feet well.
- Great care should be paid to made-to-measure footwear with insoles if appropriate. This should be checked at each visit to ensure that the foot shape or gait has not changed. New shoes may be needed.
- Patient education for self-care.
- Diabetic foot patients may have problems with concordance with health care and should be included in community case management systems if locally available
- Health care staff education for foot and general diabetes care of *this* patient
- Work with the patient to reduce all risk factors for diabetic glucose instability and tissue damage
- Reassess the whole patient for tissue damage regularly (📖 p.324, p.42)
- React fast if any further foot problems appear (same day referral to diabetic foot team)

Summary

- Diabetes foot problems are preventable.
- The consequence may be amputation.
- Educate the patient about daily foot care.
- Take a personal interest in their feet. Check at least annually.
- Examine high-risk feet at every visit.
- Respond urgently to any foot problems. A small ulcer may eventually kill the patient.
- Refer all patients with diabetic foot problems to the specialist diabetic foot team or diabetologist.
- Institute full risk factor preventive care.
- Be alert for other diabetic tissue damage.

Useful reading

Assal JP, Gfeller R, Ekoe JM. Patient education in diabetes. In *Recent trends in diabetes research* (ed. H. Bostrom), pp. 276–90. Almquist & Wiksell, Stockholm, 1982.
Website about foot testing—patient leaflets in 30 languages. www.diabeticfoot.org.uk

Chapter 16

Diabetes in young people

Diabetes in young people

This chapter is about teens to early twenties—adolescence. The care of pre-teen children with diabetes is sometimes different and has not been included in this book.

Young people with diabetes are often challenging to care for and need specialized diabetes care. Under-18s should be managed in secondary care. Children under teenage should ideally see a formally trained paediatric diabetologist. If not, they should be under joint supervision by a paediatrician and a diabetologist. Teenagers should have joint care from paediatric and adult diabetes services to provide wide expertise and continuity of care as they move into the adult service. This is often called a young diabetic clinic (YDC). If this is not possible, formal transition arrangements should be made. Few hospitals have adolescent wards and adult diabetes teams will usually manage inpatients >16 yrs old. Their diabetes will be affected by, or will influence, most other health care issues. Diabetes may also have a major effect upon the young person's parents and siblings, and vice versa. Communication between the services involved (often many) must remain good at all times.

In the UK those <16 yrs are below the legal age for consent to medical treatment, those between 16 and 18 yrs can agree to treatment but cannot refuse life-saving treatment, and those >18 yrs old have full adult rights to consent to or refuse treatment. Adult thought processes and behaviours begin to develop in the teens, but progress to full maturity varies widely. Assume that all teenagers wish to be fully involved in their own care and have their views properly heard, and their confidentiality and personal privacy respected. Confidentiality can be maintained in those <18 yrs unless the safety of the patient or others is at risk. However, parents are responsible for them until 18 and their views should also be sought. Most clinics will see young people with and without their parents to allow young people fully to express their views. Do not examine them without a chaperone.

Health professionals caring for patients <18 yrs old should be aware of responsibilities and procedures for child protection should concerns arise.

Presentation and assessment

Presentation

Most patients with new diabetes under the age of 30 yrs will have type 1 diabetes. However, variants of type 2 diabetes are becoming more frequent, especially among patients of South Asian and African Caribbean origin, particularly if overweight. In the USA nearly half the diabetes in young people is now type 2. Diabetes presents with the same symptoms as in adults (📖 p.2, 15). Additional features may include growth retardation, difficulties at school, behavioural problems, and bed-wetting (even in teenagers). Weight loss can be dramatic. In type 2 diabetes more gradual symptoms and onset may lead to delayed diagnosis and symptoms not being taken seriously.

Assessment of newly diabetic young people (📖 p.19)

- Full history and examination.
- Height and weight—plot on centile chart.
- Pubertal stage.
- General clinical state—ill or not? Admission required?
- Is diabetes the only problem? Has the presentation been triggered by infection?
- Remember that diabetes is more frequent in a variety of chromosomal disorders, and in other conditions such as cystic fibrosis. About 4% of patients with coeliac disease have diabetes.
- Investigations as for adults including tissue transglutaminase, islet cell, and antiGAD antibodies

Management

Treatment

What type of diabetes is it? (📖p. 14, 15)

Definition can be difficult. The following are practical suggestions. Seek expert specialist advice same day. If in doubt as to whether type 1 or 2 diabetes use insulin and monitor very carefully until expert help arrives. I would now advise sending blood for islet cell and antiGAD antibodies on all newly diagnosed diabetic patients <20 yrs of age. Only a positive result is really helpful. Negative results do not disprove a diagnosis of type 1 diabetes—merely make it less likely.

- Ill ± severe symptoms ± ketones present (≥1mmol/l in blood or >+ in urine) ± venous bicarbonate <15 mmol/l = type 1 diabetes—needs insulin
- Not 'ill' ± milder symptoms ± minimal ketones (<1mmol/l in blood or ≤+ in urine) ± overweight ± South Asian or African Caribbean origins ± strong family history of diabetes = type 2 diabetes. May manage with tablets (or may be early type 1 and actually need insulin).

Most young people now start treatment at home without hospital admission. Some centres still admit type 1 patients for a few days. The home start approach can be achieved only by a dedicated diabetologist/paediatrician who provides personal care, or by a diabetes specialist nurse (preferably paediatrically trained). Other members of the team may be seen at the hospital or at home. The patient and their family are visited once or twice a day until they are confident in insulin injection technique and diet. A 24 hr telephone diabetes helpline is essential.

Insulin

Basal bolus regimens are first choice (📖 p.190). No other intermittent injection pattern achieves the same flexibility of control. CSII works well for motivated young patients. These patients will have diabetes for the rest of their lives with ample time to develop tissue damage and must be encouraged to aim for good glucose control from the start. It is *not* kind to undertreat them. However, it is very difficult to obtain good control in many patients. Young people are as capable of injecting insulin as adults, but also have the same range of anxiety about injections. Encourage them to do their own injections from the start—overprotection by staff or parents is not helpful. 'Pinch and prick' techniques are best to avoid IM injections in slim patients. The Novopen[R] Demi, which gives half units, may be needed for smaller patients. The lunchtime injection is difficult in patients who are unable or unwilling to give it themselves. Young people usually feel embarrassed about injecting insulin at school, and this may be difficult to arrange. Schools should provide a room in which this can be done. Patients and parents need to be warned about the honeymoon period of diabetes (📖 p.192). Lipohypertrophy is common, especially abdominal. Seek it. Avoid injections in these areas (📖 p.186).

Non-insulin treatments

Most pharmaceutical manufacturers have not caught up with the increasing need for treatment for type 2 diabetes in young people. The relevant SPCs state the following.

- Metformin: 'In children from 10 yrs of age and adolescents, Glucophage® film-coated tablets may be used as monotherapy or in combination with insulin.'
- Slow-release metformin: 'In the absence of available data, Glucophage® SR should not be used in children.'
- Gliclazide: not for 'juvenile onset diabetes.'
- Glibenclamide: 'As non-insulin dependent diabetes is not usually a disease of childhood, Daonil® is not recommended for use in children.'
- Glipizide: 'Use in children: safety and effectiveness in children have not been established.'
- Repaglinide: contraindicated in children <12 yrs of age.
- Nateglinide. 'There are no data available on the use of nateglinide in patients under 18 yrs of age, and therefore its use in this age group is not recommended.'
- Rosiglitazone: 'For children aged 10 to 17 yrs, there are limited data on rosiglitazone as monotherapy … The available data do not support efficacy in the paediatric population and therefore such use is not recommended.'
- Pioglitazone: 'There are no data available on the use of pioglitazone in patients under 18 yrs of age, and therefore its use is not recommended in this age group.'
- Sitagliptin: 'Januvia® is not recommended for use in children below 18 yrs of age due to a lack of data on its safety and efficacy.'
- Exanetide: 'There is no experience in children and adolescents below 18 yrs.'

Paediatricians are less familiar with oral hypoglycaemic agents than adult diabetologists—another reason for joint clinics for diabetic teenagers. A common-sense approach, which would conform to the licensed use, is to give metformin to all teenagers with type 2 diabetes and add repaglinide at meal times, adjusted according to food intake. However, it should be noted that most centres would probably add gliclazide if metformin alone failed, and slow-release metformin has a better side-effect profile and greater practicality with once-daily administration. Also, most people are not good at taking lunchtime medication, and the fewer pills the better the concordance. Weigh the dangers and misery of persistently high glucose vs the risks of using medications not tested on teenagers but widely used on those a few years older.

Diet

Refer all young people with diabetes to a dietitian used to caring for this age group. Advise a healthy diet which everyone should follow (📖 p.69). It helps if the whole family has the same diet. Quantities should be enough to maintain appropriate weight for height and continued normal growth and development. Food is the most common battleground between the diabetic teenager and his/her parents. Teenagers like to 'graze', and formal family mealtimes are increasingly uncommon. Chocolate, crisps, and burgers are often what their peer group eats. Banning sweets at home increases secret outside consumption. It is better to include sugar/chocolate as part of meals; this will reduce its impact on the blood glucose and reduce the desire for guilty extras. Young people need to eat enough to grow properly—the 'diet' must not be interpreted as weight restricting unless the child is actually obese. Teenage boys eat a lot, and those who do a lot of sport will need more. There is no place for 'diabetic' foods, and fatty and salty foods should be discouraged. Introduce the new diet gradually and help the child to learn about different types of food and how they might affect diabetes. For patients and families who wish, carbohydrate counting makes insulin adjustment easier long term and helps to improve glucose balance.

The patient must carry glucose if on insulin, and have snacks immediately available (agreed beforehand with the school or college if necessary).

School lunches can be prepacked if that is what peers do. If lunch is provided, encourage healthy options. However, once out of parental view teenagers will eat what they want. The patient may need to 'jump the queue' for food to avoid hypoglycaemia—risking embarrassment.

By the time the school day finishes a teenager often arrives home hungry, and possibly hypoglycaemic. This leads to a large snack, followed by the full evening meal later. An extra dose of insulin may be needed to cover the snack to avoid high glucose levels later.

Teach teenagers how to shop economically for healthy food before they go away to university or college. Basic nutritional principles and cooking skills are also essential.

Weight and body image

Obesity

More than one in four <16-yr-olds in the UK are overweight. This has contributed to the increase in type 2 diabetes in young people and to adult obesity. Young people reflect family lifestyles, health beliefs, and eating patterns. Obese teenagers are often bullied and may be depressed. A prolonged combined psychological, family, and dietetic approach is needed. Set realistic goals—first not gaining more weight. Diet and exercise are both important.

Weight loss or limitation

Some authors suggest an increased frequency of eating disorders in diabetes (these can affect adults too). Both anorexia nervosa and bulimia occur, and may explain bizarre fluctuations in blood glucose control (especially the latter). Laxative abuse also occurs and can cause dangerous hypokalaemia in insulin-deficient patients.

A more common form of self-abuse, usually in girls (up to one in three), is insulin omission as chronically high glucose levels cause weight loss. Suspect this in slim girls with persistently high HbA_{1c}.

Any eating disorder or deliberate insulin omission needs specialist psychological and psychiatric advice from multidisciplinary teams familiar with caring for such patients and their families. A first step is to elicit the problem non-judgementally (e.g. 'Lots of people worry about their weight. Sometimes they cut their food or their insulin. Have you ever thought about doing that?'). Show that it is safe to talk about it. Discourage parental nagging which is understandable but counter-productive.

All these patients are at increased risk of diabetic tissue damage (e.g. retinopathy) and must be monitored closely. Follow NICE 2004 guidance for eating disorders (guidance.nice.org.uk/CG9/niceguidance/pdf/English).

Exercise

The computer generation spends increasing time in front of their PCs and less time on physical activity. This may lead to reduced face-to-face friendship, but intense Internet communication. It reduces overall fitness and may cause repetitive strain injury in hands/wrists. School sports and gym can help maintain exercise, but these activities have been reduced in some schools. Obese young people feel embarrassed in sports or swimming kit and try to avoid activities. Encourage any safe physical activity which the young person is happy about. Even walking further from the parental car to the school gate can help. The paediatric DSN can talk to the physical education teacher at school. Those who enjoyed sport at school may find that they have no time or opportunity for this at university. Encourage them to find a practical physical activity which fits their new timetable.

Glucose should be checked before a sports session. Follow the rules for exercise (📖 p.259). The physical education teacher or trainer should carry glucose tablets or glucose drink and know how to recognize and treat hypoglycaemia.

Home blood glucose monitoring (HBGM)

- Often finger-prick blood tests are more unpopular than the insulin injections.
- Find the finger-pricking system and part of finger which hurts least. Consider needle-less methods.
- Safety tests (before bed, before sport, when ill) should be insisted upon.
- Ideally the tests should be more frequent to allow insulin and dietary adjustment.
- New meters and 'cool' electronics are popular, and may improve testing.

Diabetes kit

- Small bag/bum bag/pocket bag
- Fast-acting insulin pen
- Compact glucose meter with integral strips
- Small finger-pricker
- Dextrosol ± Glucogel®
- Durable snack
- Diabetic card

Complications start in childhood

It is not true that only diabetes after puberty 'counts' towards the development of diabetic tissue damage. This dangerous myth led to undertreatment of childhood diabetes for years. In fact, children as young as 10 yrs old can develop retinopathy. Patients whose type 1 diabetes began in childhood are much more likely to have proteinuria than those diagnosed as adults but with similar duration (*Diabetic Med* 2001; **18**(suppl. 2):35). We have to improve diabetes care in children and teenagers. Failure to do so may seriously impair quality and quantity of life. This requires intensive patient and parent education and support, with good access to out-of-hours help. Sadly, adult diabetes services still see 20-yr-olds with multiple diabetic tissue damage.

Microvascular disease (retinopathy or nephropathy) is the most likely complication, but note that hypertension and macrovascular disease can occur in young people. Even young diabetic children may have abnormal vascular resistance. The accepted limits for blood pressure readings in those <15 yrs old (systolic is thought to be most reliable) are <95 centile for gender, age, and height; checked on three occasions. Patients <18 yrs old should certainly have systolic blood pressures <130. The Diabetes NSF advises digital photographic retinal screening for children >12 yrs old. Retinopathy can occur at younger ages. Microalbuminuria should be screened annually, as for adults (📖 p.104).

For microalbuminuria and hypertension in young people reduce dietary salt and tighten blood glucose control. Many snacks (e.g. crisps) are high in salt. Weight normalization is also important.

In those >16 yrs treat persistent microalbuminuria or hypertension as for adults. There is no consensus about treatment for those <16 yrs. It would seem logical to treat them as for adults. Thiazides, captopril, and atenolol have been used in teenagers (see SPCs). Girls over menarche (mean onset at 13 yrs old) are often sexually active and at risk of pregnancy (📖 p.283).

Lipids are not routinely measured in paediatric diabetic clinics, yet this will identify those with concomitant familial hyperlipidaemia who are then at much increased risk of cardiovascular disease. They should be monitored in YDCs. Treat young patients with significant hyperlipidaemia as for adults (seek specialist advice). Statins are contraindicated in pregnancy.

Growth

- All diabetic young people <20 yrs old should have a growth chart (height and weight) in their hospital and GP records. Mark parental heights on the chart. Use age-related BMI charts as well.
- Note menarche and pubertal staging.
- High glucose levels suppress growth hormone release and stunt growth. Improve glucose control to avoid permanent shortness.
- Normoglycaemia with a healthy diet containing sufficient calories is essential for normal growth.
- Obesity is increasing. About a million chldren <16 yrs in the UK are obese, and about one in four of 2–15-yr-olds are overweight.
- If weight starts to rise inappropriately, ask the patient 'to get back to the right weight for your height' with the dietitian's help. Do *not* just say 'lose weight' as this may fuel an eating disorder.
- This commercial website allows you to plot BMI, height. and weight on national standard charts electronically: www.healthforallchildren.co.uk/?SHOP=HFAC4&DO=USERPAGE&PAGE=PLOTCHART

Puberty and sex

Puberty, with its changing hormonal balance and metabolic demands, usually needs insulin dose increases. Blood glucose balance may become erratic. Food intake usually increases around puberty. Beware excessive insulin fuelling hunger and excessive eating.

Use standard Tanner charts to assess pubertal stage. Many young patients find genital assessment embarrassing. A Tanner self-reporting system is available.

Menstruation (mean onset of menarche is 13 yrs in non-diabetic girls) can cause cyclical hyperglycaemia (sometimes hypoglycaemia). Menarche may be delayed if diabetes is diagnosed before this would normally be expected. Tell diabetic girls who have started to menstruate about sexual intercourse, the possibility of pregnancy, and the need for family planning in diabetes. Parental presence may sometimes inhibit discussions about sexual issues, although many parents are supportive. With the recent AIDS prevention campaigns and ready availability of condoms in shops, sexual ignorance is less common than before. However, everyone thinks 'It won't happen to me'! An unsuspected pregnancy can precipitate diabetic keto-acidosis, and it is particularly important to avoid unwanted pregnancy in diabetic girls. Both genders need to understand the need for protection from sexually transmitted diseases (including thrush).

Partners can be very supportive in diabetes self-care and some young patients bring them to clinic

The Family Planning Association has helpful leaflets for young people on its website www.fpa.org.uk/information/

Parents and siblings

Diabetes is a frightening condition. Some parents with diabetes will be consumed by guilt—'I gave it to him!' Health care staff do not have to live with the child and his diabetes every day. No one likes their child to have injections. Many parents are so frightened of possible adverse consequences that they adhere rigidly to the guidelines they were given on diagnosis without realizing that some flexibility is possible. Many need a lot of support in introducing flexibility. The paediatric diabetic specialist nurse's role is crucial. Parents may be terrified of hypoglycaemia and run the glucose too high to avoid this. Conversely, anxieties about tissue damage may lead to over-stringent glucose control and hypoglycaemia. Siblings may receive less attention that the person with diabetes, causing jealousy—but they may also be frightened that their brother or sister may die.

Staff in the YDC need to help the family move away from the model of paediatric consultation with the parents to talking with the patient. Some parents find this hard. Some young people also find being asked direct medical questions threatening and clam up. Give them time and have a more general discussion first. Ensure that they have enough opportunity to ask questions. The need to allow a teenager to speak to the doctor or nurse on their own may make the parent feel excluded and angry. Listen to parents too.

Alcohol and recreational drugs

Alcohol

Alcohol is cheap and readily available, even to under-age teenagers. Most teenagers start drinking before the legal age and many drink to excess in their teens and older. This exposes them to the risk of injury and unwise sexual behaviour. Remind them of the law, but make sure that they are aware of advice for safe drinking when you have diabetes (📖 p.83) as they are likely to avoid your advice to drink only legally.

Alcohol poisoning can cause ketosis and may mimic DKA.

Recreational drugs

In one study 28% of diabetic patients aged 16–30 yrs had tried or were using recreational drugs (*Diabetic Med*, 2003; 21: 295). Ask all young patients about recreational drug use (parental presence may inhibit reliable answers about alcohol and drug use). Ensure that your patients know that recreational drugs are dangerous in anyone, but especially so if you have diabetes.

Recreational drugs can have direct effects on glucose control or impede ability to self-care. Cannabis causes mood change which may mask hypoglycaemia, although the 'munchies' it induces may raise glucose. Ecstasy reduces urinary water loss and could worsen the hyponatraemia associated with high glucose, especially if a lot of water is drunk. Both cocaine and amphetamines can raise glucose. Opiates may affect insulin and glucagon release. Drugs use may precipitate an admission with DKA and should be sought in the history.

Psychological issues

Psychiatric disorders are two to three times more common in diabetic adolescents than in their peers. In one study 37% adolescents met criteria for formal psychiatric diagnosis, particularly young women. Psychiatric disorders were present in half those with a history of poor diabetes control vs a quarter of well-controlled patients. Those with poor glucose control were more likely to have had pre-diabetic behaviour problems (*Diabetic Med* 2005; **22**:152–7).

Many adolescent patients are anxious. Patients may seize on a small comment in clinic and worry about it for months. Specifically seek worries in each consultation.

❶Depression is common among young people. Believe them when they say that they are depressed or have considered suicide. Sadly, people may think they are exaggerating because they are teenagers.

Seek expert help immediately if the patient is depressed. Suicidal ideation requires an immediate phone call to your local mental health service for young people.

Unfortunately, specialist adolescent mental health services may be difficult to access in some areas. Young people may be too old for children's mental health services and too young for adult services. Clarify local arrangements for adolescents before they are needed. Websites for young people with diabetes include:

- www.youthhealthtalk.org
- www.diabetes.org.uk/Guide-to-diabetes/My-life/

Brittle diabetes

One unstable diabetic young woman can generate multiple admissions for DKA and/or hypoglycaemia and massive hospital records, and engage the attentions of the diabetes team, every on-take medical team in the hospital, mental health teams, social services, GP, and practice staff. Her parents may require psychiatric and medical help, and some staff may need psychological support. Although the dramatic behaviour of the 'brittle diabetic' is memorable and time-consuming, remember that there are few such patients in most districts.

Most such patients have complex psychological ± diabetes education issues. They are at risk of early death. They must remain under diabetologist care. If problems arise, contact the diabetes team immediately to reduce duplication and manipulation. One member of the diabetes team (e.g. DSN) should coordinate care, but may need back-up as such patients can be emotionally draining to care for.

Remember that there may be a non-psychological cause for her problems.

Concordance vs non-concordance

Adolescence is a time of experimentation with one's personality, sexuality, family, and the outside world. It is often 'make or break' time—examinaton results determine further training, apprenticeships further careers, marriage partners may be chosen. Boundaries are tested—parental authority, school or college rules, health and fitness, relationships. Parents must start handing over diabetes care to their children, if they have not already done so. This can be difficult. The worries that parents experience waiting for a child to come home from a late-night disco are compounded when that child has diabetes. Has she eaten enough? Drunk too much? If late, has she gone hypo? It is hard to relinquish care of a potentially dangerous disorder when a young person is rebelling against authority and appears least capable of taking care of themself.

Health professionals' and parents' views of the aims of diabetes care do not always match the patient's. Teenagers want their diabetes to be as inconspicuous as possible. They often run a high glucose because hypoglycaemia is frightening, and they want to avoid embarrassing behaviour in front of their friends. Clarification of the patient's goals can help acceptance of overall care.

Many YDCs have a 25% non-attendance rate. Phone calls, texts, e-mails, letters have all been tried and may work for some. The DSN is most likely to succeed in re-establishing contact. From the young patient's point of view clinics may be frightening, boring, and confusing places that smell of hospitals, where you are told off for not doing something, and asked embarrassing questions in front of your parents by a doctor you have never seen before. The following steps may help.

- Try to maintain continuity of care however 'difficult' the patient's behaviour.
- Maintain contact with the patient in whatever way works for them.
- Listen properly. Respect the patient's opinions. Be non-judgemental.
- Ensure that they know that rescue will always be provided (and how to access it) if the glucose goes badly wrong (e.g. DKA).
- If the 'lost sheep' returns, welcome them in a friendly way, manage any emergencies swiftly, and then apply a constructive approach to future improvements in care.
- Seek depression or anxiety, or other psychological issues.
- It is very important for young people to 'save face'.
- Insulin may be genuinely or deliberately forgotten. Any insulin injections are helpful; the right injections at the right time are excellent. Ask 'How are the insulin injections going?'
- Provide opportunities to admit lapses: 'Are you managing to do any blood tests?' Any blood glucose tests are helpful; the right tests at the right time are excellent.

- Encourage the use of glucose meters from which results can be downloaded onto a PC. Teenagers hate writing down glucose results. Ask them to bring the meter to the clinic and download it there.
- Faked blood test results are common, as is omission of high readings. If suspected try: 'Lots of people forget to write all their sugars down and try to remember them later. Does that ever happen with you?' Or 'I don't quite understand this result—might it be a mistake?'
- New gadgets and technology may encourage more tests and more injections.
- Concordance may improve when a driving licence application is needed!

Education and diabetes

Young people spend much of their time at school or in further education. Schools often have rigid rules and staff may not understand the needs of diabetic teenagers. There is no coordinated training for teachers and school staff about diabetes and there is considerable individual variation in the way in which young people with diabetes are supported at school. DSNs will teach staff about diabetes and the needs of individual students. Nowadays teachers may not be allowed to assist with medical care and there may be no school nurse or first-aider. Less support is provided in secondary schools than in primary schools. A study in Wales (2006) describes the situation there:
www.diabetes.org.uk/Documents/Reports/Support_for_children_english.pdf

The Diabetes UK schools pack is essential reading for parents and teachers of diabetic students. Areas of self-care which can make diabetes easier to manage at school are dietary knowledge, blood glucose testing, awareness of the symptoms of hypoglycaemia and how to treat them, and knowledge of how to cope with exercise. Self-injection means that the child can go on school trips. Everyone (including fellow pupils) should be aware that he/she has diabetes—otherwise there may be accusations of drug abuse if injections or blood tests are observed.

Time off school should be rare and repeated school absences because of diabetes must be investigated promptly so that diabetes care can be improved. There is a complex interrelationship between poor glycaemic balance, the psychological effects of diabetes, school work, and behaviour. Resolution may require the combined efforts of parents, teachers, child psychologist, paediatrician, diabetologist, diabetes team, and GP—clear communication is vital. Most diabetic students do as well as their non-diabetic peers academically, and there is some suggestion that they may do better, perhaps because of greater pressure to succeed.

Most young people complete their training unimpeded by their diabetes. Occasionally diabetes develops around examination time or interferes with a crucial time at school or university. Prompt diagnosis and treatment focused on a return to academic or practical activities as soon as possible can minimize the damage. Rarely, the young person may be unable to perform up to their usual standard for a few weeks or occasionally months. A formal letter to academic or training authorities may be needed to help the patient to gain another chance.

Leaving home

This section relates to any move from home. Going to university is the most common—exciting but worrying for students and parents.

- Students should locate and inform university medical services about their diabetes.
- Visit the medical centre and doctor on arrival.
- Book holiday visits to the familiar YDC.
- Tell students they can still phone/text/e-mail their usual DSN if necessary.
- Liaise with university town specialist diabetes services in complex cases.
- Ensure sufficient supplies of insulin, testing strips etc.
- Ascertain arrangements for re-supply while at university.
- Teach self-catering and economical shopping (family and dietitian).
- Take a mobile phone with unlimited calls.
- Ensure accommodation is clean, warm, and secure.
- Find a secure place for back-up diabetic kit.
- Carry daily diabetes kit around.
- Tell personal tutors about the diabetes.
- Tell new friends about the diabetes.
- Ask the DSN and YDC staff about adjusting diabetes treatment to new way of life.

Summary

Issues to consider when caring for young people with diabetes

- What the patient wants and fears
- How best to stay in touch—phone/text/e-mail/letter
- Family (parents—together or not, siblings, others)
- Friends
- Home environment—emotional and physical
- School or further education
- Hobbies
- Sports
- Career planning—diabetes precludes some careers (📖 p.432)
- Work (📖 p.425)
- Learning to drive/driving (📖 p.440)
- Financial issues
- Emotions—look out for depression or anxiety (📖 p.452)
- Alcohol
- Recreational drugs
- Sex
- Anything which may require Child Protection investigation
- Growth and pubertal development
- What type of diabetes do they have?
- Home blood glucose testing
- Diabetes treatment—insulin or non-insulin
- Food—home, school, eating out
- Exercise (📖 p.259)
- Diabetic tissue damage—prevention, detection, and treatment (📖 p.269)
- Other health problems
- Clinic attendance

Further reading

Children's NSF. Available at:
www.dh.gov.uk/en/Policyandguidance/Healthandsocialcaretopics/ChildrenServices/Childrenservicesinformation/DH_4089111

Chapter 17

Diabetes in women

Effects of diabetes in women

All the changes of womanhood can influence, and be influenced by, diabetes.

Menstruation

Menarche may be delayed if diabetes is diagnosed around puberty. About one in three diabetic women experience some menstrual abnormalities, most commonly infrequent or irregular periods. This is thought to be due to hypothalamic dysfunction.

The hormonal changes before and during menstruation can cause both hypoglycaemia and hyperglycaemia in different individuals. The most frequent change is hyperglycaemia on the last day or so premenstrually or, most often, during the first 2 days of bleeding. Some women are hypoglycaemic premenstrually or as bleeding subsides. Others have unpredictable oscillations in glycaemic balance. Some women increase their insulin for the first 2 days of bleeding. Hyperglycaemia can cause menstrual irregularity or amenorrhoea, especially in untreated diabetes.

Polycystic ovary syndrome (PCOS)

- PCOS is common.
- Symptoms and signs
  - overweight
  - irregular or absent periods
  - anovulatory infertility
  - acne
  - hirsutism
  - acanthosis nigricans
- Glucose intolerance in approx. one in ten PCOS patients—the greater the BMI, the more likely the glucose intolerance
- Type 2 diabetes—two to four times more likely than in general population
- Hyperinsulinaemia
- Increased risk of uterine cancer.
- Diagnosis requires two out of:
  - menstrual abnormalities
  - hormone abnormalities (raised testosterone, reduced sex hormone-binding globulin, raised LH)
  - polycystic ovaries (e.g. on ultrasound)
- Note that actual ovarian cysts are not essential for the diagnosis

Treatment

- Weight loss is the key treatment which will improve clinical features.
- Use metformin to control glucose.
- Metformin is used off-license in PCOS without diabetes as it may aid weight loss in conjunction with dietary advice, improve ovulation and menstrual regularity, reduce hirsutism, and prevent diabetes. Not all studies showed these effects with metformin, and weight loss alone may be as effective. Some patients had side effects (📖 p.138).
- Sibutramine has been used in these patients.

Infections

- Thrush (candida)—may be a presenting feature. Use standard anti-fungal—combining single-dose oral fluconazole and vaginal/perineal imidazole creams may provide cure and comfort more reliably. Treat the partner as well. Improve glucose control. See genitourinary clinic advice if it fails to resolve.
- Urinary tract infection is common. Use antibiotics from local guidelines. Check clearance with a urine dipstick for blood, protein, nitrite, and leucocytes a week after antibiotics finish.
- Pyelonephritis may be severe in diabetic patients.
- Vulval or groin abscess may precipitate DKA. Groin or genital infections can precipitate multiple organism necrotizing fasciitis which is more common in diabetic than in non-diabetic patients.
- Seek genitourinary clinic advice for the following which are more common in diabetic than in non-diabetic women:
  - herpes simplex
  - vaginal warts.

Fertility and contraception

Fertility

Diabetic women can conceive but may have reduced fertility in some situations. Factors which affect fertility are:

- late menarche
- menstrual irregularity
- PCOS
- increased risk of primary ovarian failure (and other autoimmune conditions in type 1 diabetes).

Contraception

Oral contraceptive drugs

Consider each patient's needs individually. Do not deny effective contraception on theoretical grounds. Diabetic women should use the most reliable form of contraception.

The combined oral contraceptive pill (OCP) (pregnacy rate <1/100 woman-yrs if used properly) is often used. Advise current first-choice OCPs for the general population. Monitor blood pressure, glucose control, and lipids; and increase alertness for thrombo-embolic diagnoses. Small studies have not shown worsening of metabolic control or increased likelihood of tissue damage. The BNF advises avoiding these drugs in diabetic women with complications, and those >35 yrs who have any additional cardiovascular risk factor. The WHO is more specific about their use in women with diabetes.

- History of gestational diabetes: no restriction on use.
- Non-vascular disease and type 1 or type 2 diabetes: a condition where the advantages of using the method generally outweigh the theoretical or proven risks.
- Diabetic nephropathy or retinopathy, or diabetes > 20 yrs duration: a condition where the theoretical or proven risks usually outweigh the advantages of using the method or which represents an unacceptable health risk if the contraceptive method is used

However, all these women are also at greater risk of complications of pregnancy. Balance the risks.

A combined oestrogen–progestagen patch may has the same risks as the OCP but can be removed if the patient has an adverse reaction. Patches are changed once a week. Some patients find these easier to remember than daily pills. Used properly the pregnancy rate is the same as an OCP but patches may fall off.

Some centres advocate the progesterone-only OCP for diabetic women as there is less effect upon lipids and thrombosis risk. There may be irregular or unexpected 'periods'. Pregnancy rate is 1/100 women-yrs.

Progesterone-only contraceptive implants or injections may be used in patients unable to remember to take OCPs and unsuitable for an IUCD or IUS. Once injected, the effect lasts fr 12 weeks. The implant lasts for up to 3 yrs and can be removed if there are problems. It may not be so effective in women with a BMI >35 kg/m^2.

Intra-uterine contraceptive devices (IUCDs) have a pregnancy rate of <1/100 women-yrs. In any woman there is a risk of pelvic infection, rarely leading to infertility. This risk is greater in women with diabetes because of their propensity to infection generally. Nowadays, more women are using a progestogen-coated intra-uterine system (IUS) Mirena^{R}. This has a pregnancy rate of <1/100 women-yrs and lasts for 5 yrs. Periods are lessened or even stop.

Barrier methods have no metabolic or thrombotic sequelae but have a greater failure rate than the methods above (pregnancy rates: male condoms, 2/100 women-yrs; female condoms 5/100 women-yrs). They are also harder to use properly. The addition of a spermicide which does not damage the condom improves contraceptive effect. Condoms protect from sexually transmitted diseases. They can also easily be bought in a wide variety of shops, supermarkets, and garages. A diaphragm or cap requires gynaecological assessment for fitting and there may be an increased risk of vaginal and urinary infection. Pregnancy rate is 4–8/100 women-yrs. .

All barrier methods are useless if not used properly, and planned conception and the avoidance of unwanted pregnancy are particularly important in women with diabetes. Some patients, especially those with multiple sexual partners, use both an OCP and a condom.

The rhythm method and withdrawal are not effective and cannot be recommended for diabetic women.

Post-coital contraception using levonorgestrol can be initiated within 72 hrs of unprotected intercourse. An IUCD may also be used for up to 5 days after unprotected intercourse.

There is clear information for patients on the Family Planning Association website: www.fpa.org.uk/information/leaflets/

Pre-pregnancy counselling

Refer all diabetic patients planning pregnancy to a specialist pre-conception diabetic clinic promptly.

Tell teenage diabetic girls to plan pregnancy when they do decide to have a family, and to use contraception, if necessary, until then. All health professionals, especially GPs and practice nurses, should consider the possibility that a girl or woman with diabetes of child-bearing potential might become pregnant. This includes women with type 2 as well as type 1 diabetes. Discuss contraception or pregnancy plans with women at annual review.

Half the pregnant women in pregnant diabetic clinics in London have type 2 diabetes, and half of those are from non-white ethnic backgrounds. A high proportion of type 2 diabetic pregnant patients live in areas with high social deprivation. CEMACH 2007 (www.cemach.org.uk) audited pregnancies in diabetic women and noted that under half the women surveyed had had pre-pregnancy counselling, under half had been given folic acid, and a third had had no measure of glucose control in the 6 months antepartum. Two-thirds had evidence of poor glucose control antenatally or during the first trimester. Suboptimal glucose care was linked with poor pregnancy outcome, as was suboptimal antenatal care. Half the women had suboptimal post-natal diabetes care. 29% of babies had a congenital anomaly.

Congenital malformations are most likely if women are hyperglycaemic in the first 8 weeks of pregnancy. Strict normoglycaemia pre-conception reduces the likelihood of congenital malformation to near that of the non-diabetic population.

As few women know when they conceive, the usual advice is to maintain contraception, adjust treatment to achieve normoglycaemia, and then stop the contraception. It is easier to use barrier methods here, as menstrual cycles may be erratic after stopping OCPs and it is helpful to be able to date the last menstrual period if pregnancy occurs. Normoglycaemia is continued until after the baby is born. It is hard work and means 4–7 finger-prick glucose estimations daily, sometimes for years if conception is slow to occur.

Medication

Hypoglycaemic therapy

Nowadays, many diabetic women of child-bearing age take oral hypoglycaemic drugs. This is more common in women of Asian and African Caribbean origin. There has been concern that these drugs may be associated with fetal malformation. In South Africa glibenclamide and/or metformin have been used in pregnancy for years. In New Zealand retrospective analysis showed no adverse effect on pregnancy outcomes with metformin (*Diabetic Med* 2006; **23**:318–22). The Hyperglycemia and Adverse Pregnancy Outcome (HAPO) study of 25 000 pregnant women (*Int J Gynaecol Obstet* 2002; **78**:69–77.) is due to report in 2007–2008 and should answer this, among other questions. NICE CG 063 (2008) advises stopping oral hypoglycaemic drugs and transfering the patient to insulin treatment. Some diabetologists use metformin in very overweight women who are resistant to insulin after explaining that it is not licensed for use in pregnancy (it does cross the placenta).

Folic acid

Prescribe folic acid 5 mg daily for diabetic women planning pregnancy.

Other drugs

Most hypotensive drugs, especially ACE inhibitors, are contraindicated in pregnancy. If the patient is hypertensive, convert her to methyldopa until after pregnancy and breastfeeding are complete and contraception is in use but see 📖 p.283.

Statins are teratogenic and must be stopped at least a month before trying to conceive. Do not restart until breastfeeding is finished and contraception is in use.

Overall fitness for pregnancy

The woman's fitness to withstand pregnancy and her prospects of healthy survival to care for her child until grown up must also be considered. Nowadays, women with severe tissue damage are surviving pregnancy with normal infants, but this requires 9 months very intensive effort, and the harsh reality is that they may become severely disabled or die before their child grows up.

Retinopathy can worsen in pregnancy, and digital photographic screening should be part of the pre-pregnancy screen as should assessment of renal function. Renal failure may also worsen considerably during pregnancy, and such women should be managed jointly by obstetrician, renal physician, and diabetologist from pre-pregnancy onwards.

Diabetic women may have cardiovascular disease. If there is any suggestion of this refer the patient for formal cardiological assessment.

Education

Provide structured diabetes education for women planning pregnancy.

Pregnancy

- If pregnancy is suspected, proceed as if the patient is pregnant.
- Patients attending a preconception clinic should contact their diabetes team the same day if they suspect pregnancy (individual discussion is required for those with irregular periods).
- Send a blood sample for quantitative beta human chorionic gonadotrophin analysis. Often the patient has made the diagnosis herself using over-the-counter tests.
- Refer pregnant diabetic women the same day by telephone to the diabetologist and obstetrician who provide joint care (most diabetologists will contact the obstetric services themselves). An urgent fax with full details is very helpful.
- Prescribe folic acid 5 mg daily until 12 weeks gestation (some clinics say longer).
- Check calcium levels in patients with dark skin or dietary problems. Give calcium and vitamin D if low.
- In the joint diabetic–obstetric clinic.
  - Full clinical assessment, including BP check and renal function.
  - Arrange formal ophthalmological review
  - Check HBGM, before and 1 hr after each meal, and occasionally during the night.
  - Basal bolus insulin regimens are best.
  - Adjust insulin to achieve blood glucose concentrations:
    3.5–5.9 mmol /l fasting
    4.0–7.7 mmol /l 1 hr after meals
    ≥6 mmol/ at bedtime to reduce the risk of hypoglycaemia.
  - HbA_{1c} 4.0–6.0% if safe
  - Prescribe glucagon and show her partner how to use it
  - ❗Hypoglycaemia is common as patients strive for normoglycaemia and patients and their partners must be warned of this. The patient should always carry glucose on her person and needs to be particularly careful to avoid hypoglycaemia if she is already caring for small children.
  - Insulin dose rises during pregnancy and may have more than doubled by term.
  - Hypoglycaemia and the need to reduce insulin dose near term indicates placental underfunction—admit immediately.
- A dietitian and diabetes specialist nurse or midwife trained in diabetes care should see the patient. The diabetes specialist nurse or midwife can also see her at home.
- Obstetric care will include frequent checks (e.g. fortnightly for the first two trimesters and weekly in the last) and serial ultrasound scans, including examination for anomalies.
- Many obstetricians deliver diabetic women at 38 weeks and may have a low threshold for Caesarian section.
- Cover Caesarian section with prophylactic antibiotics as there is high risk of infection.

- During labour and delivery, insulin and glucose need to be infused intravenously according to a sliding scale.
- Within hours of delivery the insulin requirements will fall to the pre-pregnant dose.
- Check thyroid function 2 months post-partum

Risks in pregnancies of diabetic women

Most complications of pregnancy are increased for mother and fetus in diabetic women. They include:

- pregnancy-induced hypertension
- polyhydramnios
- ketoacidosis
- fetal malformation
- poor fetal growth
- macrosomia
- sudden intra-uterine death
- respiratory distress syndrome
- post-partum hypoglycaemia (mother and fetus)

These complications can be reduced by intensive diabetes and obstetric management, but some women who have been normoglycaemic through–out pregnancy still have macrosomic babies. NICE 063 (2008) reviews this: www.nice.org.uk/guidance/index.jsp?action=by ID&o=12014

Full evidence awaited

One of the difficulties with care of the pregnant diabetic woman is that we are awaiting a full evidence base for optimal management.

The most important factor appears to be frequent care by a team experienced in the management of diabetes in pregnancy, with close attention to detail, and 24 hr availability of immediate help (by telephone or in person) if problems arise.

Gestational diabetes (GDM)

Diabetes may arise during pregnancy, especially in the third trimester. Previously there was debate about whether treatment was of benefit. The ACHOIS study confirmed that treatment of GDM with diet, and insulin adjusted according to HBGM, greatly reduces perinatal complications (*N Engl J Med* 2005; **352**:2477–86). The study also suggested that this treatment improved the women's quality of life.
NICE CG 63 (2008) advocates screening for GDM.

Screening

- Women with past GDM should be offered HBGM or an OGTT at 14–16 weeks
- At 28 weeks screen patients with:
  - BMI >30 kg/m^2
  - non-white ethnic group
  - previous GDM (if OGTT nomal earlier)
  - previous big baby (>4.5 kg)
  - family history of diabetes.
- Screen by performing a formal 75g OGTT(📖 p.9). Diagnostic values are in Table 17.1.
- Once diagnosed, women with gestational diabetes are treated like any other pregnant diabetic woman.

Table 17.1 Oral glucose tolerance test in pregnancy (ACHOIS)

	Venous plasma glucose concentration (mmol/l)		
	Fasting		**2 hrs after glucose load**
GDM	>7.0	*and*	>7.8

Post-partum in patients with GDM

After delivery, glucose tolerance may revert to normal, or remain impaired. In GDM it is usual to stop insulin treatment immediately post-partum. Continue HBGM for 2 days post-partum and contact the diabetes team if it remains high. Check a fasting glucose 6 weeks post-partum. Some clinics do a formal OGTT at 6 weeks.

Over a third of women with gestational diabetes will eventually develop permanent diabetes. This is especially likely in Asian women. The maintenance of a diabetic diet and regular exercise (📖 p.70) may delay or prevent the reappearance of diabetes. There is a high likelihood of gestational diabetes in further pregnancies.

A fasting glucose once a year or once every 2 yrs, or opportunistic screening when the patient attends the GP, will provide earlier diagnosis of diabetes in these women.

Breastfeeding

Diabetic women can breastfeed. They may need to eat more carbohydrate (about 100 g more a day) and reduce their insulin dose according to blood glucose levels. They should snack before feeding and drink more fluid (e.g. milk). With disturbed nights and erratic exercise patterns, there is a risk of hypoglycaemia. Aim for HBGM levels of 6–9 mmol/l during this time. Restart contraception unless further pregnancies are planned.

All non-insulin hypoglycaemic drugs are contraindicated while breastfeeding. See SPCs. However NICE CG 63 says that metformin and glibenclamide can be used if patient consent is obtained.

Motherhood

Women sometimes forget about themselves as they rush around, cooking, cleaning, picking Johnny up from nursery school, delivering Suzanne to ballet, and more. It is even harder work if the woman has an additional paid job. The diabetes can be the last item on the agenda, and the aim may be seen as 'keeping a little sugary to avoid hypoglycaemia and not testing too much because I'm busy'. The diet may be erratic, including remnants from the children's plates. 'I know what I ought to do. I'll focus on the diabetes when the children are older.' A family of two can occupy a woman for 18–20 years, long enough to develop all the complications of diabetes. Mothers should be encouraged to give themselves some time for daily body maintenance, perhaps at a time when their partner is at home and can look after the children. The GP and practice nurse can keep an eye on the way in which the patient is coping with her diabetes when she attends with her children, as well as ensuring that she attends for her own check-ups.

Menopause and hormone replacement therapy

Blood glucose balance occasionally becomes erratic during the menopause although afterwards insulin requirement may fall. This may not apply if the woman is given hormone replacement therapy (HRT).

The MHRA (2007) states: 'use of HRT increases the risk of breast cancer, endometrial cancer and ovarian cancer in a duration-dependent manner. There is no evidence for a beneficial effect of HRT on cardiovascular disease—in fact HRT has been shown to increase the risk of myocardial infarction and venous thromboembolism, especially in the first year of use, and to increase the risk of ischaemic stroke. The risk of most of these conditions increases with age, therefore increasing the overall risks the longer HRT is taken.' The MHRA concluded:

- 'for the treatment of menopausal symptoms, HRT is beneficial for the majority of women in the short-term;
- 'when used in the long-term the balance of risks and benefits of HRT is such that it should be restricted to second-line therapy for the prevention of osteoporosis.

'The decision to use HRT should take into consideration a woman's age, history, risk factors, and personal preferences, and for all women the minimum effective dose should be used for the shortest duration. Continued use of HRT should be regularly re-assessed (e.g. at least annually).'

Diabetes increases the risk of cardiovascular disease and thus HRT should be used with particular caution.

Summary

- All the changes of womanhood can influence, and be influenced by, diabetes.
- Menstrual irregularity is common.
- Glucose control may vary around period time.
- Diabetes is common in PCOS.
- PCOS is common in overweight diabetic women.
- Use the best contraception for each individual. OCPs are commonly used in diabetic women.
- Fertility may be impaired in some diabetic women.
- Pre-pregnancy counselling and care is essential to reduce the risk of congenital malformation.
- Diabetic pregnancy is associated with increased risk of most complications for mother and fetus.
- Normoglycaemia and very careful glucose monitoring avoiding hypoglycaemia is crucial.
- Diabetic pregnant women should be cared for only by specialist diabetic–obstetric services.
- Screening for GDM is essential as treatment is proven to reduce maternal and fetal risk.
- GDM may persist as diabetes post-partum, and increases long-term diabetes risk. These patients should have diet and exercise advice and be followed up.
- Glucose levels may alter around and after menopause.
- HRT is more risky in diabetic patients than in non-diabetic women and MHRA advice should be followed.

Further reading

NICE CG 63 www.nice.org.uk/guidance/index.jsp?action=byID&o=12014

Chapter 18

Diabetes in men

Fatherhood

The diabetic father is under many of the same pressures as the diabetic mother. He may be the one looking after the children. In many cases, he may be the breadwinner. He may worry that his diabetes is going to stop him working and make him let his family down. As with working women, he may be working so hard that he neglects himself and his diabetes. He may ignore check-ups because he does not wish to take time off work. Diabetic fathers may be difficult to contact, but they may be prepared to attend an evening or Saturday clinic. Being self-employed can be particularly stressful.

Infections

Diabetic men may develop candidal balanitis. Both the man and his partner should be treated with antifungals. As in women, the critical factor is returning the blood glucose toward normal.

Fertility

There are conflicting reports about whether or not diabetes alters sperm quality, quantity, or motility. Some diabetic men may have retrograde ejaculation. Fertility does not appear to be impaired unless there is significant erectile dysfunction. There appears to be no problem for the fetus if the father has hyperglycaemia at conception

Libido

Untreated diabetes or hyperglycaemia can temporarily reduce libido. The psychological stress and distress of the new diagnosis and subsequent difficulties may also reduce libido.

Erectile dysfunction

30–50% of men with diabetes may experience erectile dysfunction (ED), either temporarily or permanently. ED may be under-reported as the ambience of many diabetic clinics or busy surgeries is not always conducive to such sensitive discussions. Bearing in mind that it may have taken considerable courage on the patient's part to reveal this symptom, any mention of sexual difficulties should be followed up, if necessary at another appointment with appropriate privacy and time, and preferably with his partner.

Define the patient's problem. ED is the inability to develop and maintain a penile erection sufficient for sexual performance. Although some men with diabetes do have permanent ED associated with diabetic tissue damage, many have reversible ED. Reversible factors or those suggesting another condition requiring investigation and treatment should be sought, but a final decision that the ED is due to diabetes does not mean that the patient and his partner cannot be helped.

Assessment of a man with ED

- Take a full history, including prescribed and non-prescribed drugs and alcohol
- Examine the patient including genitals
- Check for penile deformity which may make drug treatment of ED dangerous
- Check for evidence of the causes of ED below
- Seek evidence of vasculopathy and neuropathy in particular
- Cardiac status should be assessed to inform treatment decisions
- Consider his emotional state

Blood tests

- 9 a.m. testosterone, LH, FSH, and prolactin
- Usual annual review blood tests if not done recently

Causes of erectile dysfunction in diabetic men

- Psychological, including anxiety and depression
- Drugs, including antihypertensives, antidepressants, fibrates, statins, NSAIDs, H_2 blockers, psychotropics, allopurinol
- Alcohol (acute or chronic intake)
- Neuropathy (peripheral and/or autonomic)
- Vascular disease
- Endocrine–hypogonadism

All patients will have some psychological problems either causing or due to the ED. ED due to psychological factors may start suddenly, be associated with reduced libido, and be patchy, i.e. present with one woman and not with another, or present during masturbation but not when intercourse is attempted. However, all these can apply to ED due to diabetic tissue damage.

Evidence of diabetic tissue damage elsewhere, such as retinopathy, nephropathy, neuropathy, and peripheral vascular disease, make it more likely that the ED will be related to diabetic tissue damage. Improve blood glucose control as hyperglycaemia can cause non-specific malaise which may be associated with ED. An erectile response to alprostadil injection demonstrates adequate vascular supply. In unresponsive patients angiography may identify treatable vascular disease. If autonomic neuropathy is evident elsewhere (e.g. with postural hypotension or problems with bladder emptying), the ED is likely to be neurogenic.

Endocrine causes can be suspected by finding other evidence of hypogonadism clinically. It is also more common in patients with other endocrine disorders.

More detailed studies can be undertaken in specialist centres—ideally, by a diabetologist or endocrinologist with a special interest in ED, or urology or genitourinary medicine—check local arrangements.

Treatment of erectile dysfunction

Provide psychological support as needed. Some patients will need specialist psychosexual counselling. Some districts have psychologists trained in assessment and treatment of psychosexual problems. In the UK men whose ED is due to diabetes are entitled to NHS prescriptions for drug treatment for this.

Phosphodiesterase type-5 inhibitors

Phosphodiesterase type-5 inhibitors are the most popular. They include sildenafil (Viagra®), tadalafil (Cialis®), and vardenafil (Levitra®).

Before prescription consider that sudden resumption of sexual activity may increase exertion at night, causing hypoglycaemia, and may precipitate angina or a cardiac event in those with severe coronary atheroma.

Avoid these drugs in patients with:

- blood pressure <90/50
- recent history of stroke
- ischaemic heart disease or cardiac failure
- hepatic failure
- renal failure—adjust the dose according to SPC
- known hereditary retinal degeneration
- nitrates, doxazosin and other vasodilators, cimetidine, ketoconazole, and erythromycin.

These drugs are effective in a high proportion of diabetic men. Tell patients that they work only after sexual stimulation. Side effects include headache, flushing, dizziness, dyspepsia, nasal congestion, and visual changes.

Alprostadil

There are two versions: an intra-urethral dose via an applicator (Muse®) and intracavernosal injection (now less popular). The first dose of alprostadil should be given in the ED clinic teach the patient how to give it and to assess response.

Avoid in men with:

- penile deformities and those susceptible to priapism
- urethral infections, i.e. balanitis or urethritis (intra-urethral version)
- urethral abnormalities (intra-urethral version).

Warn all patients of the risk of priapism and provide written information to bring to their nearest A&E department. The BNF has specific guidance on the treatment of priapism. Other side effects include penile pain, bruising and scarring with injection, urethral burning (Muse®), hypotension, dizziness, and headache.

Testosterone and androgen analogues

Hormone treatment works only in patients with proven testosterone deficiency and should be started only by a specialist service (e.g. endocrinology). Testosterone treatment should not be used in patients who are not testosterone deficient.

Summary

- Diabetic men may struggle (as women do) to balance their responsibilities to work and family with their need to care properly for their diabetes.
- Diabetes does not appear to cause infertility in the absence of ED.
- ED is common and multifactorial. Proper assessment to define cause is important.
- Control the blood glucose.
- Phosphodiesterase type-5 inhibitors are effective in many patients.
- Only prescribe testosterone in patients with proven deficiency.

Chapter 19

Older people with diabetes

Diabetes is predominantly a disease of older people in whom type 2 is much more common than type 1 (although this can present at any age). Prevalence varies according to ethnic variation within a population and increases with age. In the UK diabetes is found in ~10–30% of those >65 yrs. The combination of old age, diabetes, and diabetes tissue damage can require complex care from many agencies. The potential role of preventative care is considerable, but its delivery can be difficult. Patient education is as important in the elderly as in the young, but it may take longer and health care professionals may not have enough time. It is well worth making time.

Factors for the increased frequency of diabetes in the elderly include increased insulin resistance and reduced glucose clearance, as well as obesity and lack of exercise. Thiazides, steroids, and other drugs are diabetogenic.

Presentation and assessment of diabetes in older people

Presentation

Patients >65 yrs are highly likely to fulfil requirements for screening (📖 p.7) and so should have a blood glucose test annually—fasting venous plasma glucose if practical, opportunistic random venous plasma or capillary glucose otherwise.

Screen for diabetes in elderly patients if:

- unwell with no apparent cause
- thirst (but this lessens with age)
- polyuria, incontinence, or any urinary symptom
- ulcers or wounds
- recurrent infections
- cardiovascular disease
- falls
- confusion
- depression
- 'off legs'
- difficulty coping
- repeated attendances.

Assessment

Try to allocate at least 40 min to see an older new diabetic patient. If the patient permits, see them with a partner or relative. Follow the assessment in Chapter 2 (📖 p.19), with particular emphasis on a functional assessment. This includes ability to cope with activities of daily living, social support, accommodation, and careful drug history. Consider excess alcohol and seek comorbidities. Assess vision, dexterity, mobility, and cognitive function. Review their health care arrangements. Who co-ordinates care? How easily is it accessed?

Management

Who supports the older diabetic patient?

- Most older diabetic patients function normally on their own.
- Older patients who have problems with self-care or are vulnerable may have a partner or caring relative or friend. If not who will provide care?
- Every older person should have a phone that they can use easily, and ideally one that they can carry around the house.
- Vulnerable older diabetic patients who live alone should have an alarm button on a wrist band or pendant and practise using it (e.g. Call Aid® www.ageconcern.org.uk)
- Advise wearing a warning pendant or bracelet notifying diabetes and other conditions (e.g. www.medicalert.org.uk). Consider a refrigerator Green Cross Datalink canister scheme or similar (try your local council).

Easy to read, easy to use, easy to access (?)

Written information

Most people finds larger text easier to read as they get older. Many diabetic patients have visual impairment. This sentence is written in 8 point. It is too small for most older people to read easily. Use lower-case black text in 12–14 point on a plain white background. Use plain fonts aligned to the left margin. Use one font (not many) with bold for emphasis if needed. Use matt, not glossy, paper of ≥90 g weight. Follow the RNIB guidelines: www.rnib.org.uk/xpedio/groups/public/documents/publicwebsite/public_printdesign.hcsp

Note that current disability legislation requires that information provided for patients is easy to use. RNIB also has guidelines about websites.

Easy to use

- Packs are harder to open if one has any upper limb, coordination, or visual problem. Child-proof tablet bottles are a particular challenge. Provide easy access medications. Consider pharmacy pre-packed daily dosage blister packs or boxes.
- Electronic devices are often small and fiddly. Numbers are hard to read. So are instructions. Ensure that patients can use any devices (e.g. HBGM meters, insulin pens).
- There are many 'silver surfers', but the older generation were not brought up in an electronic world and find it hard. A simplified list of specific instructions may be needed for electronic equipment.

Easy to access

- Complex telephone answering systems, answer phones, busy receptionists, and complex rules about appointments are all barriers to care. Consider giving vulnerable elderly diabetic patients a direct line to someone who can deal with their concerns. Passing patients from one person to another increases their confusion.
- Complex systems in the currently fragmenting NHS make it hard for everyone to understand who does what, when, and how in a patient's care. Provide the patient with a list of who does what for them and how to contact them.
- Physical access to primary or secondary care is a huge issue. Plan how the patient is going to get to their diabetes appointments. Does transport need to be booked? Prepare the patient for possible long journeys and waiting times if using NHS transport. They should carry food, drink, and daytime medications to avoid hypoglycaemia or other glucose fluctuations.
- Can the patient hear? Remind them to bring their hearing aid. If they need one and have not been assessed yet, arrange an assessment.
- Does the patient need an interpreter? If so, book one or bring one. Older patients from ethnic minorities are less likely to speak English than their younger relatives.
- Don't waste the patient's time and effort. Combine appointments if possible—doctor, nurse, dietitian, podiatrist—but remember that older patients tire easily. Provide food and drink if they need it.
- Remember that a 15 min clinic visit, simple for the doctor, can be a whole-day nightmare for a disabled elderly person.
- Home visits are very helpful and provide much more information and educational opportunity than a clinic or practice appointment. Can the local diabetes specialist nurse do one?

Diet

This is as important as in younger patients, but introduce change gradually. The patient has had 70 yrs on their previous diet and so is unlikely to want to change. One danger is of starvation because of overstrict interpretation of sucrose reduction or vague memories of the old low-carbohydrate diet. Sudden introduction of fibre can cause abdominal discomfort. Regular meals of sufficient calorie content but not too much sugar are the most important advice for thin elderly people. Include snacks between meals. A practical weight-reducing diet with less fat and sugar is needed for overweight patients.

Ensure that the dietitian meets the person who does the shopping and cooking if this is not the patient. If the patient needs insulin (other than daily long-acting) the food must be linked with insulin injections which is hard when an outsider (e.g. the district nurse) is giving it.

Exercise

- Keep the patient moving, even if limited by joint stiffness or pain
- Any exercise is helpful—walking, gardening, housework
- Patients can exercise while sitting.
- Daily exercise is best
- Beware undue pressure on neuropathic feet
- Protect injury-prone areas—legs or hands
- Refer to physiotherapy if the patient has severe mobility problems
- Help carers to implement simple and appropriate exercise programmes

Medication review

- Review all medication
- Reduce polypharmacy where appropriate (you are about to add more drugs)
- Stop thiazides and replace with less diabetogenic agent
- Review steroids—are they really needed, and in that dose?
- Other glucose-affecting drugs (e.g. antidepressants)?

Glucose targets in older people

- As for younger people if safe and practical.
- If the patient lives alone, has problems with self-care, or if hypoglycaemia is a risk aim for HbA_{1c} 7.5–8.5% or glucose levels 8–11 mmol/l.
- In frail elderly patients unable to maintain good glucose balance safely the aim is symptom prevention without hypoglycaemia. This can be hard to achieve.

Non-insulin treatments in older patients (see Chapter 8, 📖 p.129)

Metformin

- Safe and practical for many elderly patients.
- Long-acting preparation easier to remember and fewer side effects.
- Monitor U&E regularly.
- Risk of lactic acidosis in hypoxic patients or those with renal failure.

Sulphonylureas

- All cause hypoglycaemia (📖 p.214).
- Long-acting drugs convenient but can cause prolonged hypoglycaemia.
- Gliclazide M/R 30 mg initially with monthly increments if needed. No need for dose reduction in elderly.
- Patients who eat at variable times might benefit from tolbutamide or glipizide with the meal.
- Multiple drug interactions (📖 p.142).
- Familiar to most doctors.

Meglitinides

- Repaglinide could be useful with variable meal times and quantities.
- SPC advices against use of repaglinide in patients >75 yrs old as there have been no studies.
- Nateglinide—experience in patients >75 yrs old limited.

Incretin-effect enhancers

- Sitagliptin—no need for dosage adjustment but limited safety data in patients >75 yrs old.
- Exenatide—very limited experience in patients >75 yrs old. Needs injection (easier than insulin pens for most patients).

Non-insulin treatments ineffective?

- Prescribe insulin. Persistent hyperglycaemia makes patients feel awful.
- Add insulin to oral agents where SPC allows.

Insulin in older patients (see Chapter 9, 🕮 p.159)

Most older patients are completely capable of giving their own insulin and adjusting the dose according to blood glucose concentration.

Potential problems

- Visual impairment
- Reduced dexterity
- Cognitive impairment (which may vary)
- Erratic timing and quantity of meals eaten
- Risk of hypoglycaemia

Practical issues of insulin in older people

Type 1 diabetes, which may be slow onset, can occur in older patients (🕮 p.14). They will be insulin-dependent.

Most patients needing insulin are type 2 and already on tablets. These should be continued as they may still be providing some glucose lowering. Adding glargine or detemir insulin once daily morning or evening may be sufficient to achieve glucose aims. Twice daily 30/70 analogue insulin mixtures may be required in patients in whom once-daily insulin fails to cover post-prandial high glucose. Some patients may transfer to basal bolus regimens. District nurses are rarely able to provide more than twice-daily support.

If an insulin-treated patient has a very variable eating pattern, or refuses food, it can be extremely difficult to control their blood glucose. Carers can be given an insulin pen and a simple sliding scale and inject analogue insulin (e.g. lispro or aspart) after food has been eaten. A single small dose of longer-acting insulin can be given in the morning if needed.

- Who is going to give the insulin? Patient? Carer? District nurse?
- If more than one person is caring for the patient do they all know about diabetes and how to manage the insulin?
- When is it going to be given?
- Who is going to buy and prepare the meals? Does the patient need Meals on Wheels or home-delivered foods?
- Is glucose available, e.g. Dextrosol® tablets, Glucogel® (but this is hard to open), Lucozade® (also hard to open)? A dish of sugar lumps may be simplest.
- Are carbohydrate snacks available? Easy to unwrap.
- Are the insulin and food going to coincide? District nurses have busy schedules and may not arrive at the patient's usual meal time.
- Where will the insulin be kept? If the patient is confused they should not be able to access the insulin.

Diabetes education in older people

'Does he take sugar?' (BBC Radio 4, 1995) was about disability. In diabetes this translates to 'He doesn't take sugar, does he?' Older diabetic people are often bypassed and patronized in this way. One 65-yr-old man told me he had been given a booklet about 'Mr Insulin and Mrs Sugar'!

Most older people with diabetes are fully able to run their own lives and manage their own care, and must be treated with courtesy and respect. Every patient with newly diagnosed diabetes should have an explanation in terminology appropriate to that individual. Follow the steps in Chapter 4, 📖 p.57. If the patient permits, include the partner or close relative in the discussion.

Hypoglycaemia

See Chapter 10, 📖 p.199.
Hypoglycaemia impairs cerebral function, which is what a person requires to recognize and treat it. Older diabetic patients often have cerebral atheroma and may find it hard to recognize, and even harder to initiate appropriate treatment. It takes about 45 min for normal cerebral function to return after hypoglycaemia in younger people, but this time may be twice as long or even longer in the elderly.

Symptoms of hypoglycaemia in the elderly include:

- vaguenes
- malaise
- confusion
- forgetfulness
- inactivity
- sleepiness
- inattention
- being difficult to care for
- irritability
- paranoid behaviour
- coma.

Carers should have a high index of suspicion. If in doubt give oral glucose. Hypoglycaemia can kill elderly patients and must be avoided.

Tissue damage

No new symptom should be attributed to 'just old age'. Tissue damage is common in the elderly. Some patients have had decades of diabetes; others have had a long duration of diabetes pre-diagnosis. Seek tissue damage at diagnosis as most older patients will have some (Chapter 14, 📖 p.269).

Visual symptoms

Investigate. Cataract is common in the elderly and more so in diabetes. Cataract extraction can give a new lease of life. The retina cannot be assessed with severe cataracts, and so treatable retinopathy or age-related macular degeneration may be missed. Laser treatment should be given if required (📖 p.299).

Hearing (📖 p.300)

Deafness is common in the elderly and may act as a considerable barrier to care. Check for wax then refer for audiometry.

Dexterity and mobility

Musculoskeletal damage (📖 p.320), alone or with arthropathy, limits dexterity and mobility. Clarify the problem and arrange orthopaedic or rheumatological referral if appropriate. Treat Dupuytren's contracture, trigger finger, and frozen shoulder—all complications of diabetes.

Type 2 diabetes is a disease of overweight sedentary people. Diabetes may limit mobility in many ways—stroke, foot problems, vascular disease, neuropathy, osteoarthritis, poor vision, or the breathlessness of cardiac disease.

Cardiac disease

Have a high index of suspicion for cardiac ischaemia, which may be difficult to detect in a diabetic elderly person in whom silent cardiac events are common.

The management of cardiac failure may be a balancing act between resolution of cardiac symptoms and biochemical derangement. Over-diuresis risks renal failure. Ankle oedema increases the risk of ulceration.

Nephropathy

Renal damage may develop insidiously, and the first sign may be hypoglycaemia. Diuretics, recurrent UTI, NSAIDs, dehydration, and hypertension may worsen the situation.

Postural hypotension

Remember that autonomic neuropathy can cause postural hypotension and may precipitate falls. Hypotensive drugs can worsen this, so monitoring of blood pressure treatment in someone with diabetes should include lying and standing values. Modern target-oriented care with rewards for attaining a number may increase the risk of inadvertent over-medication and falls.

Pressure sores

Sadly, these are common in the chair-bound or bed-bound diabetic patient and can rapidly turn into large holes. Major steps must be taken to prevent them by obtaining suitable seating or mattresses, and by teaching relatives or carers about pressure care. Hyperglycaemic urinary incontinence may contribute.

Feet

Foot care is vital. Most patients who need amputation are elderly. All diabetic patients >60 yrs old should have regular chiropody. Everyone caring for them should be taught about the risk of foot problems and how to prevent them. It is good practice for all health care professionals to look at the patient's feet on every visit.

Bladder and bowel problems

Bladder and bowel problems can be due to autonomic neuropathy or other factors. Incontinence may be precipitated by UTI. Thrush may cause severe perineal soreness. Urinary retention is less common, but diabetic neuropathy may add to the effects of prostatism. Constipation can be stubborn despite a high-fibre diet and may require laxatives or enemata. Diabetic neuropathic diarrhoea may cause urgency and faecal incontinence.

Risk factors for falls in diabetic patients

- Obese
- Sedentary
- Visual problems:
  - retinopathy or maculopathy
  - cataract
  - laser treatment (reduced visual field and night vision)
- Neuropathy
  - peripheral sensory painless (especially position sensory loss) and painful
  - autonomic—postural hypotension
- Foot problems
  - ulceration
  - dressings or clumsy special boots or shoes
  - deformity
  - surgery (e.g. toe or limb amputation)
- Hypertension—hence hypotensive therapy and postural drop
- Oedema (cardiac or renal) affecting walking
- Stroke
- Frequent urination and nocturia (high glucose, urinary tract infection)
- Dementia
- Diabetic diarrhoea and urgency (often early morning)

Diabetic patients are more likely to have osteoporosis than non-diabetic people (📖 p.320), more likely to fall, and more likely to sustain fractures. Women have about twice the risk of fractures of the hip, proximal humerus, and (if on insulin) foot (*J Clin Endocrinol Metab* 2001; **86**:32–8).

Mental effects

Cerebral atherosclerosis is more frequent in people with diabetes than in the general population. Patients may have one obvious stroke but multi-infarct dementia may be more common than is generally recognized.

Dementia is about twice as common in patients with type 2 diabetes as in the general population (*Am J Clin Epidemiol* 1997; **145**:301–8, *Neurology* 1999; **53**:19–37) Vascular dementia is two to three times more common, and Alzheimer's disease is also more common.

Carers may miss the transient cognitive problems of hypoglycaemia in patients known to be confused. Teach them to check for this. Occasionally, prolonged frequent hypoglycaemia can cause confusion or memory defects, or a state of paranoia which can be very hard to manage.

Depression is about twice as common in people with diabetes as in those without. The diagnosis may be less obvious in older patients and should be sought, particularly in those with poor glucose control or who are 'not coping'.

Drugs in the elderly

Diuretics

Diuretic therapy can cause raised urea and may add to the effects of early nephropathy. Diuretics can also cause hyponatraemia (worse in those on chlorpropamide) and hypokalaemia. Thiazide-induced impairment of glucose tolerance, although minor in many patients, may be sufficient to cause failure of maximal oral therapy to control the blood glucose and an alternative diuretic or antihypertensive should be found. Loop diuretics can also impair glucose tolerance.

Beta-blockers

Loss of warning of hypoglycaemia can be a disaster at any age, but especially in the elderly. Beta-blockers can worsen the symptoms of peripheral vascular disease and must be used with care in cardiac failure.

Vasodilators

Drugs such as nitrates and calcium-channel blockers can exacerbate postural hypotension, as can ganglion blockers, although these are less often used. The ankle swelling induced by nifedipine can be uncomfortable.

NSAIDs

These are one of the most commonly prescribed drugs in the elderly. They interact with sulphonylureas to cause hypoglycaemia. Aspirin also reduces mortality after coronary thrombosis and the likelihood of stroke in patients with transient ischaemic attack, and possibly slows the development of retinopathy. It can reduce the blood glucose but this is rarely clinically relevant. NSAIDs should not be used in patients with nephropathy as they may precipitate renal failure.

Carers and care homes

Often diabetes care in an elderly person is provided by a relative or professional carer. Therefore it is essential that they accompany the patient to the clinic or surgery. Diabetes education should be provided for both the patient and the carer. The combination of diabetes and old age can place considerable burdens on carers, and their health and well-being must also be considered. Ensure that they obtain appropriate attendance allowances if relevant. Carers must know how to manage diabetes emergencies such as hypoglycaemia or a foot infection, and whom to call in an emergency.

Up to a quarter of patients in care facilities have diabetes. People with diabetes in care homes should have a formal care plan agreed with the patient, diabetes team, and care staff. They should have regular HBGM, and medication should be given as prescribed. Staff must know the signs of hypoglycaemia and how to treat it. A healthy diet should be provided in appropriate quantities and snacks should be readily available. Exercise options should be available. Patients who have the capacity to decide about their own care should be allowed to make their own choices of food (healthy or not) and other diabetes management. Patients should have at least annual formal diabetes checks by a doctor and diabetes nurse. Podiatry should be arranged at appropriate intervals and they must not miss out on retinal screening. Arrange an annual dietetic review.

Summary

- Diabetes is a disease of the elderly.
- The presentation may be subtle.
- Perform a full assessment, including functional aspects.
- Check support.
- Ensure good access to information, help, and clinic/practice.
- Tailor the treatment to the person.
- Encourage a healthy diabetic diet.
- Everyone can exercise in some way.
- Review medication.
- Use non-insulin treatments appropriately.
- Do not delay insulin if needed.
- Do not strive for normoglycaemia if this is going to be dangerous.
- Provide full diabetes education.
- Diabetes tissue damage is common in elderly people.
- Increased diabetic and non-diabetes-related health problems may hinder care and impair quality of life.
- Falls are common in diabetes and risk fracture.
- Dementia is more common in people with diabetes than in those without.
- Choose your drugs carefully.
- Provide carers with diabetes education.

Further reading

Sinclair AJ, Finucane J (ed.) *Diabetes in old age* (2nd edn). John Wiley, Chichester, 2001 (new edition pending).

Chapter 20

Diabetes in different ethnic groups

Introduction

The International Diabetes Federation (IDF) estimates that the number of people with diabetes worldwide will increase from 246 million in 2007 to 380 million in 2025. The prevalence of diabetes varies according to ethnic background and the country in which the person is living (Tables 20.1 and 20.2). It also varies according to city and social situation. Inner-city communities have a higher prevalence than some more rural areas (Table 20.2). This also applies to the UK. Changes in incidence and prevalence make it hard to plan health care. In the UK diabetes is particularly common in the South Asian community and there is an increased frequency in the African Caribbean community. There are communities from many different backgrounds in the UK, including refugees from recent conflicts. These include Somalia and other African nations, Afghanistan, and Eastern Europe. Modern UK populations are mobile and continuity of health care may be interrupted.

Table 20.1 Prevalence (%) of diabetes (known and previously undiagnosed) in people of African Caribbean, Asian, and European origin (1996)

Age (yrs)	Asian		African Caribbean		European	
	Men	Women	Men	Women	Men	Women
20–39	2.5	1.5			0.5	0.5
40–59	12.5	9.5			3.5	6.0
60–79	25.5	20.0			6.5	8.0
≥40			16.7	17.7	5.0	3.1

The male female ratio appears to be changing. In UKPDS (📖 p.39) the ratio of newly diagnosed men to women was 3:2.

Data from summaries in *Diabetes in the United Kingdom—1996* (British Diabetic Association, now Diabetes UK)

Table 20.2 Age-standardized prevalence (%) of type 2 diabetes (known and newly detected, WHO criteria (📖 p.9)) among people of African Caribbean, Asian (Pakistani), and European origin in Manchester (2001)

Age (yrs)	Asian		African Caribbean		European	
	Men	Women	Men	Women	Men	Women
35–79	29.9	35.7	23.4	20.8	20.8	19.9

Communication

Good communication is essential for good diabetes care. The patient must learn what diabetes is, how to care for him/herself, and how to stay fit. Communication can be difficult if the patient and the health care team have different ethnic and cultural backgrounds. Diabetes and its care are particularly influenced by cultural beliefs and practice. Some barriers to communication include:

- staff ignorance of the patient's correct name and status, and vice versa
- gender difference
- differences in non-verbal signals
- lack of a common language—the patient's incomplete or non-existent understanding of spoken and/or written English, and the doctor's inability to speak or write the patient's language
- interpreter from family modifying full disclosure of concerns or symptoms (e.g. husband or child)
- some patients may not read their own language
- different social conventions
- different dietary habits
- different perceptions of health and ill-health
- lack of knowledge of human biology and belief in folk myths (e.g. sugar makes semen)
- different understanding of the reason for seeing the health care team
- different expectations of the outcome of the consultation.

Ensure that the patient understands when and where to come for their appointment. Try to reduce anxiety before and during the appointment. Arrange an interpreter—preferably an independent professional. Otherwise, ask patients to bring a trusted friend or relative, but beware limitation of answers or modification of questions and replies. Would the patient prefer to see female staff—particularly if they are going to be examined? (Many Muslim women would.) Men may prefer a male doctor.

During the consultation make sure that the patient understands you. Invite feedback. Ask the patient to repeat what you have said—what is wrong with him/her and how it can be put right, and, most importantly, what action he/she needs to take to get better.

The treatment of diabetes is always tailored to the individual's needs. The patient must accept treatment for it to succeed. In a condition in which tissue damage develops silently until it is well advanced, it can be hard for any patient who feels well to understand the need for careful diet, regular medication, blood glucose testing, and regular self-care and health checks. A diabetes specialist nurse or practice nurse who speaks the patient's language can be a considerable help in teaching patients about their condition.

Information is available in a variety of languages, e.g.

- Diabetes UK http://www.diabetes.org.uk/Other_languages/
- Foot care leaflets written by a podiatrist, Richard Hourston, are available in 30 languages at: www.diabeticfoot.org.uk
- National Register of Public Service Interpreters (www.nrpsi.co.uk/)
- Some NHS organizations use the commercial interpreting service Language Line (www.languageline.co.uk/)

The Asian community

In the UK diabetes is more common in the adult Asian community than in the general population. In some communities up to one in four Asian people of working age have diabetes. The frequency increases with increasing age, and older Asian patients are up to seven times as likely to have diabetes as the general population. The likelihood of diabetes appears to vary according to the place of origin and other factors such as diet.

Most Asian people with diabetes, even those <30 yrs old, have type 2 diabetes. Type 1 diabetes is uncommon, although up to 50% of patients with type 2 diabetes eventually need insulin to control their blood glucose level.

Diabetes may go undetected until the patient attends their doctor for another reason. It may be difficult for any patient to accept that he/she has a disease and should therefore modify his/her lifestyle and diet, or take medication when he/she does not feel unwell. A community nurse spent one day a week at an Asian day centre. Within a couple of months she had discovered previously unrecognized diabetes in 20 people.

Beliefs about the causation of diabetes may be unusual (e.g. lack of sweating). Patients may believe that the cause is external rather than internal. Beliefs about behaviour and family pressures may counteract health advice. Clothing, modesty, and social pressure may limit exercise (*BMJ* 1998; **316**:978–83).

Diet

People of Asian origin living in the UK eat a wide variety of diets. Many eat a Western diet which may have contributed to the increased frequency of diabetes in the Asian population. Take a dietary history and talk with the person who actually does the cooking. Ideally, the dietitian should speak Asian languages and have a clear understanding of Asian diets.

The main carbohydrates in Asian diets are breads (nan, chapatti, bhatura), rice, and pulses such as lentils and beans. The breads can be made with wholemeal flour, and brown rice can be used, although this may be considered inferior. Butter or ghee is often used in breads, pilau rice, and curries. Patients may not count fat in cooking when trying to reduce dietary fat. Sugar is used in sweetmeats and festival foods (e.g. Mithai, Laddoo, Jalaibi, Gajer halwa, Karah parshad). Patients may not realize that ghor (brown sugar) needs to be included in sugar totals.

Suspicion that a food breaches religious rules may mean that the whole meal is thrown away (Table 20.3). Asian patients may prefer to eat food brought into hospital by their family. People vary in the strictness with which they observe religious rules, but their wishes must be respected. Vegetarians may be vegans who risk vitamin B_{12} deficiency. Other vegetarians eat dairy products. The use of ghee has religious significance. Different foods may have different significance under varied circumstances. Many foods are believed to cause allergies, and particular foods may be avoided in certain illnesses. Some foods are considered hot and others cold, and are taken to treat certain conditions. Some foods are strong (e.g. sugar, ghee, beef, lamb). Raw foods and those which have been baked or grilled may be regarded as indigestible. Karela, a vegetable used in some Indian dishes, reduces the blood glucose and can cause hypoglycaemia. Ensure adequate calcium and vitamin D intake (📖 p.82).

The African Caribbean community

Diabetes is more common in this community than in white Europeans (see Tables 20.1 and 20.2). African Caribbean patients usually have type 2 diabetes. They are more often overweight and are more insulin resistant than Europeans, but have a less unfavourable lipid profile than South Asian patients and are more physically active (*Int J Epidemiol* 2001; **30**:111–17, *Int J Obesity Relat Metab Disorders* 1999; **23**:25–33, *Heart* 1997; **78**:555–63). Perhaps because of this they have a lower rate of coronary disease than one might expect, although they are prone to resistant hypertension.

Diet

In some African cultures overweight people are viewed as more prosperous or more attractive. Feeding people is a sign of love in most cultures. Traditional foods may be very sweet with extra sugar, and many foods are fried. Salty foods (e.g. salt fish) are enjoyed. Carbohydrate foods include potato, sweet potato, yam, cassava, rice, cereals, breads, dumplings, beans (e.g. kidney beans), plantain, and noodles. Sauces may include coconut milk. Encourage a reduction in sugar and salt (e.g. using dried cod which is not salted), and steaming, baking, or grilling rather than frying.

Ketosis-prone type 2 diabetes

In the USA and increasingly in the UK a small proportion of patients with DKA have subsequently been found to be producing insulin long term (albeit suboptimally) and to be able to manage without insulin for some years although they may ultimately require it. Most of these patients are African Caribbean and half are overweight. There is often a family history of type 2 diabetes. This has been labelled type 1b diabetes (📖 p.14). It occurs in up to half of African Caribbean patients admitted with DKA (*Ann Int Med* 2006; **144**:350–7, *Arch Int Med* 1999; **159**:2317–22). Such patients must be assessed and monitored by the specialist diabetes team. Use diet, metformin, and sulphonylureas once the acute episode is over.

Table 20.3 Dietary restrictions practised by religious and ethnic groups

Hindus	No beef	Mostly vegetarian, fish rarely eaten, no alcohol	Periods of fasting common
Muslims	No pork	Meat must be 'halal', no shellfish eaten, no alcohol	Regular fasting, including Ramadan for 1 month
Sikhs	No beef	Meat must be killed by 'one blow to the head', no alcohol	Generally less rigid eating restrictions than Hindus and Muslims
Jews	No pork	Meat must be kosher, only fish with scales and fins eaten	Meat and dairy foods must not be consumed together
Rastafarians	No animal products, except milk may be consumed	Foods must be 'I-tal' or alive, so no canned or processed foods eaten, no salt added, no coffee or alcohol.	Food should be 'organic'

Halal meat is dedicated to God by a Muslim present at the killing. Kosher meat must be slaughtered by a Rabbinical-licensed person and then soaked and salted.

Reproduced from Table 36, *Manual of nutrition*. HMSO, London, 1995.

Medication issues in different ethnic groups

Patients in all cultures may add complementary or alternative treatments, prayer, or spiritual treatments to medical advice. Some groups advocate garlic, honey, cinnamon, ginger, and coconut. Unknown herbal mixes are sold, or water is drunk from vessels made of special wood. Sometimes patients will stop medical treatment altogether. Ask about other care in an open way.

Many Asian patients will also consult an alternative practitioner. Western doctors should not take offence as alternative medicine is usual in the East and implies a 'belt and braces' approach to health care rather than lack of trust in a doctor's treatment. A variety of approaches include the advice of a hakim or vaid, Ayurvedic medicine, Hikmat, astrotherapy, urinotherapy (drinking urine is thought to help diabetes), herbal medicine, and homeopathy. Prayer is often used to support care.

African Caribbean patients often use complementary remedies which may include teas (e.g. dandelion, a diuretic), lemon juice, or vinegar. Prayer can be particularly important—most patients will seek divine help for their illness. The support of a church or other religious group can be a great comfort for patients.

Problems may arise when the alternative practitioner advises stopping the Western medicine so that it does not interfere with his medicine (or vice versa), or when the alternative medicine causes toxic effects or interacts with the Western pharmaceuticals. Ask the patient what other treatment or advice he/she is using.

Oral hypoglycaemic agents and a diabetes diet can control diabetes in many patients. Those who need insulin should be offered biosynthetic human insulin, as pork-derived or beef insulin may be against their religious beliefs. Even insulin itself may be viewed as inappropriate and stopped. This can lead to repeated admissions with severe hyperglycaemia as the patient may not wish to upset the doctor by telling him that they have not taken the treatment.

Fasting and Ramadan

Ramadan is the month of fasting observed by Muslim communities. The timing is based on a lunar calendar and so it varies each year. Patients on medication for their diabetes do not have to fast and may wish to discuss this with their religious leader (imam). Some will wish to fast regardless of medication. Some patients will avoid all food and fluids.

Food and fluid is permitted after sunset—the first meal is Iftar—and during the night. The last meal is Sehri, just before sunrise, although in some communities Sehri is earlier in the night. In people with diabetes it is better just before sunrise.

Traditional foods for Iftar may contain high quantities of sugar and fat (both as fried food and as oil added to cooked dishes). Advise patients to reduce these and eat more rice, chapatti, naan, and daal, with plenty of fruit and vegetables. Feasting follows during the celebrations on the first day of the next month—Eid ul-Fitr.

Patients on diet alone rarely have adverse sequelae from fasting. Nor do those on metformin, who should simply take this after the meal(s) if multiple dose, or once after the largest meal if on the modified-release version.

Patients on sulphonylureas are at risk of hypoglyacemia. They can be taken with the nocturnal meals but the dose taken at Sehri may need to be reduced. Modified-release gliclazide may be taken with Iftar. Glitazones can be taken once a day; again, it may be sensible to take them with Iftar. Meglitinides can be taken with meals, perhaps reducing the dose at Sehri. Exenatide must be taken close to a meal. Sitagliptin could be taken once daily as usual. There is little experience of using exenatide or sitagliptin during Ramadan fasting.

Once-daily long-acting insulin may be continued, although the dose may need reducing depending on the usual level of glucose control. Multiple injections are more difficult. Analogue insulin can be taken with each meal during the night but care needs to be taken to avoid morning hypoglycaemia. The dose of long-acting insulin may need reduction.

Patients should be aware that their insulin may need increasing if they are eating more during Eid ul-Fitr.

Exercise during the day can precipitate hypoglycaemia and patients who are observing the fast strictly may not treat it with oral glucose. This potential issue should be discussed beforehand. In this context glucose is an essential medicine (e.g. Glucogel®).

Complications of diabetes

Ischaemic heart disease is common in Asian people. In a series followed for 11 yrs in Southall, the all-cause mortality of South Asians (242/730 died) aged 30–54 at baseline was 1.5 times that of the European cohort (172/304 died). The mortality ratio for circulatory disorders was 1.8 and that for heart disease was 2.02. In South Asians, circulatory disorders in total accounted for 77% of deaths vs 46% in Europeans (*Diabetic Med* 1988; **15**:53–9). South Asian people experience greater delays in obtaining appropriate specialist help and investigation for heart disease than Europeans, even though they are more likely to seek help for chest pain (*Lancet* 1997; **350**: 1578–83). Compared with Europeans, South Asian patients are more likely to be overweight and to have a high waist-to-hip ratio, unfavourable lipid profiles, and poorer glucose control. Asian women are less likely to be physically active.

In addition to greater cardiovascular risk, South Asian patients are more likely to develop microalbuminuria, and they are more likely to have retinopathy and hypertension (*Diabetic Med 1998;* **15**:672–7). Nephropathy occurs more often and earlier in South Asian diabetic patients, and they may need renal transplantation. Retinopathy and neuropathy are often severe when they are discovered, perhaps because there is a longer duration of diabetes before it is diagnosed. Foot problems do not seem as common as in other ethnic groups, possibly because they have less constricting footwear and better personal foot care than other patients.

Both South Asian and African Caribbean patients are more likely to need renal replacement therapy than the general population and may form up to half the patients requiring this in some clinics.

African-Caribbean-born patients with diabetes have a higher mortality from diabetes than the national rate (3.5× for men and 6× for women) (*BMJ* 1997; **314**:209–13). The same applies for mortality from hypertension. Blood glucose control may be difficult in African Caribbean patients, and they appear to have a greater risk of hyperosmolar non-ketotic hyperglycaemic states. They may have resistant hypertension which contributes to worsening their risk of endstage kidney disease. Calcium-channel antagonists appear particularly useful in this group, but multiple hypotensive agents are usually needed to improve blood pressure.

Foot ulcers are most common in White European diabetic patients 5.5/100 person-yrs vs 1.9 for South Asian and 2.7 for African Caribbean (*Diabetes Care* 2005; **28**:1869–75).

Refugees

Increasing numbers of people from many nations are seeking asylum in the UK. They may have known diabetes or it may be diagnosed during health checks. Refugees have often fled atrocities and may have been badly injured—both physically and emotionally. They may have had minimal diabetes care in their country of origin—erratically available impure insulin of unknown type, dilute insulin (e.g. U40 i.e. 40 units/ml), infected or scarred injections sites, and no knowledge of diet or tissue damage. Some have extensive diabetic tissue damage. The new diagnosis of diabetes is yet another shock, as is the discovery of established tissue damage. Such patients may have little family or other support and be living in basic conditions. Their uncontrolled diabetes puts them at particular risk of infections such as tuberculosis, and injuries (gunshot, machete, torture) may not have healed properly. They may also have malaria, intestinal parasitaemia, HIV, and hepatitis B and C.

Find the right interpreter, perform a full assessment, treat any associated problems, and control the diabetes. Find and use local appropriate support groups. It is very rewarding to see someone who has never had proper diabetes care change from a terrified emaciated teenager into a smiling well-nourished healthy young woman.

Further information

Summary

- Good communication is essential for full diabetes education and care.
- Respect religious and cultural wishes.
- Diabetes is very common in South Asian people, and is also common in African Caribbean people.
- Reduce delays in diagnosis and appropriate treatment.
- Screen for, and treat, risk factors and tissue damage.
- South Asian patients are at increased risk of cardiovascular disease, retinopathy, hypertension, and nephropathy.
- African Caribbean people are at increased risk of hypertension, nephropathy, and hyperosmolar non-ketotic hyperglycaemic states.
- White European patients have an increased risk of foot problems.
- Dietary advice must be tailored to the person's individual needs. Also talk to the person who prepares the food.
- Remember you may not be the patient's only health adviser.
- Refugees may have physical and emotional injuries and other health problems, often with poor previous diabetes care.
- Refugees may have continuing problems in obtaining proper diabetes care and appropriate standards of living.

Further information

IDF 2006 Diabetes Atlas (3rd edn) Available at: www.idf.org

Chapter 21

Work

Introduction

Legal issues

Diabetes is not a problem in most jobs. However, people with diabetes may experience difficulties at work. The job may make it hard to care for the diabetes optimally, or the diabetes may cause glucose or tissue complications which interfere with the job. Colleagues and employers attitudes vary widely and misunderstandings about diabetes and its effects can lead to problems.

People with diabetes may feel insulted to be regarded as disabled, but diabetes counts as a disability under the Disability Discrimination Act 1995 (DDA) in most circumstances. It does not apply to the armed forces, private clubs and some transport vehicles.

The Disability Rights Commission informs employers that:

'You cannot discriminate against someone with a disability or health condition:

- in the recruitment process
- in their terms and conditions of employment
- in chances for promotion, transfer, training or other benefits
- by dismissing them
- by treating them less fairly than other workers
- by subjecting them to harassment or victimization'

Under the DDA employers have a duty to make reasonable adjustments for a disabled person. This requirement is interpreted variably by different line managers or employers, and people with diabetes still experience problems. Fear of difficulties may lead people with diabetes to conceal their condition. Concealment of a problem which could interfere with how the job is done is likely to prevent any later claim against the employer under the DDA. If the patient is on drugs which could cause hypoglycaemia, or has tissue damage which may impede their functioning, they should tell employers that they have diabetes, especially in any post in which hypoglycaemia or any disability from tissue damage could place them or others at risk. Any employee who drives in relation to his work must inform his employer of his diabetes. Failure to do so is likely to invalidate insurance cover. Solely diet-treated diabetes is not a barrier to employment unless the person has tissue damage which impedes function relevant to the job.

Practical issues

People with diabetes can apply for, and successfully deliver, most jobs. The DDA protects them against discrimination in the workplace. However, each person with diabetes needs to make an individual decision about the job—whether it is the right job for them, and whether they personally can cope with it. Patients' abilities to manage their diabetes vary widely, and this will influence their job satisfaction and effectiveness. They will need to make their own balance between happiness, pay, and health. Factors to consider are:

- the hours
- normal working day
- shifts—fixed or variable?
- journey to and from work
- travel for work
- physical activity
- working environment (e.g. temperature)
- clean or dirty job and access to handwashing
- access to food and drinking water
- meal and snack breaks
- access to mobile or other telephone
- hazard to self or others
- responsibilities to and for organizations, things, or people
- support at work
- colleagues at work
- access to help.

Effects of the job on diabetes

Sedentary work

This poses few problems (other than lack of exercise). However, if the person is more active at home at weekends, he/she may need a different dose of tablets or insulin for weekdays and weekends. If someone is normoglycaemic during a sedentary working day, unexpected exercise needs to be covered by extra carbohydrate. A change from an active to a sedentary job may need a reduction in food eaten and/or a reduction in hypoglycaemic treatment. Patients may need to guard against weight gain.

Physical work

The person needs to eat enough to fuel the work. This is not usually a problem, but some people with newly diagnosed diabetes are frightened of eating the wrong foods and reduce their diet. Insulin-treated patients, and many on sulphonylureas, need regular snacks. People working on building sites and in similar industries must wear protective footwear and gloves and have up-to-date tetanus immunization.

Shift work

This can prove difficult for patients on insulin, and sometimes for those on sulphonylureas. They need to balance the timing of food intake, exertion, and insulin. One regimen is to have evenly spaced meals and snacks when awake, including one before going to sleep. A long-acting insulin is given every 24 hrs and analogue very-short-acting insulin is given before meals. Encourage patients to discuss their work pattern with their doctor—many do not do so and find it difficult to resolve their glucose balance.

Dirty jobs or work involving protective clothing

Many jobs involve dirt or grease, or infection risk (e.g. gardening, building). Finger-prick glucose testing is impossible (ensure that tetanus immunization is up to date). Insulin injections may also be impossible, e.g. if impeded by protective clothing or dirt. Glucose or food is difficult to eat safely. Glucogel® can be ingested using a non-touch technique, but this is harder when someone is hypoglycaemic. Handwashing facilities and a clean place to inject and eat food should be arranged.

Work involving travelling

Driving is discussed on 📖 p.440. Patients must not become hypoglycaemic while driving. If long journeys are involved, insulin-treated patients should snack and test blood glucose at least every 2 hrs. If possible the patient should take packed meals as it may be hard to find the components of a diabetes diet on the road. In any case, anyone who travels frequently or for long distances should carry sufficient carbohydrate for an emergency full meal in the car.

The businessman or woman

Some of the hazards of the traditional business life are smoking, alcohol, and rich food. Smoking is now banned in the workplace and restaurants. People with diabetes can drink in moderation (21 units a week for men and 14 units a week for women), but must never drink on an empty stomach. To reduce intake alcohol can be alternated with non-alcoholic drinks or diluted. Eating out may place a strain on the diabetes diet, but most restaurants will grill meat or fish and provide plain potatoes, rice, or pasta, with bread to top up. Salad or vegetables and fruit are usually available and there is no need to have butter, dressing, sugar, or cream.

Colleagues at work

People with diabetes on insulin or drugs which may cause hypoglycaemia should tell their work colleagues that they have diabetes. Insulin-treated patients should teach close colleagues what to do in the event of hypoglycaemia. Everyone on insulin should carry glucose, and a supply at work is essential. Some patients keep a supply of insulin and a blood-testing kit at work—this must be locked away. People who give insulin injections at work should do so openly in a clean environment with explanations to avoid stigmatization as a drug abuser. The same applies to finger-prick blood glucose testing. Many people do not test at work at all and miss essential information this way.

Effect of diabetes on the job

Glucose problems

High glucose levels may cause tiredness and lethargy, and increase urination. Risk of infection in small wounds increases.

Hypoglycaemia impairs concentration and may cause overt confusion and collapse. As well as endangering the patient and anyone for whom he/she is responsible, a severe hypoglycaemic attack alarms work colleagues and employers and may lead to job restriction or dismissal, although this can be challenged via the DDA. Patients may forget or minimize hypoglycaemic episodes at work and fail to appreciate the effect they have on those at work. Urgently address prevention of hypoglycaemia.

Diabetic tissue damage

This may be present when a person applies for a job, or may develop during employment. People with diabetes may fail to appreciate the existence or significance of complications. Visual loss from diabetic eye disease, retinopathy, or cataracts can obviously affect someone's job. Cataracts should be extracted promptly. Retinopathy or its treatment can cause visual loss: new vessels may cause vitreous haemorrhage, maculopathy can cause severe visual loss, and laser photocoagulation can reduce peripheral vision. Peripheral vascular disease may limit walking distance; cardiac disease may limit exertion. Nephropathy may require time-consuming treatment. Autonomic neuropathy may be embarrassing (e.g. gustatory sweating or diabetic diarrhoea) or dangerous (e.g. postural hypotension which may limit where the person may work with safety). Neuropathy in the hands may limit jobs requiring fine finger work, and in the feet may cause problems for those relying on foot work. Diabetic foot problems may cause months off work and may be repeatedly exacerbated if, for example, the job involves standing all day. Amputation or the need for crutches or a wheelchair may limit where a patient can work and what he can do. Fears about work may delay a patient seeking or accepting treatment for foot disease and other complications.

Hazardous occupations

Diabetes UK has produced 'guidelines to help employers decide whether a person with diabetes can work safely in a hazardous occupation:

- You should be as physically and mentally fit as people without diabetes.
- You should visit your diabetes care team for regular (at least annual check ups.
- Your diabetes should be well controlled.
- You should test your blood glucose levels and be well informed and motivated to care for your condition.
- There should be no cases of disabling hypos and you should be aware of your own hypo warning signs.
- You should have no advanced diabetes-related eye disease (retinopathy), kidney disease (nephropathy) nor severe nerve damage (neuropathy).
- You should have no significant circulation disorders of the heart (eg coronary heart disease), legs or brain
- Your suitability for employment should be reviewed annually by both an occupational physician and a diabetes specialist. The review should be based on previous criteria.
- You may find that if you develop diabetes whilst in employment, the organization may change the nature of your job. This could be sensible and may be worth considering.'

Limitations on employment

Patients treated with oral hypoglycaemic drugs

Patients may find that there are differences in employment for those on metformin (and probably incretin-effect enhancers) compared with those taking sulphonylureas. There is little risk of hypoglycaemia for people taking metformin alone, and if this controls the diabetes, changing to metformin may help a patient's employment prospects. Patients with tablet-treated diabetes are not usually permitted to join the armed services or to pilot aircraft. Merchant seamen who develop diabetes requiring tablet treatment are usually allowed to remain at sea, subject to a regular medical check. Patients may be allowed to drive large goods vehicles, passenger-carrying vehicles, or main-line trains, if they can prove that their diabetes is well controlled and that they have no tissue damage impairing relevant functions (e.g. poor vision, numb feet).

Patients treated with insulin

There are more limitations here because of the greater risk of hypoglycaemia. People with insulin-treated diabetes are not permitted to join the armed services, become professional divers, work on an offshore oil rig, become merchant seamen, drive large goods vehicles or passenger-carrying vehicles, drive rapid-response emergency vehicles (e.g. police), or control trains or aeroplanes. They may also be barred from working in some high-risk areas alone (e.g. supervising an electricity generating station or substation, signalman). Jobs in which hypoglycaemia could be fatal, such as steeplejack or scaffolder, or in which a hypoglycaemic person could be injured or cause injury by machinery are also inappropriate. However, people who develop the need for insulin-treatment whilst employed in some of these areas may be allowed to stay. The patient will have to prove that he/she is in full control of his/her condition, that there is no risk of hypoglycaemia, and that he/she has no tissue damage that limits relevant function. Such patients (and those on tablets) should be referred to a consultant diabetologist for assessment.

Sometimes patients face the dilemma of health or work.

> Bill was a diabetic bus driver. Oral hypoglycaemics were not sufficient to control his blood glucose. He was advised to start insulin treatment. He refused because he would lose his job. Over the next 2 yrs his hyperglycaemia increased. Diabetic retinopathy developed and worsened. He steadfastly refused to consider insulin despite warnings that his health might be permanently damaged.

A changing situation

The situation is changing as better methods for self-monitoring became more widely available and employers become better informed about diabetes. Cases must be assessed individually, and it is prudent to advise reassessment or regular checks as diabetes is a progressive disease. Advise patients to check with individual employers for up-to-date information.

One of the problems faced by people with diabetes is the different backgrounds of occupational medical officers. Diabetes is a rapidly moving field and occupational physicians may not always be aware of the extent to which people with diabetes can now monitor and control their condition. A patient who is experiencing difficulties with gaining employment or with their employer should ensure that any medical officer appointed by the company communicates with his GP and with his consultant diabetologist.

Work record and time off

American statistics (*Diabetes in America* 1995; XXVIII–1–22, National Diabetes Data Group, National Institutes of Health 85–1468) indicate that, among people aged between 20 and 64 yrs, 17% of the general population and 50% of people with diabetes considered themselves limited in some way in the kind or amount of work they could do about the house or in employment.

Most studies have shown an increase in sick leave. A Finnish study (*Diabetic Med* 2007; **24**:1043–8) found that diabetic employees had about double the risk of physician-certified sick leave of those without diabetes. They had 59 extra sickness absences per 100 person-yrs vs non-diabetic colleagues, equivalent to 4 days off sick a year. The excess was predominantly due to pre-existing non-cardiovascular diseases: asthma, chronic bronchitis, prolapsed intervertebral disc, osteo- and rheumatoid arthritis, peptic ulcer, fibromyalgia, depression, and other psychiatric disorders.

In an American survey of people aged ≥25 yrs, 6 months work disability secondary to illness/disability occurred in 26% of those with diabetes and 8% of those without. People with diabetes earned less than those without (*Diabetes Care* 1999; **22**:1105–9).

A Scandinavian study compared people with diabetes with those without diabetes but with either hypertension or musculoskeletal problems, and with people with no health problems. People with diabetes had lower incomes and were more likely to be on a disability pension than those with hypertension or no problems. Diabetic patients had more sick days and were more likely to have psychological problems than healthy people (*Scand J Soc Med* 1997; **25**:39–43).

Some people with diabetes with recurrent admissions for glycaemic instability or who develop major tissue damage (e.g. foot ulcers) may have prolonged sick leave. This may enhance an employer's negative image of diabetes.

Retirement, superannuation, and pensions

Retirement planning and pensions arrangements are complex and the situation is changeable. Patients may seek early retirement on health grounds. Diabetes may entitle patients to an enhanced annuity on health grounds. Remind patients that their GP and diabetes consultant can help by providing accurate up-to-date information about their health. They should also be aware that it is in their interests to shop around for insurance and pension schemes. Diabetes UK will provide up-to-date advice.

Summary

- Diabetes rarely impedes the opportunity or capacity for employment.
- Diabetes is a disability covered by the Disability Discrimination Act 1995 in most instances
- Factors which do influence employability and safety are the risk of hypoglycaemia and its consequences, and tissue damage which may reduce function.
- People with diabetes have more sickness absence than those without. Diabetes-related issues may be improved by specialist care, but much of the excess absence is due to non-cardiovascular comorbidities.

Further reading

Palmer KT, Cox, Brown I (ed) 2007. *Fitness for work: the medical aspects* (4th edn). Oxford University Press.

Chapter 22

Travel

Walking

Increasing the walking done daily—at home, to shops or work, and at work—is the most accessible form of exercise for most patients, young or old. This is a good form of exercise for elderly patients.

Patients on insulin or tablets which could cause hypoglycaemia should have glucose on their person. A longer or more vigorous walk than usual, or one in unfamiliar surroundings, should be preceded by either reduction in insulin or tablets (unless the glucose is high) or a carbohydrate snack.

Expeditions on foot (e.g. mountain walking) require a substantial insulin reduction (~20–50% of the daily dose) and huge amounts of carbohydrate to fuel them A rule of thumb is to double the carbohydrate in snacks and meals. For strenuous walking, advise two double snacks between each meal, and between the evening meal and bed. Nocturnal hypoglycaemia is a risk. An emergency meal should be carried. Mountain walkers should not go alone, and the group should file a route plan with a responsible person.

Good foot care is vital (📖 p.329). Any blister or rub should be treated immediately and protected from further damage.

Cycling

Cycling is increasingly popular. Many people now chose to cycle to work. It provides good exercise—sprint or endurance. Hypoglycaemia risks a road traffic accident. Again, glucose must be carried and be accessible. Long cycle trips should be treated like a mountain-walking expedition in terms of insulin and food. Liquid carbohydrate is useful.

Driving

Patients must satisfy the licensing requirements of the country in which they are driving. These vary. In the UK, the Driver and Vehicle Licensing Agency (www.dvla.gov.uk/drivers.aspx) requires people with diabetes holding any licence to inform them of their condition and treatment (the guidance is updated regularly, so check the website for current advice). Document all advice given to patients about driving.

All drivers (Group 1—car or motor cycle)

Diet alone, or tablets and diet

- Normally able to retain their 'till 70' licence.
- Must inform DVLA if they:
  - require treatment with insulin
  - require laser treatment to both eyes for retinopathy, or remaining eye if one eye only
  - if both eyes, or remaining eye if one eye only, affected by other eye problems (diabetic drivers must comply with usual vision checks for driving)
  - develop problems with the circulation or sensation in the legs which makes it necessary to drive certain types of vehicle only (e.g. automatic vehicles or modifications to a vehicle, hand-operated accelerator/brake)
  - an existing medical condition deteriorates or any other condition which may affect safe driving at any time in the future develops.

Insulin-treated (including inhaled insulin)

- Must inform DVLA.
- Those on insulin temporarily (e.g. for gestational diabetes) may retain their licence but should stop driving of they experience disabling hypoglycaemia. Tell DVLA if treatment continues beyond 3 months.
- Those on long-term insulin must recognize warning symptoms of hypoglycaemia and meet usual visual standards. They are granted a licence for 1, 2, or 3 yrs.
- ❶Hypoglycaemia
  - Frequent hypoglycaemia likely to impair driving—STOP driving until satisfactory control re-established and confirmed by doctor.
  - Impaired awareness of hypoglycaemia—STOP driving. May only drive again if doctor's report confirms that awareness has been regained.
  - As such patients may be hypoglycaemic in clinic, check their finger-prick blood glucose and record it before telling them to stop driving. Write to them formally afterwards to reiterate this advice (copy to GP/other health care staff involved with the patient).
  - Patients experiencing recurrent hypoglycaemia may become aggressive, especially if you tell them to stop driving.

All diabetic patients—diabetic tissue damage

This often occurs gradually and patients may not realize that it could interfere with their ability to drive safely. Rules for Group 2 drivers are more stringent than those for Group 2. The list below applies to Group 1.

- Visual problems—must be able to read in good light (with glasses or contact lenses if worn) a registration mark fixed to a vehicle and containing letters and figures 79 mm high and 50 mm wide (number plate font after 1 September 2001) at a distance of 20 m.
- Eye problems—cataract, retinopathy, maculopathy, glaucoma. The patient should ask the ophthalmologist about driving. Does visual acuity still comply with DVLA regulations? Has there been any laser therapy? DVLA notification may be required.
- Heart problems—DVLA guidance is very specific for each situation. Read it carefully. In general, driving should stop if there is a cardiac problem which could lead to collapse at the wheel. Treatment for this usually allows resumption of driving under cardiological guidance. This section includes implantable cardiac devices. Various periods without driving are advised after cardiac events or interventions.
- Peripheral vascular disease does not usually require stopping driving or notification, but some aortic aneurysms do. Amputation—vehicle likely to need modification. Notify DVLA.
- Foot ulceration—patients must be able to use the pedals safely and promptly. They may be unable to drive until the ulcer has healed.
- Renal disease—no need for notification unless disabling symptoms e.g. dizziness.
- Peripheral neuropathy—patients must be able to feel the controls (e.g. brake, clutch, accelerator) and operate them promptly and safely. If this is not possible, the vehicle must be modified and the DVLA notified.
- Stroke and TIA—stop driving for a month and then review.

Vocational drivers

Fear of losing one's licence stops many patients starting much-needed insulin treatment.

- Vocational (Group 2) is for large goods vehicles (LGV) or passenger-carrying vehicles (PCV). Insulin treatment precludes holding an LGV or PCV licence. The other diabetes rules are as for Group 1 but there are differences in rules for other conditions (e.g. the complications of diabetes), so drivers must check the DVLA website.
- Groups C1 (vehicles weighing 3.5–7.5 tonnes) and D1 (minibuses carrying <16 people): existing diabetic drivers may continue providing they satisfy the general health requirements until the licence expires or is medically revoked. Nowadays theses licences are included in Group 2.
- Taxi drivers are usually subject to Group 2 rules via their local licensing body.
- Police, ambulance, and health care drivers cannot drive if on insulin treatment. Group 2 rules apply.

Advice for patients

Avoid hypoglycaemia

Doctors or nurses who prescribe drugs (insulin or tablets) which can cause hypoglycaemia must warn the patient specifically about the risk of hypoglycaemia. Check if the patient holds a driving licence (whether driving at present or not). If so, warn them about the need to inform the DVLA (give them the website address if they use a computer) if they satisfy the conditions above. Specifically warn them about the need to avoid hypoglycaemia while driving.

The DVLA receives 27 police notifications a month about driving incidents associated with hypoglycaemia. Drivers have received a custodial sentence for causing death whilst driving and hypoglycaemic on insulin.

Motor insurance companies regard diabetes as a material fact. All diabetic patients should notify them of their diagnosis and ascertain their rules for further notification. Failure to do so may mean that they are not covered if there is an accident.

Box 22.1 Driving and diabetes: guidance for patients on insulin or glucose-lowering tablets

- If you take insulin or glucose-lowering tablets check the DVLA website (www.dvla.gov.uk/drivers.aspx) to see if you need to tell them about your condition.
- Everyone on long-term insulin should notify the DVLA.
- Some people on tablets need to notify the DVLA of their condition.
- Some people with diabetic complications such as eye problems or heart problems need to notify the DVLA. Check with your doctor and the website.
- Inform your motor insurance company.
- It is against the law to continue driving if the DVLA advise against this.
- Always carry glucose within arm's reach in the car.
- Carry food and drink, including water, in the car.
- Test finger-prick blood glucose before every journey, whether short or long.
- Do not drive if glucose <5 mmol/l. If <4 mmol/l treat as hypoglycaemic. If 4–5 mmol/l eat a sugary snack and re-check in 15 min.
- If any suspicion of hypoglycaemia while driving:
    - STOP safely immediately
    - Switch off engine
    - Remove keys from ignition
    - Eat or drink glucose
    - Leave driver's seat if safe to do so (it rarely is—never get out into the road while your glucose is low). Slide across to the passenger seat if possible
    - Do not drive until blood glucose is >5 mmol/l *and* you have waited 45 min since treating your hypo. Brain function takes 45 min to recover from hypoglycaemia—longer in older people.
- If starting insulin for the first time or changing the insulin treatment (e.g. a new insulin type or treatment pattern), do not drive for a week or longer if your doctor advises.

Travel at home and abroad

People with diabetes can travel wherever they wish. To reduce problems they should:

- ensure that their diabetes control is as good as possible
- ensure that their general health is as good as possible
- obtain relevant immunizations
- ensure sufficient diabetes medication and equipment plus extra to cover loss or theft
- ensure sufficient medication/dressings etc. for other conditions
- ensure that they have planned what to do if something goes wrong
- ensure that they have travel insurance—the diabetes must be declared and the cover should include repatriation (e.g. by air)
- check the Diabetes UK website (www.diabetes.org.uk), which has good travel advice, or phone Careline 0845 120 2960

Check the diabetes control and general health

Is the diabetes stable?

Review glucose balance and attempt to stabilize. Patients with erratic glucose balance may decompensate abroad and require admission or repatriation. Travelling with recurrent severe hypoglycaemia is ill advised. One study (*J Travel Med* 1999; **6**(1):12–15) found that two-thirds of patients on insulin had glucose instability on tropical holidays but only one-third of type 1 patients increased monitoring frequency. Several had a febrile illness.

Diabetic tissue damage?

- Diabetic foot problems
  - See podiatrist/chiropodist before travelling.
  - Take well-fitting comfortable shoes—lace-ups are best.
  - Protect feet. Check noon and night for rubs, grit, blisters, sunburn and treat urgently. Wash feet often and dry well.
- Untreated retinal new vessels. Treat before flying. Take ophthalmological advice.
- Cardiac disease—check if OK to fly.
- Renal disease—avoid dehydration.
- Peripheral vascular disease—protect feet and legs, keep warm in cold.
- Peripheral neuropathy—protect feet and legs, beware sunburn.

Other health problems

Diabetes may worsen other health problems. If other conditions worsen, this can destabilize the diabetes. Review these before departure.

Supplies (and extra)

- Give the GP practice and pharmacist enough time to provide prescriptions.
- Take double the diabetes and other medical supplies they expect to use.
- Medication for diabetes and other conditions.

- Insulin (cartridges, vials, and spares). Insulated container for hot or very cold countries.
- Pens, syringes, needles, needle-clipper (and spares).
- Insulin pump (take spare pump), batteries, cannula, tubing, insertors, vials, etc. Pump patients should also carry syringes and needles.
- Finger-prick glucose testing kit—finger-pricker, strips, meter (×2), spare batteries.
- Glucose—tablets, Glucogel®, boiled sweets, snacks, bottled water.
- Glucagon with syringe and needle.
- Diabetic card stating (preferably in the local language):

  'I am a diabetic on insulin/tablets. If I am found ill please give me 2 teaspoons of sugar in a small amount of water or 3 of the glucose tablets which I am carrying. If I fail to recover in 10 minutes please call an ambulance.'
- Diabetes ID medallion or bracelet.
- Letter from doctor about diabetes.
- NB security regulations may require insulin to be in the original pack unopened. Check the situation before flying. Contact the airline if necessary. With restrictions on fluids some items may need to be in hold baggage or bought airside.
- Medical summary from doctor if long trip or significant health problems.
- First aid pack (with instructions), relevant to destination including:
  - sticking plasters, bandages, wound dressing
  - wound-cleaning wipes
  - paracetamol or similar analgesic
  - anti-diarrhoeal (e.g. loperamide)
  - motion sickness pills
  - anti-emetic
  - antihistamine
  - course of antibiotics
  - antifungal cream
  - if relevant, sterile venesection, suture, and IV infusion pack
  - sunscreen
  - insect repellent
  - antibacterial hand-cleaning wipes or gel
  - copy of sick day rules (📖 p.233)

Immunization and prophylaxis

People with diabetes should have every appropriate immunization. It may temporarily upset glucose control, but not as much as the actual condition would!

- Annual influenza immunization
- Pneumococcal immunization
- All standard childhood vaccines
- Anti-tetanus immunization
- All immunizations for destination
- Antimalarials if relevant

The journey

Patients on diet alone or metformin only for diabetes have little difficulty travelling unless they have symptomatic tissue damage. Patients on glucose-lowering treatment must avoid hypoglycaemia while travelling. They may end up in the wrong place or be arrested for behavioural problems.

Patients should get a clear travel itinerary with local and actual timings. Insulin-treated patients should test their blood glucose every 4–6 hrs while travelling (every 2 hrs if driving themselves). Consider the day of travel as being from breakfast at home until breakfast in the destination. Patients should eat every 2–3 hrs. During the day they should reduce the insulins which are acting when travelling but be prepared to take a small extra dose (e.g. 2–6 units analogue fast-acting) immediately after any extra meal if the breakfast-breakfast time is >24 hrs and the glucose is >11 mmol/l. Before sleeping check that the HGBM is >6 mmol/l and have a bed-time snack.

All diabetes medication should be carried personally in hand baggage, bags, or pockets (ideally split about the person). It should never be entrusted to baggage handled by outsiders or out of sight of its owner.

Problems abroad

Food

Patients may worry about getting the 'right' food. A few weeks of a less than perfect diet is not a disaster. However, it is usually possible to find a local staple carbohydrate—bread, potato, pasta, rice, maize, yams, beans, etc. Obvious fat and sugar can be avoided. Cooked vegetables and fruit are usually available. Uncooked fruit and vegetables should be washed in bottled water or peeled carefully to reduce the risk of gastroenteritis. Advise bottled water or diet drinks (patients should break the seal themselves and clean the top of the can first). Alcohol is self-sterilizing but advise moderation (📖 p.83). It is advisable to carry some food but beware local regulations (e.g. Australia and Canada ban import of some foods).

Heat

- Britons are not always used to heat
- Increases insulin absorption from injection sites risking hypoglycaemia
- Increased sweating + hyperglycaemia may cause dehydration
- Neuropathic areas can sunburn
- Advise a cool-bag for insulin (📖 p.172)

Cold

- Cold slows insulin absorption—it is released when the patient warms up, risking hypoglycaemia
- Hypoglycaemia prevents shivering (📖 p.218)
- Patients with peripheral vascular disease must keep extremities well-wrapped to avoid frost bite
- Cold may precipitate angina

Infection

- Monitor HBGM four times daily if any infection. Increase glucose-lowering treatment if necessary.
- Minor wounds must be cleaned promptly and covered with a sterile dressing. Sepsis is common, especially on the feet.
- Fungal infections—athlete's foot and thrush are common. Use anti-fungal cream immediately. Women susceptible to thrush should take an imidazole pessary with them.
- Chest or urine infections should be treated promptly—hence the benefit of packing a course of antibiotics
- Gastroenteritis is common and may precipitate DKA. Patients should:
  - take anti-diarrhoeal and anti-emetic promptly
  - drink bottled water and non-diet canned drink
  - check HBGM every 2 hrs
  - increase insulin if necessary
  - follow sick day rules (📖 p.233)
  - get medical help promptly if the glucose rises and blood ketones >3 mmol/l (📖 p.240)

Medical aid abroad

Specialist diabetes care is available worldwide but access is variable. Local medical resources are also variable. Patients must have adequate travel insurance and have declared their diabetes. It is wise to note local emergency and ambulance call numbers and arrangements on arriving in a foreign company and program them into a mobile phone. The IDF can provide addresses of local diabetes associations (www.idf.org).

Summary

- Walking and cycling are good exercise. Ensure adequate food and reduce glucose-lowering medication if appropriate.
- Health care professionals should warn diabetic drivers of their need to check whether DVLA notification is required and to tell their motor insurance company.
- Drivers with diabetes on long-term insulin must inform the DVLA of their condition, and those on other forms of treatment must check the website (www.dvla.gov.uk/drivers.aspx) to find out if they need to notify.
- Vocational drivers face more stringent requirements and must also check the DVLA regulations.
- Patients with frequent or unrecognized hypoglycaemia must not drive.
- Patients with some forms of tissue damage must not drive and may need to notify the DVLA.
- Diabetic travellers should plan for the unexpected.
- Planning includes a diabetes and general health check.
- Immunizations and prescriptions should be obtained in good time.
- Adequate diabetes and other health supplies should be taken, along with a first aid kit.
- Patients should carry a diabetic card, preferably in the language of their destination.
- Aim to avoid hypoglycaemia while travelling.
- Aim to avoid gastroenteritis while travelling.
- Having diabetes should not prevent happy travelling—pre-planning ensures continued enjoyment.

Chapter 23

Psychological and social aspects of diabetes

Introduction

Everyone with newly diagnosed diabetes is concerned and some are very frightened, especially if they have relatives who have gone blind, had amputations, or died from diabetes. The experience at diagnosis influences the patient's attitude long term. All patients need a clear explanation in terms they can understand, an opportunity to express concerns and ask questions, and support with further opportunities for discussion from an expert. Some anxiety increases adherence to treatment regimens but excessive anxiety may hinder this.

Optimal diabetes control requires self-motivation and knowledge for self-care. A feeling of autonomy and self-sufficiency can increase satisfaction with life for diabetic patients. However, motivation for self-care has been shown to be associated with worse HbA_{1c} than in non-motivated patients (e.g. adolescents (*Diabetes Care* 2004; **27**:1517)). Self-care without knowledge of diabetes and taking action to improve will not improve glucose balance. Apathy is also associated with worse HbA_{1c}, even in the absence of depression (*Diabetes Res Clin Pract* 2007; epub: 4 8 2007).

Brain function

The prevailing glucose concentration affects brain function. This is acutely affected by hypoglycaemia, leading to changes in cognitive function and emotion, and ultimately fits or coma (📖 p.204). Evidence of longer-term effects of hypoglycaemic episodes upon brain function varies, although severe prolonged profound hypoglycaemic coma may cause brain damage.

Hyperglycaemia also alters brain function. Anecdotally, patients or relatives report increased irritability (difficult to live with) and slower thinking with higher glucose. Different studies have measured this in variable ways with variable results. One study in type 2 diabetes showed that, short-term, a glucose of 16.5 mmol vs 4.5 mmol/l impaired information processing, working memory, and some aspects of attention. Mood also changed with reduced energetic arousal, and increased sadness and anxiety (*Diabetes Care* 2004; **27**:2335–40). This suggests that teaching sessions would have greatest impact in patients with near-normal glucose levels at the time.

Dementia is discussed elsewhere (📖 p.402).

Psychiatric disorders

Psychiatric disorders, particularly depression and anxiety (see below), are common in people with diabetes. 37% of adolescents with a 10 yr history of diabetes had a psychiatric disorder. Patients with chronic poor control were twice as likely to have a psychiatric disorder, and were more likely to have pre-diabetic behavioural problems than those with good control (*Diabetes Med* 2005; **22**:152–7).

The presence of any psychiatric disorder makes diabetes care more difficult, and increases the risk of non-concordance with therapy with subsequent problems with glucose control (hyper- or hypoglycaemia) and increased risk of diabetic tissue damage. Patients in psychiatric wards may have limited access to diabetes expertise—this should be organized as fluctuations in their glucose control may worsen their emotional state.

Psychotic diabetic patients with substance abuse are four times more likely to die than similar patients without diabetes (*Psychiatric Services* 2007; **58**:270). Young people with diabetes have a similar frequency of substance abuse to the non-diabetic population (📖 p.356).

Depression

Screen for depression

- During the past month have you often been bothered by feeling down, depressed, or hopeless?
- During the past month have you often been bothered by little interest or pleasure in doing things?
- Is this something you would like help with?

www.depression-primarycare.co.uk/images/Protocol%20for%20the%20Management%20of%20Depression%20in%20Primary%20C.pdf

Patients with severe depression are more likely to develop type 2 diabetes (although more health care attention might detect this sooner). A review of 42 studies (*Diabetes Care* 2001; **24**:1069–78) found that people with diabetes are twice as likely to be depressed as the general population, women (28%) more than men (18%). 31% report depressive symptoms on questionnaires. 11% of patients formally assessed had major depression. Carers may attribute depression to a 'natural reaction' to having diabetes and some two-thirds of patients are not offered treatment. Depressed diabetic patients are less likely to adhere to their diet and treatment than those who are not depressed (*Arch Intern Med.* 2000; **160**:3278–85). Depression is associated with higher HbA_{1c}, and some studies have shown that antidepressants improve this (*Diabetes Care* 2000; **23**:934–42) Depressed diabetic patients have higher health care costs than those who are not depressed. Depressed diabetic patients are more likely to die, especially from cardiovascular causes than those without depression (*Diabetes Care* 2005; **28**:1339–45). Depression is also linked with microvascular complications. 58% of non-depressed diabetic patients and 78% of depressed diabetic patients have functional disability (*Diabetes Care* 2004; **27**:421–8). This reduces ability to work.

Tricyclic antidepressants and selective serotonin-reuptake inhibitors (SSRIs) may affect the blood glucose in either direction, although it appears that tricyclics are most likely to raise it and SSRIs to lower it. Up to half of diabetic patients with depression are unable to tolerate full-dose anti-depressant medication. Treatment of depression with cognitive behavioural therapy in type 2 diabetes improves HbA_{1c} (*Ann Int Med* 1998; **129**:613–21).

❗Assess suicide risk. Diabetic patients, especially those on insulin, have ready access to fatal overdose.

Anxiety

Anxiety is common in diabetes. A review showed that 14% diabetic patients had generalized anxiety disorder (a formal psychiatric disorder) and 40% had elevated symptoms of anxiety (*J Psychosom Res 2002;* **53**:1053–60) Elevated anxiety symptoms were more common in women than in men (55% vs 33%). Anxiety is natural but may be heightened in patients with hypoglycaemia who may run high glucose levels to avoid this. High glucose levels may also be associated with increased anxiety.

Phobias

Phobias are more common in diabetes than in the general population but <1% of type 1 patients are needle-phobic (*Diabetes Med* 2001; **18**:671–4; *Diabetes Metab Res Rev* 2000; **16**:287–93). Refer patients to a psychologist experienced in treating diabetic patients.

Eating and body image disorders

Studies have produced conflicting reports about whether eating disorders are more common in people with diabetes than those without. Diabetic patients are made to focus on what and how much they are eating as part of their care, and this may encourage abnormal fixation on aspects of eating, body image, and weight.

Refer all diabetic patients with any form of eating disorder or body image problem to the specialist diabetes team and to a mental health team specializing in eating disorders. These patients are at risk of severe illness or death from their behaviour. They tend to fail attendance, avoid help, and ignore advice. They may have other psychiatric problems and can self-harm. Try to stay in contact. Assign a key worker if possible. Non-mental-health staff should realize that such patients, who may be consciously or subconsciously manipulative, can cause distress and conflict for staff. Involve the experts early.

Up to a third of diabetic girls omit or under-dose insulin to remain slim or lose weight via hyperglycaemia and glycosuria.

Patients with a restrictive eating pattern may require very little insulin and are at risk of hypoglycaemia. They have little liver glycogen (so glucagon is unlikely to work in hypoglycaemia). Dietary ketosis is common. There is danger of fatal ketoacidosis if they also omit insulin. Those using laxatives can become severely hypokalaemic. Very thin patients may also have other hormone abnormalities.

Bulimic patients find that their glucose oscillates wildly. Those who vomit may have difficult knowing how much nutrition is retained. Those who binge and do not vomit will need extra short-acting insulin to cover this additional food.

Psychiatric drugs and diabetes

A study of Medicaid patients with bipolar disorder found that the risk of new diabetes was greatest among patients taking risperidone, olanzapine, and quetiapine—hazard ratios 3.8, 3.7, and 2.5, respectively, vs conventional antipsychotic drugs (*Pharmacotherapy* 2007; **27**:27–35). Such patients should be screened at least once a year for diabetes. Weight gain and hypertension were also linked with greater risk of new diabetes.

Summary

- Emotional factors influence diabetes self-care and outcomes.
- Primary and secondary care should liaise about individual diabetic patients with a psychological or psychiatric problem. Consider referral to the mental health service for expert help.
- Psychiatric disorders are more frequent in diabetic patients than in the non-diabetic population.
- Depression is twice as common in the diabetic population.
- About half of diabetic patients have some form of anxiety.
- Phobias may limit insulin therapy and monitoring.
- Eating disorders may be more common in diabetes than in the general population and make glucose control difficult.
- Omission or under-dosing of insulin is common in diabetic girls who are trying to stay slim.
- Substance abuse increases mortality in diabetes.
- Atypical psychiatric drugs increase the risk of developing diabetes compared with typical antipsychotics.

Useful resources

- Diabetes UK has a helpful page on tools to measure quality of life, emotional and psychological need for people with diabetes: http://www.diabetes.org.uk/en/Professionals/Information_resources/Reports/Tools-to-measure-quality-of-life-emotional-and-psychological-need-for-people-with-diabetes/
- Professor Clare Bradley has researched many psychological aspects of diabetes and has produced validated questionnaires: c.bradley@rhul.ac.uk

Chapter 24

Diabetes care in hospital

See also individual chapters

Introduction

This chapter is about the care of people with diabetes attending as emergencies or admitted as inpatients. Much of the detailed management of these conditions is described in the relevant chapters.

In 1991–1995 ~7% of hospital admissions in Wales were of patients with diabetes. They occupied 10.7% hospital bed-days with a length of stay of 10.7 days (vs 6.7 in non-diabetic patients) (*Diabetic Med* 1997; **14**:686–92). In London in 2007 ~16% of general hospital inpatients had diabetes and many more had impaired glucose tolerance. American studies show that 12–25% of inpatients have diabetes depending on the way they are identified.

In 1991–1995 ~17% of coronary heart disease admissions in Wales had diabetes. These patients were about four times as likely to require cardiac procedures as non-diabetic patients (*Heart* 1997; **78**:544–9). In the same Welsh population, 15% of admissions with foot ulceration, infection, neuropathy, or peripheral vascular disease had diabetes. Length of stay was nearly double that of non-diabetic patients. The relative risk of hospital mortality (diabetes vs non-diabetes) was 2.83 (*Diabetes Care* 1998; **21**: 42–8)

Diabetes, whether known or newly discovered, has a major adverse impact upon most inpatients. Compared with inpatients without diabetes, diabetic patients often have increased risks (Box 24.1) in addition to the condition with which they were admitted. Much of this risk is secondary to hyperglycaemia and pre-admission diabetic tissue damage.

Patients with glucose >11mmol/l are 3–4 times as likely to get infected wounds or UTIs as those with glucose in the non-diabetic range. Patients with newly diagnosed diabetes are particularly at risk. An American study showed that inpatients with newly diagnosed diabetes had a 16% mortality, vs 3% in known diabetic patients and 1.7% in those without diabetes. The newly hyperglycaemic patients also had a longer stay and were less likely be discharged to their own home (*J Clin Endocr Metab 2002;* **87**:978–82).

Risk is also increased because diabetic patients already have multiple complications on admission. The adverse effects of their primary admission diagnosis exacerbate their complications. Dehydration worsens renal failure, hypoalbuminaemia worsens cardiac failure, and infection or steroid treatment increase glucose.

Box 24.1 Risks for hospitalized diabetic patients

- ↑Infection risk (e.g. urinary tract, wound)
- ↑Risk of cannula/line/catheter site infection
- ↑Severe infections which take longer to resolve
- ↑Antibiotic-resistant or hospital-acquired infections
- ↓Healing
- ↑Risk of fistula formation
- ↑Risk of thrombosis
- ↑Risk of ischaemic events—myocardial, peripheral vascular, cerebral
- ↑Risk of renal failure
- ↑Risk of cardiac failure
- ↑Risk of pressure sores, especially heel ulcers in vasculopaths
- ↑Metabolic complexity
- ↑Hospital inpatient stay
- ↓Likelihood of returning to their own home
- ↑Mortality
- ↑Cost of care

Emergency assessment or Accident and Emergency

This is relevant to management of patients seen in emergency assessment units or A&E departments. One in three diabetic emergency attenders to one A&E had actual or compensated DKA (*Diabetic Med* 2005; **22**: 221–4).

Don't miss new diabetes. Check blood glucose, preferably venous but finger-prick if speed essential (📖 p.7) in high-risk patients:

- everyone with an acute/emergency medical problem (i.e. dealt with by physicians)
- symptoms of diabetes
- white people >40 yrs old, non-white ethnic groups >25 yrs if overweight
- overweight people
- tissue damage or conditions known to be associated with diabetes
- on medication known to be associated with diabetes (e.g. steroids, thiazides, olanzapine)
- history of glucose intolerance
- past gestational diabetes or current pregnancy (📖 p.374)
- severe mental health disorders.

See Box 1.3 (📖 p.7) for full list and Table 1.3 (📖 p.11) for diagnostic criteria for diabetes

All diabetic patients check as a minimum:

- presenting complaint
- duration of diabetes (long duration more tissue damage)
- history of tissue damage, especially cardiovascular, eyes, kidneys, nerves
- current or recent infection (may be incompletely treated)
- treatment for diabetes and other conditions
- look at medications if available, including insulin, remembering that some insulins have very similar names but different actions
- recent HBGM and HbA_{1c}—verbal report or diary or lab if available
- check injection sites in insulin/exenatide treated patients
- current finger-prick glucose—too low (<4mmol/l)? too high (>11 mmol/l)? send a laboratory sample to confirm and treat appropriately
- finger-prick glucose >11 mmol/l—check finger-prick blood ketone level
- pulse, BP, respiratory rate, oxygen saturations, temperature
- assessment of presenting complaint as appropriate
- full assessment if unwell enough to require admission (📖 p.19)
- examine emergency and elective admission patients fully (📖 p.19) including checking for foot problems and pressure areas
- urine dipstick

Box 24.2 Investigations

- Finger-prick blood:
  - glucose
  - HbA_{1c} (if available)
  - ketones if glucose >11 mmol/l (all emergency attenders)
- Urine:
  - dipstick glucose, ketones, protein, blood, leucocytes, nitrite
  - if protein dipstick negative—microalbumin, creatinine ratio (laboratory or clinic)
- Laboratory venous blood:
  - glucose (repeat fasting if diagnosis unproven)
  - urea and electrolytes
  - creatinine
  - liver function
  - calcium and albumin
  - thyroid function
  - haemoglobin A_{1c}
  - full blood count
  - consider adding C-reactive protein (?infection), urate (?gout)
  - fasting cholesterol, HDL, LDL, triglyceride next day
  - (add tissue transglutaminase/anti-mysial/anti-gliadin antibodies if <20 yrs old and not previously checked)
- Chest X-ray if chest signs or symptoms, smoker, recent immigrant, Asian (or local protocol)
- Foot X-ray if ulcer, possible infection or injury
- ECG if >30 yrs old, or diabetes >10 yrs duration, or chest pain in under-thirties
- MRSA screen for all diabetic foot patients and all admissions or day cases
- Microbiology samples–urnie, sputum, pus, blood, other

Emergencies

Hypoglycaemia

This is a brief summary—for full safety information and detailed management **read the hypoglycaemia chapter (📖 p.199)**.

- ❶Any diabetic patient on glucose-lowering treatment who behaves oddly in any way is hypoglycaemic until proved otherwise.
- Features of hypoglycaemia include confusion, sweating, shaking, blurred vision, aggression, coma, fits

In patients capable of swallowing

Glucose is absorbed most rapidly in liquid form. Give 10 g glucose. Treat hypoglycaemia as soon as it is suspected. Check finger-prick glucose if possible; if not, give oral glucose immediately. The following contain about 10 g glucose:

- three glucose tablets (e.g. Dextrosol®)
- one tube 25 g Glucogel (glucose gel)
- One-third of an 80 g bottle of Glucogel® (whole bottle contains 32 g glucose)
- 50–60 ml or one-sixth of a 380 ml bottle of Original Lucozade® (whole bottle contains 68 g glucose) (other versions contain different quantities of glucose)
- 90 ml or a third of a can of non-diet Coca Cola®
- two spoonfuls of sugar
- three sugar lumps
- three or four sweets (e.g. fruit pastilles).

In patients who cannot, or will not swallow safely

Conscious patients who refuse to swallow

- Firm encouragement to eat. Glucogel® is best in this situation as it is difficult to spit out.
- Violent patients—keep back to avoid personal injury and try to contain the patient in a safe area. Inject glucagon into whatever muscle bulk can be accessed safely. The alternative is to muster sufficient help to achieve robust venous access and give IV glucose (see below).

Unconscious patients, unsafe swallow, uncooperative

Profound hypoglycaemia is rare. It is most often seen in patients who have taken insulin overdoses, alcohol, or sulphonylureas, or in renal failure. 999 hospital admission is required.

- Risk of respiratory or cardiac arrest.
- Protect airway.
- Give oxygen if convulsing or hypoxic.
- Safeguard patient and staff from injury.
- Gain IV access, large vein, tape in cannula securely (care—extravasated glucose can cause ulceration).
- Withdraw blood for laboratory glucose, U&E, liver function, and perhaps thyroid function or cortisol.
- Give IV glucose (repeat once if not recovered within 15 min):
  - infuse 50 ml 20% glucose IV (adults)
    or
  - 25 ml of 50% glucose IV (adults).
- Flush cannula with N saline (IV glucose can cause thrombophlebitis).
- IV access impossible—inject glucagon IM (📖 p.209).
- If patient fails to recover consider steroid lack. Take blood for subsequent cortisol level and inject 100 mg hydrocortisone IV or IM.
- Monitor Glasgow coma scale, heart rate, BP, respirations, oxygen saturations.
- Feed patient if safe, or infuse 5% glucose slowly—rate depends on clinical situation.
- Monitor hourly until full consciousness regained and maintained. Keep under medical observation for at least 4 hrs and admit if any of the factors below apply.
- Do not remove IV cannula until patient ready for discharge.
- After treatment wait at least 45 min and recheck finger-prick glucose before discharge
- Hospitalize hypoglycaemia patients:
  - on sulphonylurea
  - elderly patients
  - those living alone and vulnerable
  - who have ingested alcohol or drugs of abuse
  - with renal disease, liver disease, or other significant concomitant disease
  - with psychiatric problems
  - with suspicion of overdose of insulin or glucose-lowering tablets
  - if you have concerns about their safety.
- Patients on long-acting insulin should be considered for admission unless they are fully conscious and capable of monitoring themselves and their finger-prick glucose, and adjusting their food and insulin safely.
- Why were they hypoglycaemic? Educate patient and carers.
- Diabetes team follow-up.

Diabetic ketoacidosis

This is a brief summary—for full safety information and detailed management **read the DKA/HONK chapter (📖 p.237)**.

- ❶Any suspicion of DKA requires immediate 999 transfer to hospital.
- Always consider DKA in ill diabetic patients.
- DKA is likely in vomiting insulin-treated patients and/or ill patients with glucose >11 mmol/l (📖 p.20).

Initial management (📖 p.241)

- Resuscitation : airway, breathing, circulation
- Aim door to needle time <15 min
- Good IV access
- Take venous bloods
- 1000 ml 0.9% NaCl IV over 1 hr
- One IV or IM bolus of 0.1 units/kg soluble insulin (e.g. Actrapid, Humulin S)
- Insulin infusion 0.1 units/kg/hour soluble insulin (e.g. Actrapid, Humulin S) up to a maximum of 6 units/hour.
- Inform diabetes registrar or consultant diabetologist or medical registrar on-call immediately

Tests

- Finger-prick capillary blood glucose + ketone (beware cold fingers)
- Arterial blood pH and gases
- Urgent laboratory venous glucose, U&E, creatinine, FBC
- Later LFT, TFT, lipids, blood cultures
- Dipstick urine
- MSU, throat swab, microbiology swab any lesion
- Pregnancy test
- ECG
- Chest X-ray; consider abdominal X-ray

Aims of treatment

- Initial resuscitation started within 15 min, then gradual return to normal
- Rehydrate over 24 hrs—use IV fluid and insulin to correct DKA
- Aim for a glucose fall of 4–6 mmol/hr
- Aim for arterial pH to rise gradually over 24 hrs

Actions

- Consider ICU/HDU for each patient
- Good IV access
- Consider CVP monitoring if very ill, cardiac disease, elderly
- Oxygen 35% (unless respiratory disease risking CO_2 retention)
- Nasogastric tube if severe vomiting, gastric retention, coma
- Urinary catheter if no urine within 2 hrs, elderly, immobile, coma
- IV fluids and electrolytes (📖 p.243)
- Insulin
- Treat precipitating condition (e.g. antibiotics for infection)
- Prophylactic low molecular weight heparin
- Contact seniors and diabetes team

Infection

- ❶Consider infection in every diabetic patient
- Send samples of body fluids or pus for microscopy and culture
- Do blood cultures before starting antibiotics
- Diabetic patients are immunocompromised so may have unusual infections, including fungal infections
- Intertrigo and oral and genital candidasis are common and can become secondarily infected
- CRP and WBCC may not be raised, even in the presence of significant infection
- There may be multiple organisms
- There may be little evidence of infection (e.g. slight redness, vague malaise)
- Image suspicious or painful areas (e.g. X-ray feet)
- Infected areas may have poor blood supply (e.g. PVD), which may worsen because of the infection
- Infection may recur after treatment
- MRSA and *C.difficile* are a risk in diabetic patients because they have multiple or prolonged infections and are in and out of hospital
- Diabetic patients, especially those on steroids, are at risk of necrotizing fasciitis, especially if the initial infection is between the navel and knees

Acute coronary syndromes (📖 p.279)

- Common in people with diabetes
- May accompany other presenting problems
- May have past/recurrent/extensive ACS as diffuse coronary artery disease is likely
- Atypical symptoms are common in people with diabetes
- Any chest pain, discomfort, heaviness; breathlessness, syncope—consider ACS
- Treat as for ACS in non-diabetic patients
- Proven MI:
  - use primary angioplasty or thrombolysis according to local protocols
  - active proliferative retinopathy is a contraindication to thrombolysis but is rare
  - unless on diet alone or glucose <11.1 mmol/l, start IV sliding scale (📖 p.181) but be very careful to avoid hypoglycaemia—risk of dysrhythmia
  - control glucose between 4 and 7 mmol/l
- ACS—not MI:
  - consider IV sliding scale for insulin-treated patients, and those with glucose >11 mmol/l
  - control blood glucose between 4 and 7 mmol/l
- Check for other tissue damage, especially PVD and cerebrovascular disease.
- Contact cardiology and diabetes team

TIA or stroke (📖 p.292)

- Common in people with diabetes
- May accompany other presenting problems
- Exclude hypoglycaemia which can masquerade as stroke—finger-prick glucose essential; if any doubt repeat the test on a venous sample
- May have past/recurrent/extensive strokes as diffuse cerebral artery disease is likely
- Because of previous strokes and diabetic peripheral or mononeuropathy, neurology may be confusing in new TIA or stroke
- Manage as for non-diabetic stroke/TIA patients (NICE CG 68 (2008))
- CT or MRI brain scan urgently
- Use thrombolysis if appropriate expertise is available
- Control blood glucose between 4 and 11 mmol/l without hypoglycaemia
- Use IV sliding scale if glucose >11 mmol/l
- Be extremely careful to avoid hypoglycaemia
- Contact stroke unit and diabetes team.

Diabetic foot or lower limb (📖 p.325)

Never underestimate the severity of a diabetic foot problem. Look for:

- Ulcers or wounds (including between toes)
- Infection—soft tissue, bone, systemic
- Circulatory problems
- Neuropathy
- Bone—fracture, osteopenia, deformity, infection
- Injury
- Foreign body
- All of these

Contact the diabetes registrar promptly. Refer all diabetic foot patients to the diabetic foot team. Admit if in doubt.

- Assess whole patient—there will be other diabetic tissue damage (📖 p.19)
- Investigations as in Box 24.2 (📖 p.461)
- X-ray foot indicating area of interest on request
- Treatment must be prompt and aggressive, and reviewed frequently (e.g. daily if inpatient)
- Pain relief
- Suspect infection in all patients. Treat if any evidence or strong clinical suspicion. Use your district or hospital antibiotic protocol.
- Take great care to prevent MRSA or *C.difficile* infection
- Debride dead tissue
- Remove foreign body and re-image
- Avoid further pressure on the affected area(s)
- Protect other pressure areas
- Elevation
- Prophylactic low molecular weight heparin; thrombo-embolism prevention stockings may cause heel pressure ulcers.
- Good nutrition—refer to dietitian

- Psychological support
- Optimize glucose control
- See other complications and co-morbidities and treat vigorously.
- Vascular assessment and treatment.
- Early surgery for major infection or ischaemia.

Critical limb ischaemia or gangrene (📖 p.290)

❶These patients are at risk of death. They have extensive vascular disease and usually have microvascular complications as well.

Admit immediately all patients with:
- infection with purple/blue/black ischaemic areas
- gangrene toe/foot/anywhere else
- PVD and rest pain
- acute arterial obstruction—painful, pulseless, cold leg
- note that pain may be modified by neuropathy—the situation may be worse that it seems
- local arrangements vary—all these patients require immediate vascular assessment but always have other complications of diabetes and usually unstable glucose balance so always need diabetes team input too

In hospital:
- Very detailed clerking by diabetes team including careful assessment of cardiac status (most have IHD) and renal status (risk of renal arterial stenosis or renal failure due to nephropathy, infection and dehydration)
- Investigations as in Box 24.2
- X-ray foot
- Treat infection vigorously
- Control glucose between 4 and 7 mmol/l without hypoglycaeamia
- Ensure optimal statin therapy
- Treat any intercurrent problem promptly
- Urgent arterial Doppler measurements
- Urgent arterial duplex scan for stenosis
- Refer to podiatry
- Refer to dietitian for full nutritional review
- Refer to physiotherapy for maintenance of movement and power
- Very careful protection of pressure areas—high risk of heel sores
- Angiography after discussion with vascular team and radiology
- ❶ Risk of contrast-induced renal failure; hydrate carefully before any contrast procedure
- Angioplasty or vascular procedure as indicated
- Excise slough, drain pus
- Amputate unsalvageable toes or limbs promptly
- Push for prompt effective care. There are often delays in care of diabetic foot patients—timing of radiology lists, theatre lists, availability of different staff. Delays increase risk of worsening of original problem, nosocomial infection, depression

Surgery

Both trauma and surgery cause marked metabolic disturbance, and laparascopic surgery appears no better than open surgery in this respect. Food intake and processing changes because the patient's food intake is stopped preoperatively and may be reduced for some time post-operatively, vomiting and altered bowel habit are common, and gastrointestinal and other surgery may cause long-term gastric or digestive changes. Adrenaline and steroid hormones rise and sympathetic activity increases causing insulin resistance, liver glucose release, and body fat and protein breakdown (catabolism). This process may be worse in diabetic patients, e.g. protein catabolism after colorectal surgery is increased in patients with type 2 diabetes mellitus (*Anesthesiology* 2005; **102**:320–6). Blood glucose rises.

Surgical ward nurses may not feel confident about diabetes care. The care of medical problems in surgical patients may be left to junior doctors who have no experience in managing diabetes and are unaware of the potential consequences of erratic glucose control.

There is ample evidence that peri-operative hyperglycaemia increases complication risk and impairs outcome of surgery. Diabetic patients also have tissue complications (e.g. cardiovascular disease and renal impairment) which may do this as well. However, overtreatment of blood glucose ± inadequate monitoring may be disastrous.

In a perfect world people with diabetes undergoing surgery would have non-diabetic blood glucose levels before, during, and after the operation which would occur exactly when planned with care from staff trained in surgical, anaesthetic, and diabetic management. But we all work in the real world.

Good liaison between surgeon, anaesthetist, diabetes team, and staff at all levels is essential for optimal results of surgery in diabetic patients. Current directorate structures in hospitals separate medicine from surgery/anaesthesia at all levels. There may be little contact. Doctor timetabling and different systems/locations for patient care (e.g. private treatment centres) may also impede coordinated management. Further confounding factors may be administrative (e.g. cancelled surgery because no bed is available, waiting list initiatives). Preoperative clerking is often done by very inexperienced doctors, although some units have specially trained nurses. Many factors delay surgery on the day, or for longer. This may mean ill diabetic inpatients (e.g. with infected feet) suffering fasting and sliding scales on/off for days. Diabetic clinic appointments may be scarce, and not all hospitals have diabetic inpatient specialist nurses who can see patients before admission and peri-operatively. GPs and practice nurses may not be kept closely informed. Patients may not realize that they need more than an annual diabetes review to get the best result from surgeryi—some staff may not realize this either.

Most of us could do better for these patients.

Pre-operatively

Surgery in diabetic patients should be carefully planned. Ensure good liaison between surgeon, anaesthetist, and diabetes team.

For surgical emergencies contact the diabetes registrar urgently—if he/she is not available bleep the medical registrar. Resuscitate the patient before operating. If the patient has blood glucose ≥11 mmol/l ± vomiting ± abdominal pain check finger-prick ketones. Do not operate on patients with DKA or HONK unless immediately life-threatening emergency.

For non-emergency surgery surgeons should notify the diabetes team of the operation date as soon as possible to allow intensive improvement of glucose control if required. Agree a local pre-operative clerking and investigation plan and ensure that all concerned are aware of this. Agree referral and clear communications for patients requiring improvement in glucose or management of other problems found during pre-operative clerking. The 'system' may admit patients before they are ready, who are then sent home because of poor glucose control.

Urgent surgery should not be delayed unduly. Weigh up the risk of delay (e.g. of cancer spreading/obstruction etc.) vs the potential risk of post-operative complications if sugary. Another factor to consider may be that the illness associated with the surgical condition itself could be impairing glucose control (e.g. recurrent cholecystitis).

Call the diabetic inpatient nurse and/or diabetes registrar when the patient is admitted. Outcome of surgery is often worse in people with diabetes than in those without. Complications are more likely (see 📖 p.000).

Use Box 24.2 (📖 p.461) to decide pre-operative investigations—tailor these to the patient, the situation, and the procedure. For major surgery perform all the tests in Box 24.2. In general, perform the usual investigations for your patient's particular surgical situation and procedure, and add finger-prick glucose (± ketones), laboratory glucose, U&E, LFT, HbA_{1c}, ECG, and chest X-ray.

Box 24.3 Pre-operative instructions

- Advise patient not to drive to hospital
- Ask patients to bring all their medications (including insulin and exenatide vials/cartridges and pens/syringes) to hospital
- Ask patient to keep their insulin pump on and running and bring spare infusion sets and insulin sets with them (📖 p.176)
- Ask patients to bring their HBGM records and glucose meter to hospital
- Check whether the patient has visual impairment
- Check whether the patient has other motor or sensory disability
- Add specific instructions from Box 24.4
- Add specific instructions for the planned operation
- Add specific instructions for your unit
- Example minimum fasting times for elective operations (but follow the guidance from your anaesthetist):
  - 6 hrs preoperatively - light meal
  - 2hrs preoperatively - clear fluids or water

Box 24.4 Perioperative management of diabetes

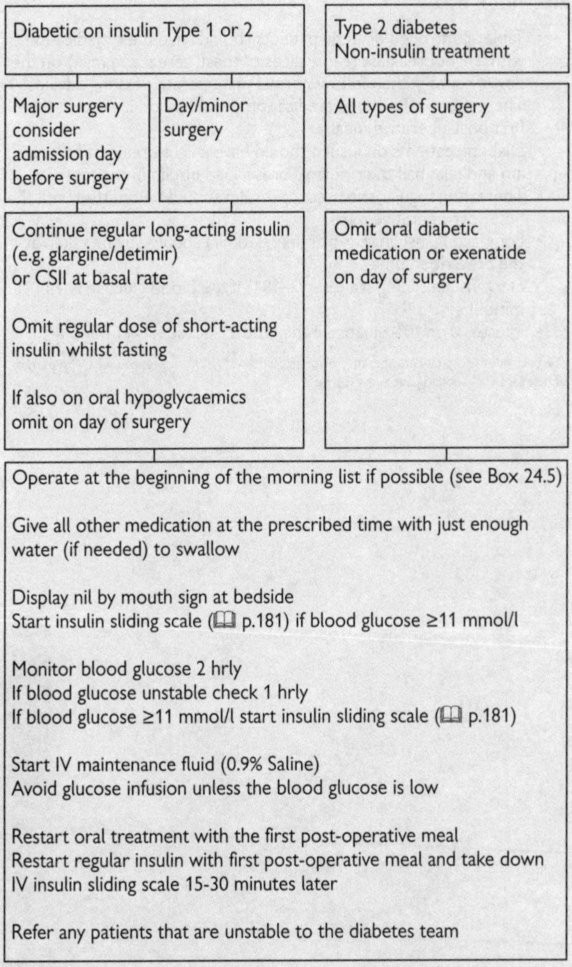

Diabetic on insulin Type 1 or 2		Type 2 diabetes Non-insulin treatment
Major surgery consider admission day before surgery	Day/minor surgery	All types of surgery
Continue regular long-acting insulin (e.g. glargine/detimir) or CSII at basal rate Omit regular dose of short-acting insulin whilst fasting If also on oral hypoglycaemics omit on day of surgery		Omit oral diabetic medication or exenatide on day of surgery

Operate at the beginning of the morning list if possible (see Box 24.5)

Give all other medication at the prescribed time with just enough water (if needed) to swallow

Display nil by mouth sign at bedside
Start insulin sliding scale (📖 p.181) if blood glucose ≥11 mmol/l

Monitor blood glucose 2 hrly
If blood glucose unstable check 1 hrly
If blood glucose ≥11 mmol/l start insulin sliding scale (📖 p.181)

Start IV maintenance fluid (0.9% Saline)
Avoid glucose infusion unless the blood glucose is low

Restart oral treatment with the first post-operative meal
Restart regular insulin with first post-operative meal and take down IV insulin sliding scale 15-30 minutes later

Refer any patients that are unstable to the diabetes team

The Hillingdon Hospital Peri-operative diabetes guidelines (2008) are reproduced with permission of Dr Bela Vadodaria and Anne Currie

Box 24.5 What if a patient's operation is scheduled for the afternoon list?

- Tablet-controlled diabetic patients should have their medication with a light breakfast (e.g. 2 slices of toast, cereal and milk) on the day of surgery, then follow normal pre-operative fasting advice. Thereafter oral diabetic medication should be omitted until the first post-operative meal.
- Diabetic patients on insulin should have a light breakfast before 7 am and take half their normal prescribed insulin in the morning.
- Thereafter, regular short-acting insulin should be omitted until the first post-operative meal.
- Long-acting insulin (e.g. glargine, detimir) should still be taken at the prescribed time.
- Start insulin sliding scale (📖 p.181) if the blood glucose is >11 mmol/l
- Infuse 5% or 10% glucose if the blood glucose is <11 mmol/l

The Hillingdon Hospital Peri-operative diabetes guidelines (2008) are reproduced with permission of Dr Bela Vadodaria and Anne Currie

Glucose, potassium and insulin (see Boxes 24.3, 24.4, 24.5)

Patients, surgeons, and administrators are keen to increase the numbers of patients managed as day cases. Unfortunately, most diabetic clinics have a mean HbA_{1c} >8%. However, if the outcome of surgery is influenced by the glucose on the first post-operative day onwards (📖 p.474) we must ensure that it is optimally controlled perioperatively. Consider admitting hyperglycaemic patients for 24 hrs glucose control preoperatively if glucose is high. Some authors would advise a longer period of admission under the diabetes team.

A much better solution, which may produce more lasting improvement in glucose balance, is intensive pre-operative glucose control as an outpatient if this can be arranged with the diabetes team.

Patients undergoing surgery often need glucose as well as insulin to counteract catabolism. Studies show that it is better to have continuous glucose and insulin rather than an intermittent regimen. Glucose with insulin lowers potassium levels. Previously GKI (glucose–potassium–insulin) was used, in which all three were combined in one 500 ml bag. Nowadays, adding concentrated potassium to infusions on the ward is not advised and there is no premixed 10% glucose with potassium commercially available. The following are suggestions to manage this, but each hospital must agree its own guidelines. It is not possible to produce guidelines to cover every patient and every situation, so seek the diabetes team's advice every time.

- Monitor blood glucose by finger-prick hourly until off insulin sliding scale:
  - once stable it may be possible to use two-hourly monitoring
  - check at least one parallel laboratory venous glucose to ensure accuracy of finger-prick readings—readings should be within 15% of each other.
- Be very alert to the risk of hypoglycaemia—if in doubt treat as if hypoglycaemic (📖 p.199).
- One peripheral cannula for glucose and insulin.
- One peripheral cannula for other fluids, one of which should include potassium.
- Check all peripheral cannulae daily and change every 2–3 days—high infection risk in diabetic patients. Follow hospital protocol for meticulous central line care.
- Most fluids can be infused via one central line but check this in the BNF or with the pharmacy.
- Use the standard insulin sliding scale and adjust it aiming for a glucose of 4–7 mmol/l (5–10 mmol/l if there are concerns about hypoglycaemia) (📖 p. 199).

- Infuse 10% glucose continuously from a 500 l bag at 50–100 ml/hr preferably via a drip counter in parallel to insulin if neded:
  - reduce infusion rate if glucose high
  - increase infusion rate if glucose low
  - use 20% glucose if volume is an issue
  - 5% glucose is usually too big a volume and too non-physiological but does come with premixed potassium
  - large volumes of IV glucose may cause hyponatraemia.
- Infuse other fluids via the other cannula, e.g. N saline with potassium chloride to maintain a normal potassium level, blood, etc.
- Monitor potassium daily—more often if abnormal. Most hospitals now have bedside blood gas analysers which also measure electolytes for instant results. Otherwise request an urgent result from the laboratory.

Post-operatively

- Control glucose well:
  - 4–7 mmol/l without hypoglycaemia, which means very careful glucose monitoring and treatment adjustment
  - 5–10 mmol/l if hypoglycaemia risk
  - see 📖 p.476 for ITU management.
- Post-operatively patients may be insulin resistant at first.
- Good nutrition—involve dietitian.

Do not use glucose-free nutrition. Use the standard nutrition (parenteral or enteral) for your hospital appropriate to your patient with dietetic input and adjust the insulin to cope with the diabetes team's help. Glucose control with intermittent enteral feeding is difficult.

- Good pressure area care.
- Thromboprophylaxis as for non-diabetic patients but note that thrombo-embolism deterrent stockings may cause pressure ulcers in vasculopaths.
- Meticulous cannula/line/catheter care.
- Meticulous wound care—increased risk of wound infection.
- Do not contaminate a clean wound from a dirty one (e.g. a surgical excision and an ulcer on the other limb).
- Neuropathy and postural hypotension may complicate rehabilitation.
- Increased exertion—walking with effort after bed-rest may cause hypoglycaemia. Reduce insulin as exertion increases

Good post-operative glucose control from day one onwards reduces the risk of hospital-acquired infection (*J Parenter Enteral Nutr* 1998; **22**:77–81). Of 100 uninfected diabetic patients admitted for elective surgery, 31% with glucose >12 mmol/l on day one post-operatively (POD1) developed an infection vs 11% with POD1 glucose ≤12 mmol/l). Excluding minor UTIs, patients with just one glucose >12 mmol/l on POD1 were 5.7 times more likely to develop serious infection. Each millimole glucose rise >6.1 mmol/l on POD1 increased risk of complications by 17% after CABG (*Diabetes Care* 2003; **26**:1518–24).

A larger study of 5259 patients (877 diabetic) found that diabetic patients had 2.2% in-hospital mortality vs 1% in non-diabetics. However, diabetic patients were more often female, with higher BMI, worse cardiac disease, and more renal failure than non-diabetic patients. Correcting for this reduced mortality to a similar level to that of non-diabetic patients. Post-operatively, renal, neurological, and gastrointestinal complications were more common in diabetic patients. Infection was not. Five-year event-free survival was less in diabetic patients and mortality greater (*J Thorac Cardiovasc Surg* 2006; **132**:802–10). Another study showed that cognitive function was worse after cardiac surgery in diabetic vs non-diabetic patients (*Thorac Cardiovasc Surg 2006*, **54:307**–12).

Diabetic patients form a high proportion of those requiring vascular surgery. In diabetic patients, increasing area under the curve for the glucose above 6.1 mmol/l over the first 48 hrs post-operatively after infra-inguinal bypass was linked with increasing risk of poor outcome (death, major amputation, or graft occlusion at 90 days) (*Br J Surg 2006;* **93:1360**–7).

Intensive care

A study in an American surgical ITU showed that intensive insulin therapy by IV infusion aiming for a glucose level of 4.4–6.1 mmol/l nearly halved mortality compared with conventional treatment, particularly in patients with multi-organ failure with a proven septic focus (*New Engl J Med* 2001; **345**:1359–67). Intensive insulin treatment also reduced overall in-hospital mortality, bloodstream infection, dialysis-requiring renal failure, blood transfusion, and prolonged ventilation for these patients. The obvious risk is hypoglycaemia

In very ill patients glucose control like this can be achieved only with very careful balance of insulin and glucose (concentration dependent on other fluid needs and clinical situation). It requires hourly or half-hourly blood glucose checks and frequent fine-tuning to avoid hypoglycaemia. Seek the advice of the diabetes registrar or consultant.

The greatest danger for glucose balance in these diabetic patients is likely to be when the patient is transferred to a general ward where one-to-one nursing is not available.

Diabetes on the wards

Diabetic patients should be cared for in a diabetes specialist ward wherever possible. Recent studies in London hospitals (personal communications) show that 14–16% of hospital inpatients have diabetes. All should be seen by a member of the diabetes team. Most should be cared for by the diabetes team either totally or with shared care. In shared care arrangements it must be clear who is ultimately responsible for the patient. Every hospital should have a diabetes inpatient specialist nurse—preferably several.

Patient plan

- These are complex patients.
- Initial assessments should be clear.
- Investigations should be recorded and easily accessed as the file gets fatter.
- Cumulative blood test results are very helpful to show trends.
- Each patient should have a clear summary of what is wrong and what the management plan is for each problem.
- There should be recognition of the interactions between facets of tissue damage, and between different treatments.
- Prescription charts should be clear (especially for insulin doses) and must be checked regularly.
- Use variable dose sections of prescription charts for insulin and other glucose-lowering drugs.
- Patients who are able to do so should control their own insulin injections and dosage in consultation with medical staff (📖 p.283).
- Patients should be seen daily by a doctor (including at weekends).
- Test finger-prick blood glucose before each meal and before bed.
- Reduce testing in stable patients (e.g. awaiting placement).
- Record blood glucose tests on a standard glucose chart used throughout the hospital and teach staff how to use it (figure 7.1, 📖 p.115).
- Monitor pulse, BP, temperature, respiration. Remember that diabetic patients can deteriorate rapidly (often after subtle signs of worsening have been missed).

Diabetes self-care

Experienced diabetic patients know much more about their diabetes and how to manage it than most health care professionals. They should be allowed to measure their glucose and administer and adjust their insulin (and other medication if this is hospital policy) with the following provisos. The patient should:

- be alert and thinking clearly
- be taught how to use the hospital's glucose meter, which should be in a quality assurance scheme
- record glucose results on the hospital chart (± his/her own record)
- have his/her readings checked occasionally
- be fully competent in insulin injection technique (check this first)
- be fully competent in self-adjustment of insulin doses (check this first)
- record doses given on the hospital chart.

The doctor should confirm that self-administration is allowed in writing on the prescription chart.

Some patients will refuse to allow staff to give or adjust insulin dose even when they are not making appropriate adjustments. If they have capacity it is difficult to stop them. Contact the diabetes team urgently to arrange some diabetes education sessions on the ward.

Some problems on the wards

- Lack of experience of diabetes in medical and nursing staff
- Failure to realize that the patient knows more about his/her diabetes than staff do
- Failure to realize that the patient is not complying with treatment or dietary recommendations
- Unfamiliarity with different insulins
- Lack of awareness of the importance of timing of food and insulin or hypoglycaemic tablets in diabetic patients
- Late meals with too little carbohydrate
- Lack of awareness of the variety of hypoglycaemic symptoms
- Overtreatment of hypoglycaemia (e.g. giving glucose when a diet-only-treated patient's blood glucose is 4 mmol/l)
- Errors in doing finger-prick glucose (e.g. wiping finger with alcohol)
- Ward glucose meter not checked or quality assured
- Failure to identify tissue damage (e.g. not noting the peripheral neuropathy which caused the fall which fractured the femur)
- Insufficiently prompt recognition and vigorous treatment of infection
- Failure to realize how ill the patient is (e.g. neuropathy may blunt symptoms, cardiac pain may be atypical)
- Failure to appreciate the severity of PVD or neuropathy
- Vulnerable feet bare on dirty floors—need slippers
- Poor ulcer hygiene—especially with multiple large oozing ulcers
- Lack of awareness of visual loss from severe retinopathy or treatment
- Failure to appreciate renal vulnerability
- Problems managing obese weak diabetic patients—insufficient bariatric equipment
- Inadequate bowel preparation for colonoscopy/radiology (dysmotility reduces effectiveness of laxatives)
- Inappropriate timing of fasting procedures or operations
- Cancellation of procedures requiring fasting, with consequent destabilization of glucose
- Many different doctors seeing patient and not always writing in the notes—good coordination is needed.
- Communication problems with patient as many staff involved
- Failure to identify the diabetes at all!

Education

Diabetes education for staff

The key is repeated education of all staff. The diabetes team should provide prompt support in managing patients. The diabetes team needs good liaison with all other departments. Link nurse programmes in which one nurse on each ward is responsible for passing on diabetes education to the others have helped in some hospitals.

Education for diabetic inpatients

A diabetic inpatient is a captive audience. Help them to understand how they came to be in hospital and how this might be avoided (if possible) in the future. Admission also provides an opportunity for revision and further diabetes education.

Box 24.6 Diabetes education for inpatients

- Assess current knowledge and understanding of their own diabetes
- Review self-care. Review previous glucose balance.
- Involve family members (with patient permission)
- For new patients—provide full diabetes starter education (📖 p.59)
- Review knowledge of general lifestyle and preventive health care
- What caused hospital admission? What actions might prevent another such admission?
- Teach about diabetes self-care and other treatment which will be needed after discharge.
- Involve the multidisciplinary team—ensure that all team members understand the current plan and have been trained in the same diabetes care protocols ('sing the same song')
- Refer all patients to the dietitian
- Explain diabetes care and education arrangements in the community
- Explain follow-up arrangements
- Explain how to get help if problems arise

Discharge planning

- Start on admission with complex and disabled patients.
- Assess family/community support available.
- Liaise with GP and community diabetes team (a phone call to the GP is often helpful).
- Set up further appointments in podiatry or wound care
- If a diabetic patient has been ill enough to require admission, at least one specialist diabetic clinic visit is usually a good idea.
- Many patients who have required admission have very complex medical problems and need continued specialist follow-up.
- Check patient's understanding of diabetes treatment and diet (admission may have been precipitated by misunderstandings or confusion).
- Go over the take-home medication very very carefully—pharmacists are usually best at this.
- Provide a timely, detailed, and legible discharge summary. Give the patient a copy and make sure they understand what it says.
- Ensure that the district nurse really has agreed to come in and give the insulin (they rarely come more than twice a day and cannot always match their visit to meal times).
- Ensure that arrangements have been made for supplies of dressings and that the district nurse or other wound care staff know exactly how to continue the right dressing (changes in dressings can lead to deterioration and re-admission).
- Ensure that arrangements for meals are in place.
- Check that equipment has been delivered.
- Check that home modifications have been made.
- Make sure that transport arrangements are in place.
- Ensure that all the staff and agencies involved know what is happening (this is much harder than it sounds).
- Ensure that everyone knows who to contact if problems arise.
- Ensure that the patient has all their appointments in writing.
- Not usually done, but seems a good idea—phone the patient over next few days to see how they are getting on.
- Educate staff about managing diabetic patients.
- Use the opportunity to enhance patient education.

Box 24.7 Summary of major recommendations for hospital management

- Good metabolic control is associated with improved hospital outcomes. Target plasma glucose levels are:
  - 4–6.0 mmol/l pre-prandial
  - 4–9.9 mmol/l peak post-prandial.
- Intensive insulin therapy with IV insulin, with the goal of maintaining blood glucose at 4.4–6.0 reduces morbidity and mortality among critically ill patients in the surgical ICU.
- IV insulin infusion is safe and effective for achieving metabolic control during major surgery, haemodynamic instability, and nil-by-mouth status.
- IV insulin infusion is safe and effective for patients who have poorly controlled diabetes and widely fluctuating blood glucose levels or who are insulin deficient or severely insulin resistant.
- IV insulin infusion, followed by multidose SC insulin therapy, improves survival in diabetic patients after myocardial infarction.
- For insulin-deficient patients, despite reductions or the absence of caloric intake, basal insulin must be provided to prevent diabetic ketoacidosis.
- Use of scheduled insulin improves blood glucose control compared with orders based on sliding-scale insulin coverage alone.
- For patients who are alert and demonstrate accurate insulin self-administration and glucose monitoring, insulin self-management should be allowed as an adjunct to standard nurse-delivered diabetes management.
- Patients with no prior history of diabetes who are found to have hyperglycaemia (random blood glucose >6.9 mmol/l) during hospitalization should have follow-up testing for diabetes within 1 month of hospital discharge.
- Establishing a multidisciplinary team that sets and implements institutional guidelines, protocols, and standardized order sets for the hospital results in reduced hypoglycaemic and hyperglycaemic events
- Diabetes education, medical nutrition therapy, and timely diabetes-specific discharge planning are essential components of hospital-based diabetes care.

From *Diabetes Care* 2004; **27**:553–91.

Summary

- 12–25% of hospital inpatients have diabetes.
- Diabetic patients do not do well in hospital.
- Diabetic patients have increased risk of severe, prolonged, and complicated infection.
- There is increased risk of thrombosis.
- There is increased risk of cardiac and renal failure.
- There is increased risk of pressure sores.
- Diabetic patients have greater mortality, longer stay, and are less likely to return to their own home that other patients.
- Do not miss new diabetes in emergency attenders.
- Assess diabetic attenders or emergency patients carefully—do not forget blood glucose.
- Manage diabetic glucose emergencies promptly and vigorously.
- Manage sepsis promptly and vigorously.
- Manage diabetic aspects of acute coronary syndrome fully.
- Plan surgical admissions and use the relevant diabetes protocol.
- Control blood glucose well post-operatively.
- Control blood glucose extremely well in ITU (but beware hypoglycaemia).
- Be aware of the problems of managing diabetic patients in a general hospital ward.
- Discharge planning must include thought about food and administration of diabetes medication, especially insulin.
- Discharge planning must include particularly clear liaison with the community multidisciplinary team and primary care.
- All diabetic patients who have required emergency admission should have at least one follow-up appointment with the specialist diabetes team in secondary or primary care.

Useful reading

Management of diabetes and hyperglycemia in hospitals. *Diabetes Care* 2004; **27**:553–91

Chapter 25

District diabetes care

Introduction

People with diabetes want the right care at the right time. They want kind, efficient, expert, and experienced care from a team they know and trust. They want their care to be easy to access at convenient times—one phone call and a prompt appointment; routine check-ups when needed to fit with their personal timetable; immediate emergency care from the specialist team. They do not want to have to keep telling their story again and again. They want good communication between the members of the district diabetes team. Best of all it should be one team 'singing the same song', friendly, and supportive.

Multiple reorganizations in health care and diabetes care in the UK have had varying impacts upon district-wide diabetes care. The Diabetes National Service Framework provides a blueprint for good diabetes district networks 📖 p.44:

http://www.dh.gov.uk/en/Policyandguidance/Healthandsocialcaretopics/Diabetes/DH_4015717

The Quality and Outcomes Framework (QOF) provides guidance about key indicators in primary care (📖 p.504). This has led to identification of diabetic patients within practices and improved outcomes. Care must be taken to note exceptions and, as with the advice in much of this book, staff should individualize care and not overtreat to target.

Planning diabetes care

Read the excellent 'Diabetes Commissioning Toolkit' agreed by the National Diabetes Support Team, Primary Care Diabetes Society, ABCD, Diabetes UK, and Yorkshire and Humber Public Health Observatory

http://www.yhpho.org.uk/diabetes.aspx
or
http://www.dh.gov.uk/en/Publicationsandstatistics/Publications/PublicationsPolicyAndGuidance/DH_4140284

This states that to plan district-wide care one needs to know:
- Where are we now?
- Where do we want to be?
- How do we get there?
- How will we know when we are there?

The cycle advised is to review local service provision, taking into account national good practice and targets, decide priorities, design services, manage supply and demand, manage referral arrangements, manage performance, seek patient and public views, assess needs, review local service provision, and repeat …

Information needed

- Available local funding for diabetes care?
- Who is in charge of commissioning diabetes care?
- Who are the local experts in diabetes able to advise the commissioners? This includes consultant diabetologists and GPs with a special interest in diabetes. Others include people with diabetes or representative bodies, public health consultants, GPs with local overview roles, those responsible for specialist nurses, podiatry, dietetics, local hospital commissioning links, hospital biochemistry/pathology leads, information technology (IT) leads, data leads in PCT and hospital.
- Local people with diabetes
  - How many people are known to have diabetes?
  - Who they are? Age, male/female, ethnicity.
  - Where they are? Diabetes densities around the district. In what accommodation or circumstance—house, care or residential home, special needs, prison, detention centre, no fixed abode.
  - Any special needs or special issue groups locally?
  - Areas of social deprivation?
  - How many people have diabetes that we don't know about (estimate ~20% of the total diabetic population)?

- Clinical issues—diabetes type, w
  specialist care?
  - Newly diagnosed annually, typ
  - Existing diabetes, type 1 or 2
  - Current prescribing patterns o
    testing materials
  - Complications—DKA or hypog
    stroke, peripheral vascular, erec
  - Pregnancy (including gestational
  - Non-diabetes—illnesses requirin
  - HIV patients on antiretrovirals
  - Psychiatric patients on diabetoger
- Local staff currently available for diabetes care
  - Diabetologists
  - Diabetes specialist nurses (DSNs)
  - Diabetes educators (if separate from diabetes specialist nurses)
  - Diabetic specialist midwives
  - Diabetic specialist podiatrists
  - Diabetic specialist dietitians
  - Diabetic specialist wound care nurses
  - GPs with a special interest in diabetes (GPwSI)
  - Practice nurses with a special interest in diabetes
  - Pharmacists with a special interest in diabetes
  - GPs with some training in diabetes
  - Practice nurses with some training in diabetes
  - Dietitians
  - Podiatrists/chiropodists
  - Health psychologists
  - Pharmacists
  - Support staff for clinics
  - Staff who could help with diabetes care if trained
- Staff expertise
  - What training? Recognized professional training? Course(s)—recognized or not?
  - What revision/update? Attends national professional diabetes meetings? Belongs to national diabetes organization, e.g. Diabetes UK?
  - What experience?
- Time available to devote to diabetes care
  - Full time (e.g. DSN)
  - Dedicated diabetes sessions as part of role (e.g. GpwSI)
  - Mixed in with other work (e.g. dietitian with no separate diabetes clinic)

abetes care

- te outpatient facilities
- l outpatient facilities
- ile facilities (e.g. caravan)
- oaming staff (e.g. visiting several clinics or practices, or homes). If roaming where is their base?
- Communications (patient confidentiality must be secure)
    - Laboratory and radiology results (paper, electronic)
    - Patient records, current and previous, diabetes and non-diabetes—within practice, across health care providers, shared with patient, etc. Paper? Electronic?
    - Communication with patients—verbal, written, electronic
    - Communication about patients—verbal, written, electronic
- About access
    - Mobile patients—pedestrian, cycle, bicycle/car parking, bus/tram/tube/train access
    - Immobile patients—care home/nursing home, hospital inpatients
    - Prison/remand homes

Where are we now?

- GP-based diabetes care—QOF
- Intermediate diabetes care
- Secondary care clinics
- Secondary care complication management—glucose emergencies and tissue damage
- Care of diabetic patients with non-diabetic illness
- Children
- Teenagers
- Adolescents
- Pregnant and pre-pregnant women
- Adults

What about the future?

- Local obesity
- Ethnicity
- Age range of population—especially elderly
- Changes in deprivation or not

Best practice

See NSF standards of diabetes care (📖 p.44)

Prevention of diabetes

The details of this are outside the scope of this book. All health care professionals should advise everyone to eat healthily, stay the right weight for their height, and exercise regularly and safely. High-risk people and those noted to have impaired fasting glucose or impaired glucose tolerance should received intensive personalized advice to prevent their condition worsening to diabetes (📖 p.11, 12).

Diagnosis of diabetes

All those in contact with patients in primary or secondary care should know who is at risk of diabetes and how to diagnose it (📖 p.7).

Comprehensive care

This means diabetes care from diagnosis to grave—from well person diabetes checks to emergency admission to ITU. To achieve this people with diabetes, those who care for them, and those who care about them need to get together. Patient care should not be impeded by artificial boundaries between care providers. People with diabetes, primary care, intermediate care, and secondary care should liaise to ensure continuity, and avoid duplication or omission of care.

Comprehensive care also means building clear pathways with other bodies such as social services, education authorities, local schools, care and residential homes, detention centres, and prisons. This includes education about diabetes and its consequences.

Initial assessment and management (📖 p.19)

There should be local protocols for initial assessment and management, and guidelines for agreed education, diet, preventive care, medication, and monitoring. Base these on national guidelines and consensus, but adapt them for the local population.

Continuing care (📖 p.502)

In a district of 100 000 people about 4500 will have diabetes, of whom about 340 will have type 1 diabetes. The numbers of diabetic patients will gradually increase as it becomes more common nationally and patients survive for longer.

Continuing care is based on annual review with more frequent contacts if any of the risk factors are uncontrolled or problems arise. There is no evidence base for annual review, but the consensus is that it is straightforward to organize and easy to remember. A year is a long time in the life of someone with diabetes, and if risk factor control is suboptimal tissue damage can develop. Therefore patients should monitor their own health and learn when to seek help.

Nowadays, many annual reviews are carried out by practice nurses in primary care. Much can be checked routinely, but it is very important that diabetic patients can ask detailed questions about their health and obtain informed replies. Therefore all practice nurses doing such checks should have training in diabetes and know when to seek further advice from a GP, DSN, or secondary care.

Diabetes education

People with diabetes and their families

Ideally, all new diabetic patients should have a formal education programme tailored to their needs (📖 p.51). They should also have annual revision and update. It takes time to teach, and many districts still cannot afford this, but it is a worthwhile and ultimately cost-effective investment.

Staff caring for diabetic patients

Those providing specific diabetes care must have training. Examples are the Warwick or Roehampton courses:
http://www2.warwick.ac.uk/fac/med/study/cpd/subject_index/diabetes
http://www.roehampton.ac.uk/pg/diabetes/
If such courses are difficult to attend, local training should be arranged, e.g. via local DSNs, diabetologists, or GPwSIs.

Specialist care

Identify local provision for the following specialist secondary care:

- diabetes
- endocrinology
- paediatric, teenage, and adolescent diabetes
- diabetic foot care
- diabetes in the elderly
- eyes
- kidney
- neurology
- cardiac
- peripheral vascular
- neurovascular
- stroke
- pre-pregnancy
- pregnancy
- erectile dysfunction
- genitourinary medicine
- gastroenterology/hepatology
- orthopaedic/musculoskeletal service
- elderly
- rehabilitation
- psychological
- psychiatric

Agree referral arrangements for emergencies and routine problems, and maintain links. Nowadays, referrals are managed, and are sometimes prevented for financial reasons. Patients should be able to choose to seek specialist advice. Similarly, patients in secondary diabetes care should be able to choose intermediate or primary diabetes care.

Who should care for whom?

There is debate about where patients should receive routine diabetes care. In the UK there is a government-led initiative to deliver most diabetes care in primary care. Each district develops referral criteria to secondary care. The presence of intermediate care is a middle step. Some diabetologists provide 'secondary care' in non-hospital settings or work entirely as community diabetologists outside hospital. For simplicity any diabetologist care has been included as 'secondary care'. In some districts individual GPs provide secondary level diabetes care—some as GPwSIs, some as clinical assistants, and some in their own practices. Suggested guidelines are given below, but each locality should produce its own based on local population needs and local health care professional availability and expertise. In some areas there is substantial expertise in primary and intermediate care, and the list below will be much shorter, e.g.:
http://www.leicestershirediabetes.org.uk/documents/Leicestershirediabetes%20Type%202%20Management%20Guidelines%202006.pdf

Box 25.1 Referral guidelines: secondary to primary/intermediate

Many patients can be shared between primary and secondary care. If so, it must be clear who is doing the annual review and communications must be excellent to avoid omission or duplication.

- All patients who ask for transfer (with appropriate warnings if they have a serious health problem which really requires specialist intervention).
- Patients with stable type 2 diabetes on diet alone or on tablets.
- Patients with stable type 2 diabetes on insulin if the practice is expert and experienced in managing this.
- Patients with minor diabetic tissue damage and risk factors within target.
- Patients with other problems for which district guidelines or protocols for intermediate or primary diabetes care have been agreed.

Box 25.2 Referral guidelines for diabetic patients: primary to secondary care

- All patients who ask for a specialist opinion.
- All new diabetic patients unless expertise is available in primary/intermediate care (it often is).
- Definitely all new type 1 diabetic patients (same day).
- Patients suitable for insulin pumps
- Children and teenagers up to age 18 yrs.
- Pre-pregnant and pregnant women (same day).
- Patient in whom primary/intermediate care cannot keep risk factors within target after intensive effort for 6 months (HbA_{1c}, lipids, BP).
- Glucose instability—lows/highs even if HbA_{1c} is within target.
- Brittle diabetes.
- Patients who may benefit from continuous glucose monitoring.
- Any patient attending hospital with hypoglycaemia.
- Any patient who has any accident because of hypoglycaemia.
- Any patient admitted with high glucose, DKA, or HONK.
- Patients with diabetic tissue damage, including microalbuminuria (if minor they can be returned to primary care, but most such patients with have tissue damage in more than one system if sought). Many districts will have protocols for specific tissue damage which is managed in primary care.
- Patients with learning disabilities (diabetes often coexists).
- Patients with psychological or psychiatric problems making diabetes care difficult. This includes significant non-concordance or suspected manipulation.
- Patients with drug-induced diabetes (e.g. steroids, psychiatric, antiretroviral drugs). It may be possible for the relevant specialist teams to reduce the diabetogenic drug in close cooperation.
- Patients with significant other disease.
- Patients requiring intensive education.
- Patients who may be suitable for exenatide or sitagliptin unless primary or intermediate expertise is available.
- Patients with unresponsive obesity. In some districts rimonabant can be initiated only in secondary care.
- Patients in whom bariatric surgery is being considered.
- Patients with eating disorders.

Gaps in diabetes care

Mobility problems (📖 p.401)

Patients with mobility problems may be unable to access GP surgeries or specialist clinics. They are likely to have multiple health problems, especially if elderly, and if possible should be seen at least once in a specialist diabetic clinic (e.g. an elderly diabetes clinic) with appropriate ambulance or hospital car transport. Their care is time-consuming (e.g. 30–40 min per appointment) and multiple resources are often required. Such patients should be discussed with their GP so that the best arrangement can be made for each patient. Home visits by the GP and primary care team members are very helpful.

Patients in care or residential homes (📖 p.404)

Ideally, a local DSN, GPwSI, or diabetologist should visit patients in the homes for an annual review. Over 10% of older patients have diabetes. People will be in this accommodation because they cannot cope at home and are likely to have multiple significant health problems. Diabetes UK produced guidelines in 1999:
http://www.diabetes.org.uk/Documents/Reports/guideline_residents.pdf

Psychiatric patients (📖 p.452)

Whether at home or in hospital, psychiatric patients have a higher frequency of diabetes than people without psychiatric disease. Their psychiatric problem often prevents access to diabetes care. Ideally, each mental health trust should have a system for identifying diabetic in- or outpatients and a planned arrangement to ensure that they are receiving annual diabetes reviews and interim care. Diabetic glucose problems or tissue damage can worsen psychiatric problems.

Patients whose first language is not English (📖 p.407)

Districts with high proportions of such patients should make appropriate provision for diabetes care. Diabetes is more common in people of South Asian or African Caribbean descent than in White European populations. A few of these patients will be seeking asylum or on temporary visas. Frequent change of address and fear of authority can make continuity of diabetes care difficult. Diabetes health workers who speak the relevant language(s) are invaluable. Establish links with community leaders, and resources (e.g. Asian day centres). An example is the Apnee Sehat Temple food project in South Warwickshire:
http://www.institute.nhs.uk/health_and_social_care_awards/h&sca_synopsis/apnee_sehat_project_team.html

Patients in prison or detention centres

All such patients are entitled to proper diabetes care. There is little in the literature. In 1992 diabetologists provided diabetes care to inmates of Walton Prison, Liverpool, and demonstrated that the strict prison routine, diet, and supervision could provide good diabetes control (*BMJ* 1992; **304**:152–5). Usual diabetes care in a Texas prison was observed. A high proportion of Texan inmates were on insulin and non-adherence was common (*J Correctional Health Care* 2001; **8**:37–53). Without specific arrangements for diabetes care, it is likely that UK experience may mirror that in Texas.

Itinerant patients

Such patients rarely have continuous diabetes care. Those who live in the streets may have infections, foot problems, and tissue damage. One suggestion is to link with bodies already working with such groups to try to provide assistance in a clearly identified location and way, and to communicate this to the patients.

Non-attenders

Every clinic/surgery has non-attenders. Such patients often have high HbA_{1c} and tissue damage. Some have psychological problems or communication difficulties. Attempts should be made to contact them and re-book them. Nowadays, secondary care patients who have failed to notify inability to attend are often discharged back to their GPs. Check that there has not been an administrative error (e.g. wrong address, failure to note patient's phone message). Do not discharge pregnant women or those <18 yrs old. Telephone, text, or e-mail them.

Inform both patient and GP of the discharge. Ensure that the patient knows that he/she can come back (tell him/her the local system for this). It may be helpful to telephone non-attenders before discharge in case an error has occurred.

Communications

Those responsible for commissioning, providing, and using diabetes care should have regular joint discussions to ensure that the care commissioned is appropriate to local needs and uses resources optimally. This means good communication across multiple organizations, often with changing structures and personnel, in response to governmental, regional, and local reforms, and financial issues. The importance of maintaining good communication, whatever the difficulties, cannot be overestimated.

Give patients full information about their condition. Those who wish should have copies of all letters. Agree the communication system preferred by the patient—telephone, text, e-mail, letter. Ideally there should be a district-wide approach. Some districts use patient-held records. Sophisticated electronic diabetes systems can provide this (but such options are expensive).

Agree communication systems between health care professionals. Ideally there should be one district-wide electronic record system. In a few districts these exist and work well, but others are fragmented by the changes in the NHS, funding problems, or IT issues. Elsewhere in the world such systems are commonplace (e.g. Prowellness in Finland).

Letters should be sent promptly and contain accurate legible information. Check addresses frequently, as those of patients and professional service change. Patients also change GP, and this may lead to letters going to a previous surgery.

Laboratory services should be accessible by primary, intermediate, and secondary care at the point of care. Diabetes is a metabolic specialty and relies on timely laboratory results. Ideally, radiology results should also be accessible district-wide.

Audit

Both process and outcome of care should be audited. To do this a full register of all diabetic patients is required. Audit is much easier if the register is electronic (clearly, it must satisfy confidentiality, data protection and Caldicott requirements). In the UK, all GP practices should have a register of diabetic patients. In some areas there is a district-wide register. There are various commercial systems and some areas have homegrown ones. All systems should suit local needs, have maintenance and update contracts, and have an identified skilled person responsible for them. Changes in government or NHS strategy, personnel, funding, and IT arrangements can cause havoc.

If possible, participate in the National Diabetes Audit:
http://www.ic.nhs.uk/our-services/improving-patient-care/diabetes
or
DiabetesE https://www.diabetese.net/Quest/

Audit topics and some methodologies are listed in:

- National Diabetes Audit reports
  http://www.ic.nhs.uk/statistics-and-data-collections/health-and-lifestyles/diabetes
- Diabetes NSF
  http://www.dh.gov.uk/en/Policyandguidance/Healthandsocialcaretopics/Diabetes/DH_4015717
- NICE publications (which are being updated):
  http://www.nice.org.uk/guidance/index.jsp?action=byTopic&o=7239

Box 25.3 Diabetes audit topics

- Define audit population, e.g. GP surgery, hospital clinic, whole district
- Number of patients with new and existing diabetes
- Demographics
- Type of diabetes
- Treatment
  - Diet alone
  - Non-insulin hypoglycaemic drugs
  - Insulin (injection, pump)
- Annual review done/not done
- Risk factors—checked. Within target? Treatment?
  - BP
  - Smoking
  - HbA_{1c}
  - Cholesterol
  - Creatinine/eGFR
  - BMI ± waist circumference
  - Eye check done
  - Foot check done
  - Urine albumin checked
- Complications
  - Cardiovascular—heart, brain (e.g. stroke), peripheral vascular
  - Retinopathy
  - Nephropathy
  - Neuropathy
  - Feet—infection, ulceration, deformity, amputation
- Emergency, A&E attendances, and/or hospital admissions
  - Diabetes-related, e.g. hypoglycaemia or DKA
  - Non-diabetes-related
- Elective hospital admissions
  - Diabetes-related
  - Non-diabetes-related
- Diabetes education
- Patient and carer experience (this should be at the top of the list!)

Annual review

See 📖 p.42.

- Who is the patient? Age? Child/teenage/adolescent/adult?
- Woman of child-bearing potential?
- How is the person feeling? Any symptoms?
- Life events? Births, deaths, marriages, separations? Moves? Job? Hobbies?
- Emotions. Check for depression or anxiety and manage appropriately if present.
- Driver? If yes, check knowledge of safe driving with diabetes. Told insurance company and DVLA?
- Diet. If unhealthy or overweight, provide appropriate advice and dietetic referral as required. Ideally everyone with diabetes should see a dietitian annually.
- Exercise? Advise if insufficient.
- Smoker? If yes, help them stop.
- Alcohol? If excessive, help them reduce/stop.
- Hospital attendances or admissions? For diabetes (e.g. hypoglycaemia, high glucose/diabetic ketoacidosis)? For non-diabetes (reason)?
- Symptoms of cardiovascular disease, eye problems, neuropathy, foot problems, sexual dysfunction, other complications.
- Woman—periods? Planning pregnancy? Contraception?
- Glucose control—HBGM, hypoglycaemia.
- BP (including home monitoring if done).
- Full foot assessment—shape, skin, pulses, sensation. Any problems—refer to podiatrist.
- Cardiovascular examination if any hint of cardiac disease.
- Examine other systems if any relevant symptoms.
- Finger-prick or laboratory glucose (± ketone).
- Laboratory HbA_{1c}, cholesterol, HDL, LDL, triglycerides, urea, electrolytes, creatinine, eGFR if relevant, LFT, thyroid function. Full blood count and vitamin B_{12} if on metformin or otherwise relevant.
- Urine dipstick, laboratory microalbumin:creatinine ratio.
- Ensure patient has had visual acuity check and digital photographic retinal screening by a recognized service. Obtain the results.
- Check patient knows what and how to monitor.
- Diabetes education and revision
- Check patient knows where and how to seek help.
- Any questions?
- Date of next appointment.
- Give the patient a copy of the annual review.

Quality and Outcomes Framework for diabetes in primary care

This series of indicators of evidence-based patient care, agreed with the Department of Health, is collected during routine patient encounters.

DM1. The practice can produce a register of all patients with diabetes mellitus

DM2. Percentage of patients with diabetes whose notes record BMI in the previous 15 months.

DM3. Percentage of patients with diabetes in whom there a record of smoking status in the previous 15 months, except those who have never smoked where smoking status need be recorded only once since diagnosis.

DM4. Percentage of patients with diabetes who smoke and whose notes contain a record that smoking cessation advice or referral to a specialist service, where available, has been offered in the past 15 months.

DM5. Percentage of diabetic patients who have a record of HbA_{1c} or equivalent in the previous 15 months.

DM6. Percentage of patients in whom the last HbA_{1c} is ≤7.4% in the last 15 months

DM7. Percentage of patients with diabetes in whom the last HbA_{1c} is ≤10% in the last 15 months

DM8. Percentage of patients who have a record of retinal screening in the previous 15 months.

DM9. Percentage of patients who have a record of the presence or absence of peripheral pulses in the previous 15 months.

DM10. Percentage of patients with diabetes with a record of neuropathy testing in the previous 15 months.

DM11. Percentage of patients with diabetes who have a record of BP in the past 15 months

DM12. Percentage of patients with diabetes in whom the last BP is ≤145/85.

DM13. Percentage of patients with diabetes who have a record of microalbuminuria testing in the previous 15 months (exception reporting for patients with proteinuria)

DM14. Percentage of patients with diabetes who have a record of serum creatinine testing in the previous 15 months.

DM15. Percentage of patients with diabetes with a diagnosis of proteinuria or microalbuminuria who are treated with ACE inhibitors (or ARBs)

DM16. Percentage of patients with diabetes who have a record of total cholesterol in the previous 15 months.

DM17. Percentage of patients with diabetes whose last measured total cholesterol within the previous 15 months is ≤5 mmol/l. Above this statin therapy should be initiated and titrated until total cholesterol is ≤5 mmol/l.

DM18. Percentage of patients with diabetes who have had influenza immunization in the preceding 1 September to 31 March.

http://www.dh.gov.uk/en/Healthcare/Primarycare/Primarycarecontracting/QOF/DH_4125653

Summary

- People with diabetes should have accessible expert diabetes care matched to their individual needs—the right care at the right time.
- Plan diabetes care on a district-wide basis.
- Involve people with diabetes, those who commission diabetes services, and those who provide them in the planning.
- Ensure good communications within the diabetes network.
- Use the Diabetes Commissioning Toolkit.
- Local care must fit local needs and circumstances but fulfil national requirements.
- Apply Diabetes National Service Framework standards.
- Apply best practice—but tailor care to the individual.
- Agree who should care for whom.
- Identify gaps in care and fill them.
- Use resources wisely—avoid omission or duplication.
- Audit the process and outcome of diabetes care.
- Follow the annual review process for risk factor management and prevention and identification of diabetic tissue damage.
- Ask patients how they are doing.

Chapter 26

Useful contacts

The author cannot take responsibility for the content of the websites listed or for advice provided by these organizations

Diabetes UK

The national patient and professional diabetes association. Professionals involved in diabetes services should join. Publishes *Diabetic Medicine*.
www.diabetes.org.uk/

Careline for patients

Diabetes UK Careline: 0845 120 2960, Monday–Friday, 9a.m.–5p.m.
BT calls from landlines should cost no more than 4p per minute. Calls from other providers and mobiles may vary. Alternatively, call 020 7424 1000 and ask Reception to transfer your call to the Careline.
Interpreter service available.

Send questions by e-mail to: careline@diabetes.org.uk

Postal address:
Diabetes UK Careline
Macleod House
10 Parkway
London NW1 7AA

Scientific enquiries:

E-mail: scienceinfo@diabetes.org.uk

Telephone: 020 7424 1020

Fax 020 7424 1001

Post: Science Information Team at address above

Membership

E-mail: customerservice@diabetes.org.uk

Telephone: 0845 123 2399 (during office hours).

Address above

Useful links

http://www.diabetes.org.uk/Professionals/Links/

American Diabetes Association (ADA)

A good source of evidence-based guidelines and free viewing of diabetes-related papers. Publishes *Diabetes Care*.
www.diabetes.org

Association of British Clinical Diabetologists (ABCD)

For consultant diabetologists and diabetes specialist registrars. Consensus statements about aspects of diabetes care on website.
http://www.diabetologists.org.uk/

British National Formulary

Up-to-date prescribing information—evidence-based or consensus.
http://www.bnf.org/bnf/index.htm

Confidential Enquiry into Maternal and Child Health

Report on diabetes in pregnancy.
http://www.cemach.org.uk/Publications/CEMACH-Publications/Maternal-and-Perinatal-Health.aspx

Department of Health

Assorted diabetes publications and links.
http://www.dh.gov.uk/en/Policyandguidance/Healthandsocialcaretopics/Diabetes/index.htm

Electronic Medicines Compendium

Full up-to-date details of drugs for professionals and patients.
http://www.emc.medicines.org.uk/

European Association for the Study of Diabetes (EASD)

Multidisciplinary scientific organization. Publishes *Diabetologia*. Free online lectures available.
http://www.easd.org/

Input (Raising awareness of Insulin Pump Therapy)

For insulin pump users.
http://www.input.me.uk/

International Diabetes Federation

Worldwide organization providing information on international diabetes associations, and data about world diabetes—'To promote diabetes care, prevention and a cure worldwide'.
http://www.idf.org/

List of diabetes associations
http://www.idf.org/home/index.cfm?node=471

National Diabetes Support Team

'The NDST was set up to support healthcare professionals as they strive to implement the Diabetes National Service Framework (NSF) standards.'
http://www.diabetes.nhs.uk/

National Diabetes Framework
http://www.dh.gov.uk/en/Publicationsandstatistics/Publications/PublicationsPolicyAndGuidance/DH_4002951

National Electronic Library for Diabetes

http://www.library.nhs.uk/diabetes/Default.aspx?pagename=HOME

NICE (National Institute for Health and Clinical Excellence)

Guidelines and technology appraisals.
http://www.nice.org.uk/

Renal Association

Kidney guidelines.
http://www.renal.org/pages/

Royal College of Physicians of London

Standards of care
http://www.rcplondon.ac.uk/

Youth Health Talk

A collection of interviews with young people about their experiences of health or illness with links to other sites for young people.
www.youthhealthtalk.org

Index

The entries appear in letter-by-letter alphabetical order.

J

K

L

M

N